Development of
the Prefrontal Cortex

This book is printed on recycled paper. ♻

Development of the Prefrontal Cortex

Evolution, Neurobiology, and Behavior

edited by

Norman A. Krasnegor, Ph.D.
National Institute of Child Health and Human Development
National Institutes of Health
Bethesda, Maryland

G. Reid Lyon, Ph.D.
National Institute of Child Health and Human Development
National Institutes of Health
Bethesda, Maryland

and

Patricia S. Goldman-Rakic, Ph.D.
Yale University School of Medicine
New Haven, Connecticut

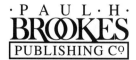

·P·A·U·L·H·
BROOKES
PUBLISHING C°

Baltimore • London • Toronto • Sydney

Paul H. Brookes Publishing Co.
Post Office Box 10624
Baltimore, Maryland 21285-0624

Typeset by Brushwood Graphics, Inc., Baltimore, Maryland.
Manufactured in the United States of America by
The Maple Press Company, York, Pennsylvania.

The conference on prefrontal cortex on which this book is based was supported by the
National Institute of Child Health and Human Development of the United States Public
Health Service.

Permission to reprint the following materials is gratefully acknowledged:

Pages 370–373: Excerpt from Pribram, K.H., Ahumada, A., Hartog, J., & Roos, L. (1964).
A progress report on the neurological processes disturbed by frontal lesions in primates.
In S.M. Warren & K. Aker (Eds.), *The frontal granular cortex and behavior* (pp. 47–52).
New York: McGraw-Hill; reprinted by permission.

Library of Congress Cataloging-in-Publication Data

Development of the prefrontal cortex : evolution, neurobiology, and
    behavior / edited by Norman A. Krasnegor, G. Reid Lyon, and Patricia
S. Goldman-Rakic.
        p.   cm.
    Includes bibliographical references and index.
    ISBN 1-55766-275-4
    1. Prefrontal cortex—Physiology.   2. Prefrontal cortex—Growth.   3. Prefrontal
cortex—Evolution.   4. Developmental neurobiology.   I. Krasnegor, Norman A.   II. Lyon,
G. Reid, 1949–   .   III. Goldman-Rakic, P.S. (Patricia S.)
    [DNLM: 1. Prefrontal Cortex—growth & development—congresses.
WL 307 D4893   1997]
QP383.17.D48   1997
612.8′25—dc20
DNLM/DLC
for Library of Congress   96-43037
                                                                                      CIP

British Cataloguing in Publication data are available from the British Library.

Contents

Introduction
Norman A. Krasnegor 1

I   EVOLUTION AND NEUROBIOLOGY

II   BRAIN–BEHAVIOR RELATIONSHIPS

List of Tables and Figures

I EVOLUTION AND NEUROBIOLOGY

1 *Evolution of Prefrontal Cortex*

2 *Synaptic Substrate of Cognitive Development: Life-Span Analysis of Synaptogenesis in the Prefrontal Cortex of the Nonhuman Primate*

4 Developmental Anatomy of the Prefrontal Cortex

5 Human Frontal Lobe Development: A Theory of Cyclic Cortical Reorganization

II BRAIN–BEHAVIOR RELATIONSHIPS

6 *Competence, Cortex, and Primate Models: A Comparative
   Primate Perspective*

7 *Language and the Prefrontal Cortex*

8 *Development of Neuronal Activity in Cortical Regions
Underlying Visual Recognition in Monkeys*

9   *Frontal and Attentional Mechanisms Regulating Distress
    Experience and Expression During Infancy*

III NEUROPSYCHOLOGY AND NEUROPATHOLOGY OF PREFRONTAL CORTEX

10 *Corticolimbic Circuitry and the Development of
    Psychopathology During Childhood and Adolescence*

11 *Frontal Lobe Dysfunction Following Closed Head Injury in
Children: Findings from Neuropsychology and Brain Imaging*

12   *Dimensions of Executive Functions in Normal and Abnormal Development*

13   *Prefrontal–Subcortical Circuits in Developmental Disorders*

14   *Cognitive and Social Development in Children with Prefrontal Cortex Lesions*

About the Editors

Norman A. Krasnegor, Ph.D., Chief, Human Learning and Behavior Branch, National Institute of Child Health and Human Development, National Institutes of Health, 6100 Executive Building, Room 4B05, 9000 Rockville Pike, Bethesda, Maryland 20892. Dr. Krasnegor is a behavioral neuroscientist whose interests include comparative evolution of the central nervous system, developmental psychobiology, and behavioral development.

G. Reid Lyon, Ph.D., Psychologist and Acting Chief, Learning Disabilities, Cognitive, and Social Development Branch, National Institute of Child Health and Human Development, National Institutes of Health, 6100 Executive Building, Room 4B05, 9000 Rockville Pike, Bethesda, Maryland 20892. Dr. Lyon specializes in developmental neuropsychology, learning disabilities, dyslexia, language disorders, and disorders of attention in children.

Patricia S. Goldman-Rakic, Ph.D., Professor, Section of Neurobiology, Yale University School of Medicine, 333 Cedar Street, New Haven, Connecticut 06510-8001. Dr. Goldman-Rakic is Professor of Neuroscience at Yale University School of Medicine. Her research interests include the development, organization, and plasticity of the cerebral cortex, in particular the cellular and circuit bases of cognition.

About the Contributors _____

Jocelyne Bachevalier, Ph.D., Associate Professor, Department of Neurobiology and Anatomy, University of Texas at Houston Health Sciences Center, 6431 Fannin Avenue, Houston, Texas 77225. Dr. Bachevalier received two bachelor's degrees, as well as a doctoral degree in clinical sciences, from the University of Montreal, Quebec, Canada. She also received a master's degree from the University of Provence, Marseilles, France, as well as a doctorate in psychophysiology from the University of Paris. She had a postdoctoral training position at the laboratory of neuropsychology at the National Institute of Mental Health, Bethesda, Maryland. Her association with that laboratory continued as Guest Researcher and Visiting Associate until 1991. She has also been a research associate professor in the Department of Psychology at George Washington University, Washington, D.C. She retains the title of Guest Researcher at the National Institute of Mental Health and is an adjunct professor in the Department of Psychology at Rice University, Houston, Texas. Dr. Bachevalier has conducted extensive research in clinical sciences, electrophysiology, neuroanatomy, neurobiology, behavioral neuroscience, and developmental psychobiology of humans and primates.

Francine M. Benes, M.D., Ph.D., Director, Laboratory for Structural Neuroscience, McLean Hospital, Mailman Research Center, 115 Mill Street, Belmont, Massachusetts 02178-9106. Dr. Benes received a doctoral degree in cell biology in 1972 and a medical degree in 1978 from Yale University School of Medicine. In 1982, after completing her residency at McLean Hospital, she established the Laboratory for Structural Neuroscience, the research of which is aimed at understanding how brain development may be disturbed in patients with schizophrenia and how postnatal ontogeny may play a role in the onset of this disorder during late adolescence. Dr. Benes also directs the Harvard Brain Tissue Resource Center and the Harvard Psychiatry Clinical Neuroscience Training Program, both located at McLean Hospital. She serves on the editorial boards of several neuroscience and psychiatry journals.

Kathleen R. Biddle, Ph.D., Research Coordinator, National Institute of Child Health and Human Development Center for Reading Research, Eliot-Pearson Department of Child Development, Tufts University, 105 College Avenue, Medford, Massachusetts 02155. Dr. Biddle coordinates intervention research in the Boston public schools for the multisite study that evaluates treatment outcomes among subtypes of impaired readers. She received her doctoral degree in applied child development from Tufts University. Her research interests include reading disabilities and developmental language outcomes following brain injury.

Jean-Pierre Bourgeois, Ph.D., Director of Research, CNRS, Laboratory of Molecular Neurobiology, Institut Pasteur, FR-75724 Paris cedex 15, FRANCE. Dr. Bourgeois was trained as a molecular biologist. His research interests are the epigenetic mechanisms of synaptogenesis and the establishment of synaptoarchitectony in the neocortex of primates.

Arun S. Dabholkar, Ph.D., Instructor, Department of Pediatrics, University of Chicago, 5841 South Maryland Avenue, MC 3055, Chicago, Illinois 60637. Dr. Dabholkar received his doctoral degree from the University of Udaipur, India, in 1977. His research interests are in cytochemistry and ultrastructure. He has been a research associate at the University of Chicago since 1991.

Martha Bridge Denckla, M.D., Professor of Neurology, Pediatrics, and Psychiatry, The Johns Hopkins University School of Medicine, Director, Developmental Cognitive Neurology Clinic, Director, Learning Disabilities Research Center, Kennedy Krieger Institute, 707 North Broadway, Suite 501, Baltimore, Maryland 21205. In addition to her affiliation with the Kennedy Krieger Institute, Dr. Denckla is also Professor of Neurology, Pediatrics, and Psychiatry at The Johns Hopkins University School of Medicine. She received her medical degree (*cum laude*) from Harvard Medical School and trained with Dr. Norman Geschwind in behavioral neurology. She is Principal Investigator of a National Institutes of Neurological Diseases and Stroke–funded Center entitled "Neurodevelopmental Pathways to Learning Disabilities," as well as the National Institute of Child Health and Human Development–funded "Mental Retardation Developmental Disabilities Research Center." Dr. Denckla has been awarded the Lucy G. Moses Prize in Clinical Neurology at Columbia University, the Norman Geschwind Memorial Lectureship at the Orton Dyslexia Society, the Rita G. Rudel Memorial Lectureship at Columbia University, the Herbert Birch Memorial Lectureship at the International Neuropsychology Society, the Soriano Guest Lectureship of the American Neurological Association, as well as being named 1996 Neurofibromatosis Scholar by Neurofibromatosis, Inc. She is serving her second term on the governing board of the International Neuropsychology Society and is a past president of the Behavioral Neurology Society. Her past positions include Director of the Learning Disabilities Clinic at the Boston Children's Hospital and Chief of the Section on Autism and Related Disorders at the NINDS.

Paul J. Eslinger, M.D., Professor of Neurology and Behavioral Science, Departments of Medicine and Behavioral Science, College of Medicine, Laboratory of Neuropsychology and Cognitive Neuroscience, The Milton S. Hershey Medical Center, Pennsylvania State University, 500 University Drive, Hershey, Pennsylvania 17033. Dr. Eslinger is Director of the Neuropsychology and Cognitive Neuroscience Laboratory and also Consulting Neuropsychologist to the University Hospital Rehabilitation Unit, the Comprehensive Epilepsy Program, and the Stanford Research Institute. In addition to providing diagnostic and rehabilitation training in clinical neuropsychology and graduate training in cognitive neuroscience, his research programs focus on the neural and cognitive architectures underlying executive functions, learning and memory, social development, recovery from early frontal lobe damage, neuropsychological rehabilitation, and applications of fMRI.

Nathan A. Fox, Ph.D., Professor of Human Development and Psychology, Department of Human Development, College of Education, University of Maryland, 3304 Benjamin Building, College Park, Maryland 20742-1131. Dr. Fox is Associate Editor of *Developmental Psychology* and is a past president of the International Society for Infant Studies. His research interest lies in the interface of biology and behavior in understanding individual differences in cognitive and socioemotional development.

Lynn M. Grattan, Ph.D., Assistant Professor, Department of Neurology, University of Maryland School of Medicine, 22 South Greene Street, Baltimore, Maryland 21201. In addition to her position as Assistant Professor at the University of Maryland Medical School, Dr. Grattan is Director of the Neuropsychology Laboratory at the University of Maryland Hospital, a member of the graduate faculty at the University of Maryland at Baltimore, and a faculty member of the Department of Psychology at the University of Maryland–Baltimore County (UMBC). At UMBC, she teaches neuropsychology to doctoral students. She also serves as a consultant to multicenter projects that examine the course of executive functions in normal aging, and her research interests focus on the neuroanatomical and neurobehavioral mechanisms of executive functions, neurorehabilitation of disturbances of executive functions and associated social disturbances, and the contributions of executive functions to stroke outcome in children and adults.

Catherine Harman, Ph.D., 2425 Stansby, Way, Eugene, Oregon 97405. Dr. Harman received a bachelor's degree from the University of Minnesota. She received a doctoral degree from the University of Oregon in 1994 under the auspices of Dr. Mary Rothbart and Dr. Michael Posner. As a graduate student, she published work on attention and visual system development, as well as work on attention and emotional development. She then pursued postgraduate work with Dr. Nathan A. Fox at the University of Maryland, during which time her chapter in this volume was written. Dr. Harman is planning a career as a clinical/applied developmental psychologist.

Peter R. Huttenlocher, M.D., Section Chief of Pediatric Neurology, Department of Pediatrics, Wyler Children's Hospital, University of Chicago Medical Center, 5841 South Maryland Avenue–MC 3055, Chicago, Illinois 60637. Dr. Huttenlocher received his medical degree from Harvard Medical School in 1957. He subsequently spent 2 years at the National Institutes of Health in Dr. E.V. Evart's laboratory, working on the neurophysiology of sleep. This was followed by training in pediatric neurology and in neuropathology at Massachusetts General Hospital in Boston. He has been on the faculty at Yale University Medical School (1966–1974) and is Professor of Pediatrics and Neurology and a member of the Committee on Neurobiology at the University of Chicago. His research interests include the development of the human cerebral cortex, both normal and abnormal, and the study of neural plasticity in the immature nervous system.

Harry J. Jerison, Ph.D., Professor, Department of Psychiatry and Biobehavioral Sciences, School of Medicine, University of California at Los Angeles, Santa Monica, California 90402. Dr. Jerison was born in Bialystok, Poland, and was educated at the University of Chicago (B.S., 1947; Ph.D., 1954). He is Professor Emeritus in the Department of Psychiatry and Biobehavioral Sciences of the School of Medicine, University of California at Los Angeles (UCLA). Prior to joining the UCLA faculty in 1969, he was Research Psychologist at the Aero Medical Laboratory in Dayton, Ohio, and Professor of Psychology and Biology and Director of the Behavior Research Laboratory at Antioch College in Yellow Springs, Ohio. As a visiting scholar, he has held appointments at the Center for Advanced Study in the Behavioral Sciences in Stanford, California; the Medical Research Council in Cambridge, England; the Rockefeller Foundation Center at Bellagio, Italy; the Max Planck Institute in Tübingen, Germany; and at universities in Italy, England, and Hawaii. He is the author of more than 150 scientific publications, including a seminal volume, *The Evolution of the Brain and Intelligence* (Academic Press, 1973). Dr. Jerison is known internationally for his innovative quantitative analyses of the evolution of the brain.

Christiana M. Leonard, Ph.D., Professor of Neuroscience, Psychiatry, and Psychology, College of Medicine, Department of Neuroscience, University of Florida Health Sciences Center, J.H.M. Health Science Center, 1600 S.W. Archer Road, Gainesville, Florida 32605. Dr. Leonard has been at the University of Florida since 1976, where she is a professor of neuroscience happily supervising a flock of students in communication processes, neuropsychology, psychobiology education, medical physics, computer science, bioengineering, and medicine. Like many other contributors to this volume, her interest in prefrontal cortex was sparked in the laboratory of Walle J.I.I. Nauta at the Massachusetts Institute of Technology (MIT). She subsequently worked on olfaction, taste, and neurobehavioral development in the rodent, birdsong in the canary, "face cells" and grooming in the macaque, and facial expression in the human. Developments in magnetic resonance imaging (MRI) and computer technology have at last afforded her techniques powerful enough to attack what was always a latent goal, understanding the neural substrate of human cognitive development and its pathological variants.

Harvey S. Levin, Ph.D., Professor and Director of Research, Department of Physical Medicine and Rehabilitation, Baylor College of Medicine, 1333 Moursund Avenue, Room A-205, Houston, Texas 77030. Dr. Levin's research since the mid-1970s has focused on characterizing the long-term neurobehavioral consequences of traumatic brain injury, including the overall impact on quality of life. His work has elucidated the relationship of the pathophysiology of brain injury, including the utilization of magnetic resonance imaging to characterize focal brain lesions and tissue loss, to the neurobehavioral sequelae in children and adults. This research has involved specific projects such as the National Institutes of Health Coma Data Bank. Dr. Levin's research has also produced widely used assessments instruments, including the Galveston Orientation and Amnesia Test to evaluate posttraumatic amnesia, and the Neurobehavioral Rating Scale, which measures behavioral disturbance after brain injury. Dr. Levin is Director of Research for the Department of Physical Medicine and Rehabilitation at the Baylor College of Medicine in Houston, Texas.

Patricia McDonough-Ryan, M.A., Graduate Student, Department of Psychology, University of Cincinnati, Dyer Hall, Mail Location 376, Cincinnati, Ohio 45221-0376. Ms. McDonough-Ryan was a graduate student at the University of North Carolina–Wilmington when she participated in the research described in Chapter 15 of this volume.

Kristy L. Nace, B.A., Doctoral Student, Center for Neuroscience, University of California at Davis, 1544 Newton Court, Davis, California 95616.

William H. Overman, Ph.D., Professor, Department of Psychology, University of North Carolina at Wilmington, 601 South College Road, Wilmington, North Carolina 28403-3297. Dr. Overman has conducted research in memory and learning processes with nonhuman primates and humans. In the 1990s, his research has concentrated on comparing the ontogeny of cognitive behaviors in infant humans and infant monkeys.

Bruce F. Pennington, Ph.D., Professor, Department of Psychology, University of Denver, 2155 South Race Street, Denver, Colorado 80208. At the University of Denver, Dr. Pennington heads the developmental cognitive neuroscience program. He was trained at Harvard and Duke Universities, receiving a doctoral degree in clinical psychology from Duke in 1977. Before receiving his doctorate, he worked as a schoolteacher and helped start an alternative school, School-Within-A-School, at Brookline High School, Brookline, Massachusetts, which has been in operation since 1970. Dr. Pennington is author of *Diagnosing Learning Disorders* (Guilford Press, 1991), as well as numerous scientific papers on dyslexia, autism, and attention-deficit/hyperactivity disorder. In an analysis of citation impact among psychologists conducted by the American Psychological Society, he ranked in the top 25 psychologists in the world for the 1990–1995 period. His honors include Research Scientist, MERIT, and Fogarty Awards from the National Institutes of Health. Dr. Pennington was selected as University Lecturer by the University of Denver for the 1996–1997 academic year.

Karl H. Pribram, M.D., Ph.D. (Hon. Multi.), Center for Brain Research and Informational Sciences, Radford University, 423 Russell Hall, Post Office Box 6977, Radford, Virginia 24142. Dr. Pribram received both his bachelor's and medical degrees from the University of Chicago. Briefly at the University of Tennessee, he was instructor in surgery. He then moved to Jacksonville, Florida, where he practiced neurosurgery and began a brain research program at Robert Yerkes Laboratory for Primate Biology. He was appointed Assistant Professor and then Lecturer in the Department of Physiology at Yale University, where he spent the next 10 years. During this period, he also served as Director of Research at the Institute of Living, a mental hospital in Hartford, Connecticut. In 1958, he was at the Center for Advanced Studies in the Behavioral Sciences, where he coauthored the influential book *Plans and the Structure of Behavior* with George Miller and Eugene Galanter. He was then appointed professor in the Departments of Psychology and Psychiatry at Stanford University, where he spent the next 30 years, having been awarded lifetime research career support from the National Institutes of Health. On becoming Professor Emeritus at Stanford, he accepted the James P. and Anna King Distinguished Professor Chair at Radford University in Virginia, where he directs the Center for Brain Research and Informational Sciences and where he published his most recent book, *Brain and Perception: Holonomy and Structure in Figural Processing* (1991).

Pasko Rakic, Ph.D., Professor of Neuroscience, Section of Neurobiology, Yale University School of Medicine, 333 Cedar Street, New Haven, Connecticut 06510-8001. Dr. Rakic's research interests are in developmental neurobiology, cellular and molecular mechanisms of neuronal migration, and axonal navigation and synaptogenesis. He is particularly interested in genetic and epigenetic regulation of neuronal interactions during development.

Allan L. Reiss, M.D., Professor of Psychiatry, Neurology, and Pediatrics, The Johns Hopkins University School of Medicine, Director, Behavioral Neurogenetics and Neuroimaging Research Center, Kennedy Krieger Institute, 707 North Broadway, Baltimore, Maryland 21205. Dr. Reiss directs the Behavioral Genetics and Neuroimaging Research Center and is Vice President of Psychiatry and Behavioral Neurosciences at the Kennedy Krieger Institute. He is also a professor of psychiatry, neurology, and pediatrics at The Johns Hopkins University School of Medicine. In addition to his interests in the genetic, neurological, and psychiatric aspects of children's developmental disorders, Dr. Reiss is developing advanced software modules for the quantitative analysis of neuroimaging data.

Hillary R. Rodman, Ph.D., Assistant Professor, Department of Psychology and Yerkes Primate Center, Emory University, 532 Kilgo Circle, Atlanta, Georgia 30322. Dr. Rodman's research interests lie primarily in studies of the development, plasticity, and comparative organization of visual cortex, especially higher areas underlying object perception and other cognitive functions. She received graduate training at Princeton University that focused on single-unit electrophysiology of primate cortex followed by several years in which she concentrated on the physiological and anatomical development of inferior temporal cortex in macaque monkeys. Subsequently, she received postdoctoral training in comparative neurobiology at the University of California at San Diego, where she had an opportunity to explore similarities and differences in vertebrate vision and brain organization using a number of approaches. Returning to primate work at Princeton, she next began a program of exploring behavioral, physiological, and anatomical parallels between the human blindsight phenomenon and preserved vision after striate cortex damage in monkeys. Dr. Rodman is an assistant professor in the Department of Psychology at Emory University, Atlanta, Georgia, as well as a member of the Division of Visual Science at the Yerkes Regional Primate Research Center. Her work focuses on mechanisms of recovery from early cortical damage and on the development of pattern recognition capacity in normal primates, that is, how the brain combines innate biases with early and later experience to determine how humans know what it is that they see.

Duane M. Rumbaugh, Ph.D., Professor, Department of Psychology and Biology, Director, Language Research Center, Georgia State University, University Plaza, Atlanta, Georgia 30303. Dr. Rumbaugh's primate research began in 1958 with comparative studies of learning in primates, ranging from prosimians to great apes. In 1971, with support from the National Institute of Child Health and Human Development, he started the LANA Project to assess chimpanzees' capacity for language using a computer-monitored keyboard, which anticipated the development of portable systems now used with special human populations. Research with Sue Savage-Rumbaugh documents that apes both understand and use symbols to communicate and count. Research with a bonobo, Kanzi, defines his speech comprehension—for both single words and novel sentences of request. Rumbaugh received his bachelor's degree (1950) from the University of Dubuque, his master's degree (1951) from Kent State University, and his doctoral degree (1955) from the University of Colorado. He was Georgia State University's first Alumni Distinguished Professor (1987) and was elected a distinguished alumnus of Kent State University (1992) and of the University of Dubuque (1993). He was the 13th distinguished member of National Psi Chi (1996), the G. Stanley Hall Lecturer on comparative psychology for the American Psychological Association (1984), and president of APA's Division on Comparative and Physiological Psychology (1988). In 1995, he was president of the Southern Society for Philosophy and Psychology. Dr. Rumbaugh and his wife were invited speakers at the XXXII Nobel Conference (1996) on Apes at the End of an Age, Gustavus Adolphus College, St. Peter, Minnesota.

Randall S. Scheibel, Ph.D., Assistant Professor, Department of Physical Medicine and Rehabilitation, Baylor College of Medicine, 6550 Fannin Avenue, Suite 1421A, Houston, Texas 77030. Dr. Scheibel's research interests include examination of the relationship between brain imaging data and the cognitive and behavioral symptoms of neurological disorders, including head trauma and intracerebral tumor. He is also the outcome monitor for a multicenter National Institutes of Health study of systemic hypothermia for the treatment of severe head injury.

Elena Schuhmann, B.A., Graduate Student, Department of Clinical and Health Psychology, University of Florida Health Science Center, Box 100165, Gainesville, Florida 32610-0165. Ms. Schuhmann was an undergraduate honors student at the University of North Carolina–Wilmington when she participated in the research presented in Chapter 15 of this volume.

Michael L. Schwartz, Ph.D., Associate Professor, Section of Neurobiology, Yale University School of Medicine, 333 Cedar Street, SHM, New Haven, Connecticut 06510. Dr. Schwartz's research focuses on the development and organization of the mammalian cerebral cortex, with special emphasis on factors regulating cellular phenotype and connectivity.

Robert W. Thatcher, Ph.D., Professor of Neurology and Radiology, VA Medical Center, Medical Research and Development Service (151), Bay Pines, Florida 33504. Dr. Thatcher received his bachelor's degree in chemistry from the University of Oregon and his doctoral degree in biopsychology from the University of Waterloo, Ontario, Canada. He received postdoctoral training in neurobiology at Albert Einstein College of Medicine and at New York Medical College. He has been on the faculty of New York Medical College as an assistant professor, New York University Medical School as an associate professor, and the University of Maryland School of Medicine as a full professor. In 1991, he joined the staff of the National Institutes of Health and the National Institutes of Neurological Diseases and Stroke as the project manager for the development of a 128-channel electroencephalogram (EEG) system. He is a full professor in the Departments of Neurology and Radiology at the University of South Florida School of Medicine and program manager for EEG and magnetic resonance imaging (MRI) analyses of head injury at the VA Medical Center in Bay Pines, Florida. Dr. Thatcher has authored 6 books and more than 150 journal articles, book chapters, and abstracts. These publications cover the fields of basic neuroscience, neurobiology, developmental psychology, quantitative EEG, quantitative MRI, environmental toxicology and multimodal integration of MRI, EEG, and positron emission tomography (PET) scans.

Preface

The rationale for this book is based on two complimentary strands of research designed to understand the role of the prefrontal cortex in human behavioral development. In 1992, Patricia Goldman-Rakic and I met in Paris while attending a conference on fetal behavioral development that I had organized for the National Institute of Child Health and Human Development (NICHD). At that time, we agreed that the expanding literature on the identification of functional relationships between brain and behavior in children offered a challenging opportunity to organize a meeting of neuroscientists and developmentalists to review such findings and consider emerging trends. We further concurred that the focus of such a meeting ought to be one in which the neuroscience and behavioral analysis were sufficiently mature that a body of research could be examined. The field of behavioral neuroscience that we chose is one that explores the functions of the prefrontal cortex early in development, an area of investigation in which Dr. Goldman-Rakic has made many basic observations and discoveries.

In 1994, Reid Lyon and I organized a conference on attention, memory, and executive function. This meeting brought together a group of leading scientists from a variety of fields of inquiry (e.g., cognition, development, education, neurology, pediatrics) to discuss the state of the art of research on the three topics listed above. These three topics are of general interest to the NICHD because they are critical for understanding normative behavioral development and may be of particular interest in understanding potential mechanisms involved in learning disabilities. This latter topic is a major focus for research programs sponsored by the NICHD, the institute at the National Institutes of Health that has given the lead to conduct and support research on this important public health problem.

Along with my colleagues, Drs. Goldman-Rakic and Lyon, I organized the meeting that led to the publication of this book. The premise behind the conference was that a review of the basic behavioral neuroscience research on the prefrontal cortex could serve to both highlight what is known about this part of the brain early in life and provide insights into the behavioral mechanisms (i.e., attention, memory, and executive function) that it subsumes and thereby shed light on the structure's putative role in children's learning disabilities.

There were three foci for the meeting that are well reflected in this volume. These are 1) the evolution of the prefrontal cortex; 2) the neurobiological and behavioral neuroscience discoveries related to the structure in terms of the ontogeny of its anatomy, physiology, and behavioral correlates; and 3) clinical neuropsychological theories and behavioral findings that relate to the consequences of damage sustained to the prefrontal cortex. The volume arose out of the conference. This meeting, sponsored by the Human Learning and Behavior Branch of NICHD, was held in September 1994. Although the volume is based in part on the conference proceedings, the contributions are in the form of individual chapters that provide overviews of the topics on which they focus. As such, they give the reader scholarly, in-depth, scientific coverage of the subject.

This book will be of interest to a number of scientific and clinical disciplines. These include the fields of neuroanatomy, developmental psychobiology, behavioral neuroscience, neuropsychology, and learning disabilities. The work will be valuable for graduate seminars in the neurosciences and as a reference for researchers interested in brain development in primates and children.

Norman A. Krasenegor, Ph.D.
April 1997

Acknowledgments

We wish to acknowledge the efforts of Dana R. Bynum and Doreen C. Haywood, who materially aided and assisted us in the many tasks associated with the logistics necessary to ensure that final manuscripts and edited proofs were delivered to the publisher. We wish to also acknowledge the contributions of Judith Rothenberg, who facilitated the multiple written, faxed, and e-mailed communications between editors and contributors, which were so vital to successfully bringing this book to press.

*To my mother, now in her 87th year of life, and
to my wife, Rebecca, and our two sons,
Dan and Josh*
Norman A. Krasnegor

*To Drs. Jack Fletcher, Louisa Cook Moats,
and Anne Willoughby for their tremendous
support and compassion, and to my son,
Matthew, who is my hero*
G. Reid Lyon

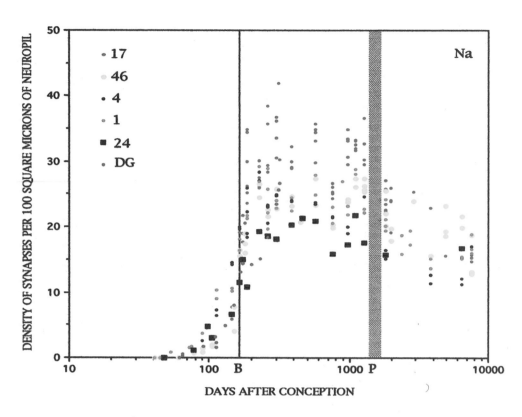

Figure 2.5. Density of synapses per 100 μm³ of neuropil in the primary visual cortex (blue dots), pre-frontal association cortex (yellow dots), primary motor cortex (black dots), primary somatosensory cortex (red dots), anterior cingulate cortex (black squares), and dentate gyrus (green dots) at various ages. Each dot represents the value obtained from a single electron microscopic probe (see Figure 2.1). The time in days after conception is represented on a semilogarithmic scale. (B, time of birth; P, puberty.) (Data compiled from Bourgeois et al., 1994; Eckenhoff & Rakic, 1991; Granger et al., 1995; Zecevic et al., 1989; Zecevic & Rakic, 1991.)

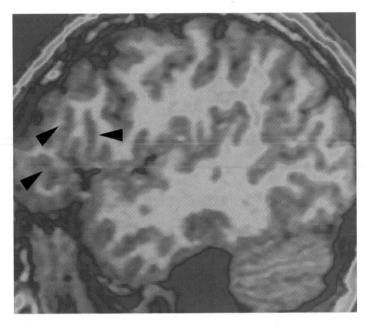

Figure 7.7. A sagittal MRI image of the left hemisphere of a child with specific language impairment. Note extra sulci in Broca's area (arrows).

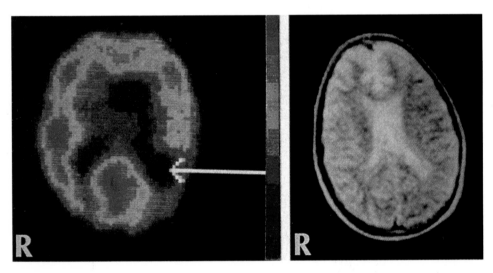

Figure 11.5. Transaxial SPECT (left) and MRI (right) images from a 10-year-old with reading difficulties 5 months after sustaining a head injury. There is a defect in the left posterior parietal region on SPECT (arrow) that is not shown on MRI. (From Newton, M.R., Greenwood, R.J., Britton, K.E., Charlesworth, M., Nimmon, C.C., Carroll, M.J., & Dolke, G. [1992]. A study comparing SPECT with CT and MRI after closed head injury. *Journal of Neurology, Neurosurgery, and Psychiatry, 55,* 93; reprinted by permission.)

Introduction

Norman A. Krasnegor _____

"Omnia Gallia in tres partes divisa est." As most people who studied Latin as high school sophomores remember, this is the opening line from Caesar's *Gallic Wars.* Karl H. Pribram (see Chapter 16) points out that the prefrontal cortex (PFC), as Gaul, can also be divided into three anatomically and functionally discernible parts. One part has been labeled *orbitofrontal.* This anatomical locus connects with the amygdala, anterior insula, and temporal pole via the uncinate fasciculus. Functionally, the region is thought to be related to the perception of novel relationships and forms the substrate for controlling *appropriate* behaviors in different contexts. A second part of the PFC is the *dorsal* sector. This locus projects to the hippocampus and its associated networks via connections through the cingulate cortex. The third part, or *middle* sector, forms the third leg of the PFC's trifurcation. It has connections with other parts of the cortex and specific linkages to areas of sensory modality representation. The middle sector "integrates the functions of the other two sectors with those of the rest of the brain . . ." (see Chapter 16, p. 360).

This volume has three main foci. These are 1) the origin of the PFC and its neurobiology, 2) the PFC's relation to behavior, and 3) the PFC's function as defined by its neuropsychology and neuropathology. The context for discussion of these three areas is development from both the evolutionary and the ontogenetic perspectives. Of particular interest is the role played by the PFC in the organization of behavior as captured by the construct *Executive Function.* Also of relevance is research designed to elucidate the function of the PFC in attention, memory, and emotion. This volume, like the PFC, is divided into three parts. The first section addresses evolution and neurobiology, and the second, brain–behavior relationships. The third is devoted to analyses of the neuropsychology and neuropathology of prefrontal systems.

EVOLUTION AND NEUROBIOLOGY

The first section of this volume is composed of five chapters that describe the evolution of the PFC and the ontogeny of this structure from the anatomical and physiological points of view. In the first chapter, "Evolution of Prefrontal Cortex," Harry J. Jerison, an expert on brain evolution, focuses on several important questions relating to the origin of the PFC. The first of these relates to *when* the PFC evolved and whether the structure in humans is unique at the cellular levels that compose it or as a structure that helps to organize the brain. Among other important issues raised in this informative exposition is a discussion of the selective pressures that may have been instrumental in establishing and shaping this anatomical locus that plays such a crucial role in organizing behaviors.

The next chapter, by Patricia S. Goldman-Rakic, Jean-Pierre Bourgeois, and Pasko Rakic, is entitled "Synaptic Substrate of Cognitive Development: Life-Span Analysis of Synaptogenesis in the Prefrontal Cortex of the Nonhuman Primate." Goldman-Rakic (a coeditor of this volume) and her colleagues are widely known for their pioneering anatomical studies of primate brain development, with a special interest in synaptogenesis. The senior author has also been at the forefront of behavior research during early development. In her research, she compared learning of human toddlers and nonhuman primates at the same developmental stage. The work is notable because her anatomical studies have been linked directly to the learning tasks, making possible inferences about necessary central nervous system (CNS) substrates for learning that are developmentally sensitive. A central question explored in this chapter relates to whether the primate cortex (both nonhuman and human) matures sequentially or concurrently across regions. The chapter also reviews assumptions about how learning and memory are supported by CNS substrates in terms of synapse formation.

The third chapter in this section, "Organization and Development of Callosal Connectivity in Prefrontal Cortex," is authored by Michael L. Schwartz. The focus of his work is on the organization of and cross-hemisphere connections between areas of the prefrontal association cortex in monkeys. The overview presented describes the topographic and laminar organization of these connections in the mature monkey and their prenatal development and maturational trajectory. Based on his studies, Schwartz concludes that "many features of the areal and intra-areal organization of callosal projections are specified prior to or just after birth" (Chapter 3, p. 62).

Chapter 4 is entitled "Developmental Anatomy of the Prefrontal Cortex." The authors, Peter R. Huttenlocher and Arun S. Dabholkar, review their early observations on synaptogenesis and synapse elimination in the developing PFC of humans. The results of the research were surprising because the findings indicated large-scale reduction in synapses during the normal development of the cortex and major changes in the cerebral cortex at ages when the anatomy was thought to be complete. Other important findings from the authors' laboratory suggest that "synaptic development in the human neocortex may not be totally concurrent, as has been found in subhuman primates" (Chapter 4, p. 73). In this regard, Huttenlocher and Dabholkar's results are in contrast to those of Goldman-Rakic et al. (Chapter 2).

The final chapter in this section, "Human Frontal Lobe Development: A Theory of Cyclical Cortical Reorganization," was contributed by Robert W. Thatcher. This chapter presents a theory of PFC development and organization that "is based on analyses of the development of human electroencephalographic (EEG) coherence that indicate that there are oscillations and cyclical growth processes that operate along the mediolateral and anterior–posterior planes of the human brain" (p. 85). In this theory, the PFC plays a necessary role because it is hypothesized to select and reduce synaptic connections during postnatal development. Thatcher describes how his theory elucidates brain development pre- and postnatally and explicates the intricate physiological and anatomical mechanisms that are thought to be responsible for the brain's organization.

BRAIN–BEHAVIOR RELATIONSHIPS

The second section of the volume consists of four chapters that describe research using experimental procedures to illuminate relationships between the PFC and various behaviors in nonhuman primates and children. The first chapter in Section II, "Competence, Cortex, and Primate Models: A Comparative Primate Perspective," was contributed by Duane M. Rumbaugh. The chapter provides an overview of a series of issues that confront researchers who employ nonhuman primates to study brain–behavior relationships in an attempt to better understand such relationships in humans. Rumbaugh considers brain evolution and competence, homology, brain size and complexity and specific effects of early environment, and both Cartesian and Darwinian ideas concerning animals and their mental capacities. He discusses the relationships between brain complexity and mode of learning and directional transfer. Rumbaugh next provides an interesting exposition concerning symbolic competence, complexity, and plasticity. He provides the reader with a useful overview of animals and language, with a particular emphasis on language acquisition in the great apes, a research topic for which he is widely known.

The next chapter, by Christiana M. Leonard, is entitled "Language and the Prefrontal Cortex." Leonard presents a tour de force overview concerning the neural substrate for language and the putative necessary involvement of the PFC in this most complex human behavior. She reviews the anatomical evidence for her thesis, along with information on brain asymmetry, handedness, and gender, to build her argument concerning the involvement of the PFC in language. She reviews language development in children and alludes to the gradual nature of subsystems of language ontogeny (i.e., phonology, semantics, syntax, pragmatics). Leonard reviews specific language impairments that accrue when the brain is lesioned through pathological processes. Such information is a basic tool of neuropsychologists to help correlate and identify brain–behavior relationships. Data from her laboratory are discussed that imply that the PFC is involved in specific language impairment and fluency.

Chapter 8, "Development of Neuronal Activity in Cortical Regions Underlying Visual Recognition in Monkeys," was contributed by Hillary R. Rodman and Kristy L. Nace. The focus of their chapter is on a review of findings from neurophysiological and anatomical studies conducted by the authors of the inferior temporal cortex of infant monkeys. The studies reported were designed to elucidate basic questions about relationships between brain structure and experience as these relationships reflect visual capacity (i.e., pattern recognition) to identify and use objects and scenes. As the authors point out,

> visual pattern recognition capacity is a complex set of abilities involving perception of identifying characteristics of stimuli, abstraction of features that reliably identify objects under varied or degraded conditions, and generation of signals indicating that a given stimulus has been seen before. In both humans and monkeys, visual pattern recognition is subserved by a ventrally coursing occipito-temporo-frontal system of interconnected cortical areas. (Chapter 8, p. 167)

The authors discuss the mounting research findings that ventral pathways mediating pattern and object recognition extend into ventral portions of the PFC. The data presented provide strong evidence concerning physiological and anatomical mechanisms that subsume behaviors, early in life, that are necessary for primates to adapt to their complex visual world.

In the final chapter in this section, "Frontal and Attentional Mechanisms Regulating Distress Experience and Expression During Infancy," Catherine Harman and Nathan A. Fox review evidence concerning putative neural mechanisms, both anatomical and physiological, for emotional expression during early development. The authors describe two different ideas concerning the control of emotion, the *valence hypothesis* (both left and right PFCs are involved in the control of emotion) versus the *unilateral hypothesis* (only one hemisphere is responsible for the control of emotion). Fox and his colleagues have argued for the valence hypothesis and present data from his and other laboratories to support this thesis. In particular, he reviews his own research concerning a longitudinal study of distressed infants in which he examines relationships between their behavior and EEG patterns. Harman and Fox discuss the development of attention and emotion in terms of the orienting response and *obligatory attention*. The authors also provide an interesting model system for studying the interaction of attention and distress.

NEUROPSYCHOLOGY AND
NEUROPATHOLOGY OF PREFRONTAL CORTEX

The third section of the book contains seven chapters that provide a perspective on the role of the PFC in the control of *executive function* and the consequences of lesions to the PFC in terms of altered behavior in those who have sustained such damage. These chapters provide unique evidence concerning functions subsumed by the PFC. In the first chapter in this section, "Corticolimbic Circuitry and the Development of Psychopathology During Childhood and Adolescence," Francine M. Benes explores two themes. The first of these relates to a comprehensive description of pathways and systems in the brain that might have a role in the expression of psychopathology in children and teenagers. The second theme relates to how corticolimbic systems may be interfered with either during gestation or postnatally, resulting in the expression of different forms of mental illness. Benes concludes by describing a strategy that employs a neurodevelopmental approach for characterizing psychopathology during childhood.

The next chapter, by Randall S. Scheibel and Harvey S. Levin, is entitled "Frontal Lobe Dysfunction Following Closed Head Injury in Children: Findings from Neuropsychology and Brain Imaging." The advent of computed tomography scans and magnetic resonance imaging has made possible noninvasive, quantitative analysis of neuropathology and has given neuropsychologists an opportunity to correlate behavioral functioning with assessment of damage to frontal structures in closed head injuries. As the authors point out, however, neurobehavioral assessment of frontal injury in children is complicated by developmental factors. Scheibel and Levin provide an analysis of what these problems are and how they increase the difficulty of answering the questions concerning frontal lobe function. The authors discuss effects of location and size of focal closed head injuries on cognitive functioning and planning abilities, and the influence of developmental stage (when the injury occurs) on behavior changes and recovery. They conclude their chapter by outlining directions for future research.

Chapter 12, "Dimensions of Executive Function in Normal and Abnormal Development," is by Bruce F. Pennington. In his chapter, Pennington discusses the "frontal metaphor" as an analogy between behavioral symptoms or test performance of children at different stages of development and similar behaviors in children with acquired frontal lesions. He also writes an overview aimed at "providing a unified account of cognitive differences by 1) examining the scope and limits of the frontal metaphor in developmental neuropsychology, 2) providing some data on dimensions of executive functions in normal and abnormal development, and 3) discussing implications for future research" (Chapter 12, p. 266). The chapter goes a long way toward buttressing the utility of the frontal metaphor and moving it from the status of an analogy to that of a homology, as well as making it an operational construct that can provide an integrated understanding of cognitive differences.

The fourth chapter in this section, "Prefrontal–Subcortical Circuits in Developmental Disorders," is by Martha Bridge Denckla and Allan L. Reiss. The focus of the chapter is on elucidating the contributions made by prefrontal–subcortical systems and pathways to cognitive dysfunctions observed in developmental disorders. The authors define areas of cognitive functioning and link them to putative prefrontal–subcortical pathways thought to subsume such functions in normal development and to be directly related to impairment of the defined cognitive domain when such subsystems malfunction. Subsequently, they discuss issues related to criteria for separating prefrontal from subcortical parts of neurological dysfunction. The chapter concludes with a review of research findings concerning two neurological diseases, Tourette syndrome and attention-deficit/hyperactivity disorder, that are used as exemplars to illustrate the potential role of the circuitry under consideration in developmental disorders.

The next chapter, "Cognitive and Social Development in Children with Prefrontal Cortex Lesions," is by Paul J. Eslinger, Kathleen R. Biddle, and Lynn M. Grattan. In this chapter, the authors review case histories of children who have documented prefrontal damage. They employ a neurobehavioral approach to explicate defined prefrontal lesions and concomitant observed behavior changes in the areas of prosocial and executive functioning. The authors next provide a useful discussion of methodological issues relevant to the type of neurobehavioral and neuropsychological research that they carry out. They summarize in detail two case histories of prefrontal lesions in children, relating the damage sustained to the cognitive and social-behavioral sequelae observed. The chapter concludes with some suggestions for future research.

The next chapter, by William H. Overman, Jocelyne Bachevalier, Elena Schuhmann, and Patricia McDonough-Ryan, is entitled "Sexually Dimorphic Brain–Behavior Development: A Comparative Perspective." The focus of the chapter is on comparative analyses of performance by male and female monkeys and young children on object reversal and concurrent object discrimination. A major question relates to whether differential performance on these tasks by males and females are biologically based or based on social/learning factors. The data demonstrate that young males (monkeys and humans) are superior to females on object reversal, whereas young females (monkeys and humans) are superior to males on concurrent object discrimination. A detailed discussion of methods and data convincingly demonstrates that these tasks are sexually dimorphic. The authors discuss their arguments for the biological bases of gender-specific performance and rule out a social-learning hypothesis.

The last chapter, "The Work in Working Memory: Implications for Development," is by Karl H. Pribram. Along with his colleagues Miller and Galanter,

Pribram was a pioneer in studying frontal association areas and pointing out that the PFC appears to serve as a site for working memory "where Plans can be retained temporarily when they are being formed, or transformed, or executed" (Miller, Galanter, & Pribram, 1960, p. 207). The author describes the anatomy of the PFC's three divisions and then discusses three functions of the PFC under the rubrics of parcelation, attention, and intention. He provides some of his own experimental data to support his functional description of the PFC. The author concludes his informative chapter by describing functional staging in the developmental trajectory of the PFC over the age span between 1 and 21 years.

REFERENCE

Miller, G.A., Galanter, E.H., & Pribram, K.H. (1960). *Plans and the structure of behavior.* New York: Holt, Rinehart & Winston.

I

EVOLUTION AND NEUROBIOLOGY

1

Evolution of Prefrontal Cortex

Harry J. Jerison

Almost all analyses of prefrontal neocortex (PFC) begin with statements about its evolution. This chapter is devoted to the basis for and implications of such statements and their relevance for the neurosciences. I begin with an overview, which provides a framework for the data presented later in the chapter and foreshadows my conclusions. Next I consider the questions that are usually posed to evolutionists, namely, when did PFC evolve, and is human PFC unique either at the cellular level or as an organ contributing to the brain's circuitry? Some of my answers depend on a quantitative analysis of the relative size of brain structures, which I discuss in the sections on uniqueness and on the surprising uniformity of the general structure of mammalian brains. In conclusion, I consider the selective pressures that may explain why PFC evolved and point out some logical and methodological limitations of my analysis.

Evolution consists of change over time in the genetic systems that determine structure and function. Aspects of theories of natural selection and genetic drift explain the facts of evolution, but it is important to keep in mind that the facts are about change itself and that theories, controversial or not, consider the reasons for change. Neural evolution poses a fundamental theoretical difficulty because of the special place of nature–nurture interactions in neural development. Because both the structure and function of the mature brain, at least in mammals, are determined by a complex interaction between the genetic blueprint and the pre- and postnatal environment in which nerves develop, the facts about mature brains are not exclusively about genetic systems and must be used with care in theoretical analysis. We now know that even such pillars of neuroscience lore as the elegant maps drawn to depict sensory and motor systems as if laid down in a blueprint are, in fact, modifiable under environmental stress (Merzenich & Kaas, 1980).

This chapter was begun while I was a visiting professor in the Department of Psychology, University College London, England. I thank my University College colleagues for their comradeship and for the facilities that they provided.

PFC was defined classically by the cytoarchitecture of the primate brain (Brodmann, 1913) and in modern neurobiology by its connections with cortical and subcortical structures. There are variations among species in these features, and there is inevitable uncertainty in decisions as to what to call PFC and what to treat as premotor neocortex. This issue has been reopened forcefully in a fine polemic by Preuss (1995), who reviewed the definition of PFC in a detailed discussion of its anatomy. I discuss Preuss briefly at the end of this chapter and indicate the modifications in my views that would be required, were I to accept his argument. However, I continue to accept the standard view (Bishop, 1994a, 1994b; Fuster, 1989; Kolb & Tees, 1990; Uylings & Van Eden, 1990) as correct and follow it in defining PFC primarily by its connection with the dorsomedial nucleus of the thalamus and secondarily by the classic "prefrontal syndrome" following ablation of PFC.

Most readers of this book are likely to be more familiar with the literature on neuroscience than with that on evolution. Although I cite sources on technical evolutionary issues in the body of this chapter, it may be helpful to recommend a general text on the subject. My favorite such volume is *The Blind Watchmaker* by Dawkins (1987),which is authoritative and well written. Thanks to Hodos and Campbell (1969), neuroscientists are properly wary of the idea of "progressive evolution." We have learned that progress does not imply an Aristotelian "scale of nature" or a teleological force toward perfection (see Lovejoy, 1936), but we may not recognize that natural selection, in fact, does imply progressive changes. The analysis of phylogenetic branching ("cladistics") is not inconsistent with the idea of progress ("anagenesis"). At the conclusion of this chapter, I present some facts of progressive cortical evolution, but these facts do not imply any mystical force in evolution. Change in a particular direction is usually interpreted as an economical adaptation, as it were, to a changing environment.

OVERVIEW

Neurobiologists conventionally describe PFC as a recent evolutionary acquisition. Many of them believe that PFC is unusually enlarged in the human brain, and they explain that this is because PFC has so much uniquely human work to do. As far as I can tell, there is no justification for these statements. In fact, were these assertions true, they would make nonsense of much research on PFC that depends on animal models.

The evidence is that PFC is an ancient part of the mammalian brain and that human PFC is the right size for a primate brain as big as ours. It seems to be put together in pretty much the way PFC is put together in other mammals, and its functions are essentially the same. The functions include "advanced" higher mental processes such as directing attention, accessing various memory systems, and coordinating sensory and motor information. Are these uniquely human control functions? Of course not. They can be and have been studied in rats (Kolb & Tees, 1990), and much of our knowledge about them is based on work with monkeys (Fuster, 1989). These processes are higher in us because of the way they work, but the way these functions work in us reflects their interaction with other specialized human brain systems, some of which, such as our language system, are in large measure unique to our species.

It is worth remembering that all species are unique in some ways. That is what makes them species. Some brain functions in every mammalian species are unique to that species, and other functions work the same way in many species. The analytic evolutionary issue is to determine the balance between diversity based on uniqueness versus uniformities based on common features. The human species is a late arrival on the evolutionary stage, notable for its behavioral specializations. Brain control of these specializations include many unique features, but the control systems are in networks distributed through many regions of the brain (Goldman-Rakic, 1988). Localized regions of these systems, such as those that are contained in PFC, may or may not contribute disproportionately to the work of the brain. The facts that I will present indicate that PFC does not contribute disproportionately.

The brain systems controlled by PFC are very extensive and involve very large amounts of tissue. Interactions with these brain systems could be maintained only if the size of PFC were related to the size of the systems with which it interacts, and, because the systems are distributed through much of the brain, the size of PFC would have to be related to the size of the rest of the brain. Our first problem is to determine whether a general mammalian relationship or a general primate relationship exists. If it exists, our second problem is to determine whether it is the same for *Homo sapiens* as for other species. The solution of these problems enables us to describe and understand the evolution of the prefrontal system as a feature of vertebrate evolution and of the evolution of the brain.

Because human brains are very large, human PFC must be expected to be very large. *Very large* does not, however, mean *disproportionately large*. The evidence at this time is that the amount of human PFC is in correct proportion for a primate brain and is possibly appropriate for mammals as a class. The general issues of uniqueness, size, and recency in evolution can be understood correctly without in any way diminishing our appreciation of the importance of PFC in human behavior and experience. A proper evolutionary perspective may also make it easier for us to think about animal models that enable us to apply to humans the results of observations and experiments on other species.

WHEN DID PFC EVOLVE?

We can begin with the question of whether PFC evolved more recently than other systems. The answer is surprisingly simple and follows from a cladistic analysis, which is a formal analysis of similarities and differences among species. Such an analysis is based primarily on gross morphology and molecular genetics, and it serves to establish the phylogenetic tree that describes the relationships of the species to one another (Cracraft & Eldredge, 1979). The assumption in a cladistic analysis is that adaptations and structures that are present in descendant groups were also present in the common ancestor of those groups. One recognizes that a particular adaptive system, such as PFC, would be unlikely to evolve independently in each descendant group; its presence in all of the groups is explained most simply as a retention of an earlier adaptation inherited from a common ancestor.

The present consensus (but see Preuss, 1995) is that PFC is present in all living mammals. Defined as the cortical system receiving input from the dorsomedial nucleus of the thalamus, PFC has been identified in marsupials (opossum: Benjamin & Golden, 1985) and monotremes, or egg-laying mammals (echidna: Johnson, 1990), as well as in placental mammals. The PFC system would, therefore, be expected to have been part of the adaptive mosaic of the ancestral species from which these groups evolved.

Kielan-Jaworowska (1992) reviewed the fossil evidence of mammalian evolution with respect to the times of branching. Figure 1.1 summarizes her conclusions in the mammalian lines. The extinct major groups, including those ancestral to all living mammals, are labeled collectively as A; monotremes are labeled as B; marsupials are labeled as C; and placentals are labeled as D. As a neural adaptation, PFC is known in living species of Groups B, C, and D and may, therefore, be assumed to have been present before the first branching. Because the first branching probably occurred about 175 million years ago, we have our answer. PFC appeared at least 175 million years ago.

Here are some details of the evolutionary scenario. Of the 40,000–50,000 species of known living vertebrates, about half are fish and another 7,500 or so are amphibians and reptiles. A large majority of vertebrate species, therefore, do quite well in the scheme of things, although they have relatively little brain and no neocortex at all. Birds, which number some 8,000 species, have brains in the same relative size range as mammals; but birds do not have cerebral cortex, although their forebrains have major regions that are possibly homologous with neocortex and function in the same way. Some forebrain regions in birds may even function analogously to PFC in mammals (Divac, 1994; Gagliardo & Divac, 1993; Karten, 1991; Macphail, 1994). It is only in the 5,000 or so living species of mammals, however, that PFC is identifiable both structurally and functionally.

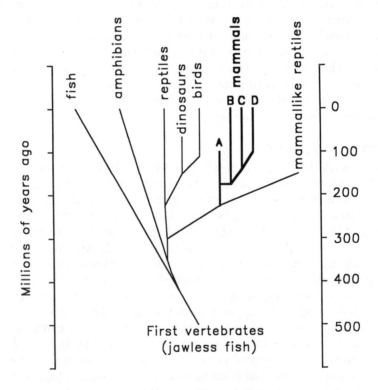

Figure 1.1.   The phylogeny of the vertebrates. (Boldface type = Mammalian phylogeny; Group A = Major groups now extinct, such as the triconodonts and multituberculates, but also the parent groups of living species. Groups B, C, D = Monotremes, marsupials, and placentals, respectively, with approximate ages at splitting from the main line indicated on the ordinate.)

The earliest mammals appeared during the Upper Triassic period of the Mesozoic era, about 225 million years ago. Although there is fossil evidence from endocasts (brainlike casts for which the cranial cavity is the mold) with regard to the external appearance of the brains of Mesozoic mammals, it is impossible to make statements about PFC on the basis of that evidence. There are no landmarks on the external surface of the brain that show the limits of the extent of PFC. Branching dates of the major groups and the presence of PFC in those groups today provide the only evidence. Kielan-Jaworowska (1992) concluded that the ancestors of living monotremes can be identified in Jurassic strata of about 175 million years ago. The earliest marsupials appeared about 140 million years ago, and the earliest placentals about 100 million years ago. This information is sufficient to indicate the latest possible date of origin for PFC. Unless it evolved independently in the three living mammalian subclasses, PFC was present in their common ancestor. The system may, therefore, be dated to at least the middle Jurassic period about 175 million years ago. It is not a recent evolutionary acquisition.

The evidence on fossil "brains" in mammals begins with an endocast of *Triconodon mordax* (Jerison, 1973), a species from Group A of Figure 1.1, which lived 150 million years ago. This "brain" is a natural cast of dorsal forebrain and olfactory bulbs. Endocasts from 75 million years ago, including some on placentals (Group D), are the oldest in which features on the lateral surface can be examined. These endocasts are from very small, shrewlike species and show a fairly clear impression of the rhinal fissure (Jerison, 1990; Kielan-Jaworowska, 1986), which is the boundary between neocortex and paleocortex in living mammalian brains. We, therefore, have direct evidence of that early date for neocortex as dorsal to the fissure.

For PFC itself, we have to rely on the cladistic analysis of Figure 1.1 and on the classic geological doctrine of uniformitarianism (Simpson, 1970), which states that present "laws of nature," such as the present structure of neocortex, were laws of nature throughout geological time. Thus, if endocasts from living species enable us to identify neocortex dorsal to a rhinal fissure, then fossil endocasts displaying the same fissure are evidence of neocortex in the fossil species. In addition, if neocortex in living mammals always receives projections from the dorsomedial nucleus of the thalamus in the prefrontal region, then fossils with neocortex are assumed to have such projections, and PFC is assumed to have been present. The two evolutionary arguments, that from cladistics and that from uniformitarianism, combine to make a strong case for PFC as an ancient adaptation.

ARE THERE DIFFERENCES
IN CELL TYPES AND CONNECTIVITY?

The issue of differences among species with respect to cell types in PFC was addressed by Powell and his group:

> From the findings of the constancy in number and proportions of cell types in the cortex between different areas and species it seems probable that early in mammalian evolution these two quantitative features of the cortex are determined genetically and this specification remains constant. (Rockel, Hiorns, & Powell, 1980, p. 236)

This "basic uniformity of structure of the neocortex" is one of several described in the report from Powell's laboratory. They also found a constancy with respect to number and proportions of cell types for the entire neocortex and, by inference, for PFC as an area of the brain.

I am aware of no evidence that connectivity within PFC or between PFC and other structures in the brain is fundamentally different from that among other nuclear centers. The qualitatively described patterns in all mammalian brains are so varied and complex (Braitenberg & Schüz, 1991) that it is not clear how one would evaluate qualitative uniqueness. We may define connectivity quantitatively, that is, as the number of connections that are made, and ignore the pattern of connections. Could one then measure connectivity to discover quantitatively unique patterns? Quantitative differences in the number of branches, number of synapses, and fiber length and diameter of single neurons have been measured. There are species differences, but these are confounded with differences in brain size. There are different constraints on neuronal growth and more opportunities for connections to be made in larger than in smaller brains, and these seem to account for the differences among the measurements (Braitenberg & Schüz, 1991). Schüz and Demianenko (1995) reported that the number of neocortical synapses per unit volume of brain tissue is approximately constant regardless of species, as expected from theoretical considerations (Jerison, 1973).

DO HUMANS HAVE MORE PFC THAN EXPECTED?

Uylings and Van Eden (1990) have published a simple analysis showing that human PFC follows the same size rule as PFC in other primates as well as in the laboratory rat. Their finding points us away from an assumption of uniqueness, that is, of some species-typical specializations that would be reflected in unusual PFC size in any species. Their analysis is summarized in Figure 1.2.

Figure 1.2, as well as Figures 1.3 and 1.4, involve methodological issues, which deserve a paragraph or two of explanation. The graphs in these figures provide comparative analysis of between-species effects of size (see Harvey & Pagel, 1991;

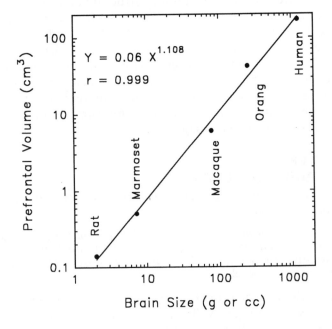

Figure 1.2.   Prefrontal neocortex as a function of brain size in five species of mammals. (Adapted from Uylings and Van Eden [1990].)

Schmidt-Nielsen, 1984). These are simple problems, but they have sometimes been misunderstood by both neurobiologists and evolutionists.

Size may work differently in biological systems than in mechanical systems. Most important, biological systems are made of cells, and a system's bulk is determined by the number of cells it contains. Cells are packed efficiently in the brain, and their number in mammals can often be estimated from the gross brain size. Increments in body and organ size occur by cell division, with each step doubling the number of cells: 1, 2, 4, 8, 16, 32, and so forth. In biological systems, the number of these steps is a natural measure of size, in which increments are multiplicative rather than additive. A measurement scale meeting the multiplicative requirement can be made with logarithms, which change the numbers to 0, .3, .6, .9, 1.2, 1.5, and so on. (With logarithms to the base 2, the new numbers are 0, 1, 2, 3, 4, 5, and so forth; with Napierian logarithms to the base e, they are 0, .7, 1.4, 2.1, 2.8, 3.5, and so forth.) Equal distances along a logarithmic scale represent equal numbers of cell divisions rather than equal numbers of cells. The graphs in Figures 1.2, 1.3, and 1.4 show phenomena scaled with logarithmic measures.

Phenomena scaled logarithmically often look simpler and easier to understand than when scaled linearly. It is occasionally assumed that there is some trick involved and that "true" variability is masked by logarithmic scaling. There is no trick. That the graphs of Figures 1.2, 1.3, and 1.4 are understandable and that they would be unreadable with linear scales is not a fault. They are not oversimplified. Scaling them linearly would unnecessarily and, in my view, falsely complicate the relationships that graphs are designed to analyze and explain.

With E as brain size, the equation of the line in Figure 1.2 as reported by Uylings and Van Eden (1990) is

$$\log(PFC) = 1.108 \log E - 1.2$$

They report the strength of the relationship (i.e., correlation coefficient) as

$$r = .999$$

The equation may be rewritten as a power-function:

$$(PFC) = .06 \, E^{1.108} \tag{Eq. 1.1}$$

Equation 1.1 and the high correlation coefficient are fundamental for understanding the evolution of PFC. That the exponent of the power function is slightly greater than 1.0 implies that as brains become diversified in size, the amount of PFC becomes a slightly larger fraction of larger brain. Equation 1.1 shows that the relationship of PFC to brain size is nonlinear but not disproportional; that is, the correct proportions or ratios of PFC to brain size are specified by the equation for all values of brain size. The equation describes a gradual divergence between larger-brained (human or not) versus smaller-brained species as a straightforward effect of changes in gross brain size.

The high correlation coefficient tells us that the size of PFC in different species is determined almost entirely by brain size. No additional unique or species-typical factors appear to determine the size of PFC. I add the "almost" to acknowledge that despite its strength, the connection expressed by Equation 1.1 and demonstrated in Figure 1.2 is correlational rather than causal. Even an almost perfect correlation leaves some residual variance, which statistical models treat as randomly distributed errors of measurement. Residuals, no matter how small, may nevertheless

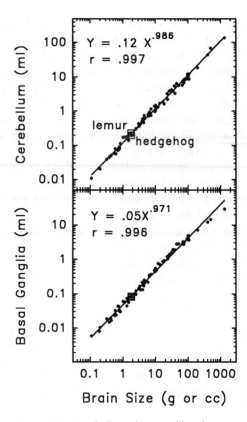

Figure 1.3.   Cerebellar volume and basal ganglia volume as a function of brain size in 76
species of mammals. (□ = Data points for the
mouse lemur [*Microcebus*] and the desert hedgehog [*Hemiechinus*].) (Data from Stephan, Frahm,
& Baron [1981].)

reflect real nonrandom effects, as is evident in Figure 1.4. There is independent
confirmation for the association between the size of PFC and the whole brain, however, at least in primates, in data from Brodmann (1913), based on older cytoarchitectonic criteria rather than on thalamic connections to define PFC. Brodmann's data lead to the same conclusions as those just presented.

For a quantitative sense of the meaning and limitations of Equation 1.1 and
Figure 1.2, consider a rat, a dog, a cow, and a person, with brains weighing 2 grams
(g), 100 g, 400 g, and 1,300 g, respectively. Equation 1.1 tells us that we should expect PFC in these animals to weigh 0.13 g, 8.7 g, 39 g, and 138 g, respectively. These
are the amounts set by the "natural law"of Equation 1.1. PFCs in these animals, as
we go from rat to human, are 6.5%, 8.7%, 9.8%, and 10.6%, respectively, of the total brain weight. One might then be tempted to conclude that PFC increased as we
"advanced" from rats to humans. But the "law" refers only to brain size and not to
anything else about a species. A horse brain that weighs 600 g should have a 60 g
PFC, and a walrus with a 1,300-g brain should have a 138-g PFC, the same as a human. The point is that species does not matter according to the "law."

To restate these conclusions qualitatively rather than quantitatively, whatever
determines gross brain size among species also appears to determine the size of

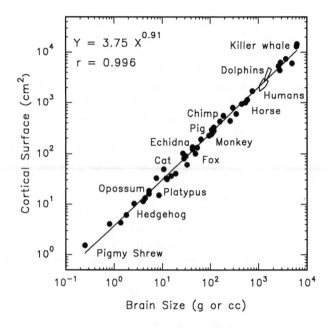

Figure 1.4.   The relationship between cortical surface and gross brain size in 50 species of mammals. Each point represents a species. In addition, two labeled minimum convex polygons indicate within-species variability in humans ($N = 23$) and dolphins (*Tursiops truncatus*; $N = 13$). Several species are labeled to indicate the diversity of the sample.

PFC. If you are a mammal, then your brain structure should obey the law described by Equation 1.1, which is the same for *Homo sapiens* as for a horse or a walrus. Based as it is on so small a sample of species, Equation 1.1 is really not much of a law, but it is the best we can do at this time. We obviously need more data on more species.

Although surprising, these results on PFC make good sense. Because PFC is known to be a kind of control organ, governing operations of other parts of the brain, its size in a species should be related to the sum of the sizes of the brain systems that it controls, and total brain size is probably a good estimator of that sum. A high correlation between brain size and PFC size is exactly what we should expect. We can, moreover, be confident that there is a true relationship between PFC size and brain size, approximately as presented in Figure 1.2, despite the small sample size, because comparably strong part–whole relations in the brain have been found in data on much larger and more diverse samples of species. When we examine the quantitative evidence, we find that, on the whole, the brain hangs together quite well. If we know its size, then we can make surprisingly good estimates of the size of the major structures within it.

THE BRAIN HANGS TOGETHER

Size relationships between major parts of the brain and the whole brain in different species are usually orderly. The orderliness is maintained in brains of different size, regardless of whether the brain in a species is enlarged because of the evolution of larger body sizes or whether the enlargement is an "advanced" feature related to the evolution of unusual neural control, perhaps associated with higher mental processes. In the analysis of brain size, the body size effect is called "allometric," and the advancement effect is "encephalization." In statistical terms, the allometric effect is determined from the regression of log brain size on log body size, and the encephalization of a species is measured as a residual, which is the deviation of the size of the brain of the species from the regression equation's prediction. All of the analysis is at a species level; individual differences within a species are treated as statistical errors of measurement.

Two sets of data based on large samples of species demonstrate the extent to which the organization of mammalian brains is comparable across species. The first relates the volumes of selected brain structure to one another and to body size and lends itself to a multivariate analysis. The second is a bivariate analysis of the relationship between total cortical surface area and brain size. Table 1.1 summarizes the structure of the first data set and charts the results of a multivariate analysis of the most extensive quantitative data on mammal brains published to date: measures of 10 brain structures, brain weight, and body weight in 76 species (Stephan, Frahm, & Baron, 1981).

The species were 28 insectivores, 3 tree shrews, 18 prosimians (lemurlike primates), and 27 anthropoids (monkeys, apes, and humans). I performed the factor analysis of the 12×76 matrix of measurements using Wilkinson's (1989) SYSTAT computer program. The outstanding result is that only two factors were required to account for almost all of the variance in this sample and that a single "general size" factor accounted for 86% of the variance. (For additional discussion, see Jerison, 1991.)

When factor loadings follow a pattern as shown in Table 1.1 and we pair two variables with high loadings on the general size factors, we find correlations close to 1.0. When graphed, the points are very close to the regression line. This is evident in Figure 1.3 and exemplifies our theme: The brain hangs together.

Like the relationship between PFC and brain size in Figure 1.2, these within-brain relationships are more or less independent of species-typical aspects of brain enlargement. There are no important quantitative differences in the data in Figure 1.3 between brains of species in which the enlargement is mainly an allometric effect of body size and those in which the enlargement is associated with encephalization, independently of allometry. Marked data points in Figure 1.3 (small squares) illustrate this in a desert hedgehog (*Hemiechinus*) and in a mouse lemur (*Microcebus*), two species that differ markedly in body size yet have brains that are about the same size. The mouse lemur, which is the smallest known primate and has about a 1.8-g brain, weighs about 50 g; the hedgehog, with a 1.9-g brain, weighs about 250 g (Stephan et al., 1981). It is clear from Figure 1.3 that, like the brain as a whole, cerebellum and basal ganglia in these two species are about equal in size. (Data for basal ganglia are so close to one another that the squares marking these points are almost congruent and may be too close to one another to be distinguished.)

The graphs in Figure 1.3 show that if you know the size of a brain, regardless of why it reached its size, you can very accurately estimate the size of the cerebellum and the size of the basal ganglia. The same would be true for all of the brain measures listed in Table 1.1, with the exception of the olfactory bulbs. The relatively low factor loading for the size of the olfactory bulbs is probably a consequence of the large number of anthropoid primates in our sample. Monkeys, apes, and hu-

Table 1.1.   Factor loadings and percentage variance explained by two principal components (Factors 1 and 2) in brain and body in 76 species of mammals

	Factor 1 General brain size	Factor 2 Olfactory bulbs
Neocortex	.991	.059
Total brain weight	.989	.137
Diencephalon	.987	.144
Basal ganglia	.987	.133
Cerebellum	.983	.168
Mesencephalon	.972	.196
Medulla	.966	.224
Hippocampus	.962	.239
Schizocortex	.954	.274
Body weight	.939	.285
Piriform lobe	.899	.399
Olfactory bulbs	.157	.985
Percent total variance	85.855	12.668

From Jerison, H.J. (1991). *Brain size and the evolution of mind.* 59th James Arthur Lecture on the Evolution of the Human Brain. New York: American Museum of Natural History.

Note: Varimax rotation.

mans are unusual among mammals in having olfactory bulbs much reduced in size relative to both their brain and body sizes.

Another data set from a more diverse sample of mammal species illustrates the significance of brain size as a measure to estimate the information-processing capacity of the brain. The analysis is presented in Figure 1.4, which combines data from Brodmann (1913), Elias and Schwartz (1971), Ridgway (1981), and Ridgway and Brownson (1984). Figure 1.4 shows the relationship between total cortical surface area (including that hidden in fissures) and brain size. The 50 species are from the orders Artiodactyla, Carnivora, Cetacea, Edentata, Insectivora, Marsupialia, Monotremata, Perissodactyla, Primates, Proboscidea, and Rodentia. (For additional details, see Jerison, 1991.)

The orderly picture in Figure 1.4 confirms how useful brain size is as a natural biological statistic. I first discuss why it shows the relationship of brain size to information-processing capacity. I then discuss other inferences from Figure 1.4 because it also demonstrates that the human brain is less convoluted than expected, below average for mammals, and implies that animal intelligence is not related to convolutedness. Finally, it provides a useful restraint on our thinking about the causal relations implicit in statistical correlation.

The relationship to processing capacity is based on our knowledge of the organization of information in the cortex. The unit of information may be defined at various levels, such as the synapse, the neuron, or, at a higher level, the cortical column, which is often identified as a higher-order unit. The number of cortical columns in a mammal's brain should be directly related to the information-processing capacity of that brain, and, because cortical columns are fairly uniform in diameter (Szentagothai, 1978), their number must be proportional to the cortical surface area. Figure 1.4 shows that total brain size estimates the surface area and, thus, the information-processing capacity of a brain.

The need to rethink convolutedness comes from an interesting detail in Figure 1.4. The regression line in this graph represents the expected amount of surface for any mammal brain. A species lying above the line has more than its share of surface, as it were, and a species below the line is underendowed. Normally, we would assume unquestioningly that the points deviate randomly from the line because of the almost perfect correlation; but, in two samples, we have enough data to test this assumption. These are 1) a cetacean sample (*Tursiops truncatus*) of 13 individuals enclosed in the minimum convex polygon labeled "Dolphins" and 2) a "Humans" sample of 23 individuals in an adjacent polygon. Although the data enclosed by the polygons are close to the regression line, all 13 dolphin points lie above the line, and 19 of the 23 human points lie below it. A point above the line signifies a more convoluted brain than average, and one below the line means a less convoluted brain. Statistically, both dolphins and humans are significantly different from what is expected, and we humans are below average relative to mammals as a whole in convolutedness. (Must one comment?)

Interesting as it is to learn that convolutedness cannot be treated as a measure of braininess (or intelligence) unless we accept the status of below-average mammals, there is also a useful statistical lesson in Figure 1.4. Even very small residuals may be significant and not simply random error effects. The computed correlation of 0.996 between log-cortical surface-area weight and log-brain weight in Figure 1.4 means that the regression explains 99.2% of the variance in this system, leaving less than 1% unexplained (i.e., attributable to the residuals). In most statistical analyses, so small an unexplained variance would be assumed without question to represent error of measurement, and one is pleased to be able to reduce errors to that extent. We know better. We know that the "residuals" in our data on humans and dolphins are not due to error. They reflect a true difference between species.

For our topic, it would be nice to have data as extensive as those of Figures 1.3 and 1.4 on PFC. Unfortunately, we do not. Those of Figure 1.2 are the best that we can do. Although its sample is small, Figure 1.2 is convincing because of the high correlation coefficient and the more or less independent confirmation from Brodmann (1913). Thus, we can properly conclude that much, perhaps all, of the size of PFC in mammals should be understood as related to its role in controlling the rest of the brain—that its size relative to total brain size follows a single rule (Equation 1.1) in all mammals. But from the significant residuals in the face of the almost perfect correlation in Figure 1.4, we have learned that there may be species-typical effects hidden in the residuals of the regression of PFC on brain size in Figure 1.2.

In applying the result to fossils, we take advantage of the fact that brain volume is easy to estimate from endocasts and is often the only available measure. Although the brain's weight is the more usual measure available for living brains, the weight of a brain in grams and the volume of an endocast in milliliters are interchangeable numbers because most mammalian brains are tightly packed in the cranial cavity, and the specific gravity of brain tissue (about 1.06) makes unnecessary a correction in the conversion from weight to volume. On the basis of the data in Table 1.1 and Figures 1.3 and 1.4, we are confident that we can make reasonable judgments about the size of important structures within a fossil mammal's brain from the size of its endocast. Information about gross size from the fossil data—the most direct basis for inferences about the evolution of the whole brain—is also applicable to the analysis of the evolution of some of the major parts of the brain.

DISCUSSION: EVOLUTION
OF BRAIN SIZE AND SELECTION FOR PFC

We have now seen essentially all of the direct evidence and some of the indirect evidence on the evolution of PFC. Because of its strong relationship to the size of the whole brain, we can relate the evolution of PFC to the fossil evidence on the evolution of brain size, which I have discussed extensively elsewhere (Jerison, 1973, 1991). Mammalian encephalization to the grade of living opossums and hedgehogs occurred early, perhaps 225 million years ago, with the appearance of the earliest mammals. That initial grade of encephalization was maintained without further increase for more than 150 million years and was a characteristic of all Mesozoic and early Cenozoic mammals. Body size followed a correlated course. The earliest Mesozoic mammals were miniaturized to about one tenth the size of their closest reptilian relatives, and there was relatively little evolution of larger species. According to the available fossil evidence, there were probably no Mesozoic species that were larger than house cats; their typical size was in the range of living shrews and rats. The main inference from these and many related facts about their skeletal structure is that, in splitting from their reptilian ancestors, mammals "discovered" nocturnal niches, and their adaptive radiation during the Mesozoic was to exploit such niches.

From a neurobiological perspective, adaptations for life in the evening or at night required the use of sensory information from distance senses other than the typically reptilian diurnal vision. The additional information was from audition and olfaction as well as nocturnal (rod) vision, according to the scenario that I have suggested (Jerison, 1973). Newly evolved mammals were only slightly modified reptiles, and the neurobehavioral systems controlling their adaptations for action in the dark would presumably have handled as much information as those controlling diurnal activity in normal reptiles. Furthermore, to integrate information from the nocturnal visual channel and each of the several nonvisual channels, specialized integrative (association) systems also had to evolve. Regardless of where in the brain the new sensory and integrative systems would be located, the amount of processing that they had to do required a larger brain than that of reptiles. The evolution of mammalian cortex, in particular sensory neocortex with the segregation of specialized regions for each sensory input, could have been part of the response to these selection pressures. Furthermore, it would have been necessary for the association systems, presumably including those localized in PFC, to evolve at the same time. Encephalization by mammals relative to their reptilian forebears would have been the response to accommodate the packaging of the new forebrain systems.

Without specifying its localization, I have suggested (Jerison, 1973, 1991) that the integrative activity of handling cortical information, including that within sensory neocortex, should be labeled as "perceptual/cognitive" and that its function was the recognition and response to objects in an external environment. Controlling that work; directing attention to various parts, objects, and regions in the external environment; correlating present information with stored memories; and selecting among possible actions while inhibiting other actions are all part of the integrative requirement. Distributed through much of the neocortex, the systems controlling these activities include primary and secondary sensory cortex and also involve association functions, such as those of PFC in living species (Goldman-

Rakic, 1988). There was, in other words, a selective requirement for brain systems such as PFC as soon as the systems that are controlled by PFC had evolved. It is this requirement that makes the early evolution of PFC almost a necessary feature of the evolution of the brain.

Although I have not outlined a scenario for comparable motor control, it must have evolved as part of the same evolutionary mosaic. Sensing and perceiving are not passive activities. They are features of the behavior of animals engaging and acting upon their environment. Thus, it is more correct to relate perceptual/cognitive activity to sensorimotor systems than to restrict it to purely sensory systems. Other functions of PFC, in particular those in connection with autonomic control and with motivation and affect, are not considered or explained in this account, nor is it clear how they fit in with the evolution of cognitive functions.

According to this evolutionary narrative, neural control centers are needed in all species, and PFC qualifies for such a role. Its special place in the human species is in the multiplicity of sensory, motor, and other systems to which it must have access, including the language system. If we accept that PFC is specialized for such work, it follows that its size has to be proportional to the size of the systems that it controls. That, I think, is the main inference from evolutionary thinking applied to the major quantitative discovery of Uylings and Van Eden (1990) and forecast by Brodmann's (1913) work on primate brains.

To be more concrete about what might have happened in evolution, we have to imagine an evolutionary scenario in which a species develops a novel specialized sensory-motor adaptation. The integration of information from that novel system into information from other neurally controlled sensory, motor, and association activities would require adding to existing neural systems in the species. If the integrative system is localized elsewhere than within the novel sensory system, we could identify the new location as an anatomically discrete association system. For further speculation, I believe that the best analogy is to computers, considering their operation when they are required to handle novel jobs. If the basic computer has only enough capacity for word processing and it is required to run computer-assisted design (CAD) programs, its required adaptation includes an increased processing capacity, an enlargement involving more memory to store information, and additional storage space for the set of instructions in the CAD program. There remains a basic uniformity in the computer's method of operation. It uses the same kind of information-handling hardware, but there is more hardware, which performs more operations, and the computer becomes a larger machine.

The analogy is straightforwardly applied to the brain (cf. Jerison, 1973, on "proper mass"). In species in which echolocation, for example, evolved as a specialized system, the brain structures that support it are enlarged, as in the inferior colliculi and auditory cortex of bats (Grinnell,1995; Suga, Niwa, & Taniguchi, 1983). Analogous changes should occur with each novel control problem faced by the brain, and another example is that described by Welker (1990) in procyonids (see below). The integration of such new information into the behavior of an animal is performed by systems such as PFC. The integrative systems must be large enough to handle all of their control functions, and they integrate the data by selecting, combining, and arranging temporal orders among the available operations of the specialized systems. The behavior measured by Rumbaugh's transfer index (Chapter 6; Rumbaugh & Pate, 1984), for example, involves this kind of integration of data from many sources. It is to be expected that species with more tissue devoted to control and integration would perform better than other species with less tissue, just as Rumbaugh has reported. This is our model for PFC functions generally. Their peculiar place in humans, I believe, should be explained by their requirement to integrate data from the language sense with other sensory and motor data.

CODA

It is not appropriate at this time to develop the argument and analysis at greater length, but there are other important points that should be made on which I have hardly touched. I have emphasized the uniformity of brain structure and function and the fact that the size of PFC in mammals may be determined by a primitive function such as Equation 1.1. I have understated the diversity that also evolved, which implies a paradox that can probably be resolved but on which there are no data. If one had measurements of the size of somatosensory cortex in procyonids (the raccoons and their relatives), including information on the distribution of mappings of the paws and rhinarium, those data would show major distinctions among species. The qualitative evidence is that raccoons have greatly enlarged paw regions and small rhinarial representations; the reverse is true for their close relatives, the coatis (Johnson,1990; Welker, 1990). If measurements were actually available and the analysis were fine enough, the orderliness evident in the graphs in Figures 1.2, 1.3, and 1.4 might disappear, to reflect these differences quantitatively. There is no information about the level of analysis at which the effect of diversity would be detected, but the inconsistency is undoubtedly there. It is a forest-and-trees problem, and we should resolve it by recognizing that both the broad analysis and the fine picture are true and important, although at this time only the broad picture has been quantified.

With respect to specialized adaptations in the amount of PFC, although I have presented the Uylings and Van Eden (1990) data in Figure 1.2 as proving a uniformity, these authors made a strong point about a differentiation. It is evidently the case that PFC in the rat is less segregated from other brain areas than PFC in primates. The full significance of this fact is not understood; it is analogous to the overlapping of sensory and motor fields in marsupials (Johnson, 1990) and suggests that PFC may function more finely in primates.

In my own work (Jerison, 1990), I have found evidence for the selective value of neocortex that has implications for the evolution of PFC. Those not involved in evolutionary analysis may not appreciate how difficult it sometimes is to demonstrate that natural selection is important. For example, when applying rigorous mathematical models such as Lande's (1976), even the increase in brain size in hominid evolution can be accounted for by genetic drift, and one need not assume any role for natural selection, although all students (myself included) believe that there was in fact selection for larger brains. With respect to neocortical evolution in mammals, I have been able to demonstrate, first, that the relative amount of neocortex actually did increase during the past 60 million years, at least in a large sample of fossil carnivores and ungulates. Second, I found that in two orders of carnivorous mammals that evolved over tens of millions of years in what appear to have been very similar environmental niches, fossil species from the surviving order, Carnivora, were more neocorticalized than those from the other order, Creodonta, which became extinct about 5 million years ago. Accepting the picture of PFC as an organized structure in mammalian cortex, its evolution had to be a feature of the evolution of mammalian neocortex, and the identifiable trends in neocortical evolution had to be, by extension, also trends in the evolution of PFC.

Finally, I address Preuss's (1995) analysis, which presented data relevant to the cladistic part of this chapter. If his identification of PFC as a structure unique to primates is correct, its age as a neocortical system would date to 60 million or 70 million years ago, when the earliest fossil primates appeared. Because his model primate is the macaque (family Anthropoidea), the branching might be even more recent, at 40 million years ago or so, when the first major Eocene branching of primates as lemuroids versus anthropoids is identifiable (Simons, 1990). The branching in this instance is evident in the brain's configuration as revealed in fossils (Jerison, 1973; Radinsky, 1979) as well as in skeletal morphology. It would remain a reasonably old discovery as a specialized *primate* or *anthropoid* adaptation. There would be only a few substantive changes in this chapter. We would replace the word *mammals* with *primates*, remove the rat datum from Figure 1.2 (the regression equation is essentially unchanged), and alter the time scale for the first appearance of PFC. I am not, however, prepared to accept Preuss's challenging ideas, in part because their evolutionary basis strikes me as not appreciating the amount of diversity of structure that can occur in homologous systems in different species and as overstating the importance of critiques of the Aristotelean scale-of-nature mystique that plagues the older literature of neurobiology. His analysis is nevertheless significant, and his evaluation and review of literature are major contributions to our knowledge of both structure and function of PFC in relation to the rest of the brain.

REFERENCES

Benjamin, R.M., & Golden, G.T. (1985). Extent and organization of opossum prefrontal cortex defined by anterograde and retrograde transport methods. *Journal of Comparative Neurology, 238,* 77–91.

Bishop, A.B. (1994a). The evolution of the dorsal pallium in the telencephalon of amniotes: Cladistic analysis and a new hypothesis. *Brain Research Reviews, 19,* 66–101.

Bishop, A.B. (1994b). The evolution of the dorsal thalamus of jawed vertebrates, including mammals: Cladistic analysis and a new hypothesis. *Brain Research Reviews, 19,* 29–65.

Braitenberg, V., & Schüz, A. (1991). *Anatomy of the cortex: Statistics and geometry.* New York: Springer-Verlag.

Brodmann, K. (1913). Neue Forschungsergebnisse der Grosshirnrindenanatomie mit besonderer Berucksichtigung anthropologischer Fragen [New research results on the anatomy of the cerebrum with special consideration of anthropological questions]. *Verhandlungen des 85ste Versammlung Deutscher Naturforscher und Aerzte in Wien,* 200–240.

Cracraft, J., & Eldredge, N. (Eds.). (1979). *Phylogenetic analysis and paleontology.* New York: Columbia University Press.

Dawkins, R. (1987). *The blind watchmaker.* New York: Norton.

Divac, I. (1994). The prefrontal system: A smorgasbord. *Progress in Brain Research, 100,* 169–175.

Elias, H., & Schwartz, D. (1971). Cerebro-cortical surface areas, volumes, lengths of gyri and their interdependence in mammals, including man. *Zeitschrift für Saugetierkunde, 36,* 147–163.

Fuster, J.M. (1989). *The prefrontal cortex: Anatomy, physiology, and neuropsychology of the frontal lobe* (2nd ed.). New York: Raven Press.

Gagliardo, A., & Divac, I. (1993). Effects of ablation of the presumed equivalent of the mammalian prefrontal cortex on pigeon homing. *Behavioral Neuroscience, 107,* 280–288.

Goldman-Rakic, P.S. (1988). Topography of cognition: Parallel distributed networks in primate association cortex. *Annual Review of Neuroscience, 11,* 137–156.

Grinnell, A.D. (1995). Hearing in bats: An overview. In R.R. Fay & A.M. Popper (Eds.), *Hearing by bats* (pp. 1–36). Heidelberg, Germany: Springer-Verlag.

Harvey, P.H., & Pagel, M.D. (1991). *The comparative method in evolutionary biology.* Oxford, England: Oxford University Press.

Hodos, W., & Campbell, C.B.G. (1969). Scala naturae: Why there is no theory in comparative psychology. *Psychological Review, 76,* 337–350.

Jerison, H.J. (1973). *Evolution of the brain and intelligence.* New York: Academic Press.

Jerison, H.J. (1990). Fossil evidence on the evolution of the neocortex. In E.G. Jones & A. Peters (Eds.), *Cerebral cortex: Comparative structure and evolution of cerebral cortex, Part I* (Vol. 8A, pp. 285–309). New York: Plenum.

Jerison, H.J. (1991). *Brain size and the evolution of mind.* 59th James Arthur Lecture on the Evolution of the Human Brain. New York: American Museum of Natural History.

Johnson, J.I. (1990). Comparative development of somatic sensory cortex. In E.G. Jones & A. Peters (Eds.), *Cerebral cortex: Comparative structure and evolution of cerebral cortex, Part II* (Vol. 8B, pp. 335–449). New York: Plenum.

Karten, H.J. (1991). Homology and evolutionary origins of the "neocortex." *Brain, Behavior and Evolution, 38,* 264–272.

Kielan-Jaworowska, Z. (1986). Brain evolution in Mesozoic mammals. In J.A. Lillegraven (Ed.), *Contributions to geology* (pp. 21–34). G.G. Simpson memorial volume. Casper: University of Wyoming.

Kielan-Jaworowska, Z. (1992). Interrelationships of Mesozoic mammals. *Historical Biology, 6,* 185–202.

Kolb, B., & Tees, R.C. (Eds.). (1990). *The cerebral cortex of the rat.* Cambridge, MA: MIT Press.

Lande, R. (1976). Natural selection and random genetic drift in phenotypic evolution. *Evolution, 30,* 314–334.

Lovejoy, A.O. (1936). *The great chain of being.* Cambridge, MA: Harvard University Press.

Macphail, E.M. (1994, December 8). Conservation of brain organization and cognition in vertebrates. In G. Roth (Chair), *Evolution of brain and cognition.* Symposium conducted at the University of Bremen, Germany.

Merzenich, M.M., & Kaas, J.H. (1980). Principles of organization of sensory-perceptual systems in mammals. *Progress in Psychobiology and Physiological Psychology, 9,* 1–42.

Preuss, T.M. (1995). Do rats have prefrontal cortex? The Rose-Woolsey-Akert program reconsidered. *Journal of Cognitive Neuroscience, 7,* 1–24.

Radinsky, L. (1979). *The fossil record of primate brain evolution.* 49th James Arthur Lecture on the Evolution of the Human Brain. New York: American Museum of Natural History.

Ridgway, S.H. (1981). Some brain morphometrics of the bowhead whale. In T.T. Albert (Ed.), *Tissues, structural studies, and other investigations on the biology of endangered whales in the Beaufort Sea* (Vol. 2, pp. 837–844). Final report to the Bureau of Land Management, U.S. Department of the Interior, from the University of Maryland, College Park.

Ridgway, S.H., & Brownson, R.H. (1984). Relative brain sizes and cortical surfaces of odontocetes. *Acta Zoologica Fennica, 172,* 149–152.

Rockel, A.J., Hiorns, R.W., & Powell, T.P.S. (1980). The basic uniformity in structure of the neocortex. *Brain, 103,* 221–244.

Rumbaugh, D.M., & Pate, J.L. (1984). The evolution of cognition in primates: A comparative perspective. In H.L. Roitblat, T.G. Bever, & H.S. Terrace (Eds.), *Animal cognition* (pp. 569–585). Hillsdale, NJ: Lawrence Erlbaum Associates.

Schmidt-Nielsen, K. (1984). *Scaling: Why is animal size so important?* Cambridge, England: Cambridge University Press.

Schüz, A., & Demianenko, G.P. (1995). Constancy and variability in cortical structure: A study on synapses and dendritic spines in hedgehog and monkey. *Journal fur Hirnforschung, 36,* 113–122.

Simons, E. (1990). Discovery of the oldest known anthropoidean skull from the Paleogene of Egypt. *Science, 247,* 1567–1569.

Simpson, G.G. (1970). Uniformitarianism: An inquiry into principle, theory, and method in geohistory and biohistory. In M.K. Hecht & W.C. Steere (Eds.), *Essays in evolution and genetics in honor of Theodosius Dobzhansky* (pp. 43–96). Amsterdam: North-Holland.

Stephan, H., Frahm, H., & Baron, G. (1981). New and revised data on volumes of brain structures in insectivores and primates. *Folia Primatologica, 35,* 1–29.

Suga, N., Niwa, H., & Taniguchi, I. (1983). Representation of biosonar information in the auditory cortex of the mustached bat, with emphasis on representation of target velocity information. In J.-P. Ewert, R.R. Capranica, & D.J. Ingle (Eds.), *Advances in vertebrate neuroethology* (Vol. 56, pp. 829–867) (NATO ASI series: Series A, Live Sciences). New York: Plenum.

Szentagothai, J. (1978). The neuron network of the cerebral cortex: A functional interpretation. *Proceedings of the Royal Society (London), Series B, 201,* 219–248.

Uylings, H.B.M., & Van Eden, C.G. (1990). Qualitative and quantitative comparison of the prefrontal cortex in rat and in primates, including humans. *Progress in Brain Research, 85,* 31–62.

Welker, W.I. (1990). Why does cerebral cortex fissure and fold? A review of determinants of gyri and sulci. In E.G. Jones & A. Peters (Eds.), *Cerebral cortex: Comparative structure and evolution of cerebral cortex, Part II* (Vol. 8B, pp. 1–132). New York: Plenum.

Wilkinson, L. (1989). *SYSTAT: The system for statistics.* Evanston, IL: SYSTAT.

Development of the Prefrontal Cortex: Evolution, Neurobiology, and Behavior
edited by Norman A. Krasnegor, Ph.D., G. Reid Lyon, Ph.D.,
and Patricia S. Goldman-Rakic, Ph.D.
copyright © 1997   Paul H. Brookes Publishing Co., Inc.
Baltimore • London • Toronto • Sydney

2

Synaptic Substrate of Cognitive Development
Life-Span Analysis of Synaptogenesis in the Prefrontal Cortex of the Nonhuman Primate

Patricia S. Goldman-Rakic,
Jean-Pierre Bourgeois, and Pasko Rakic

The synaptic architecture of the cerebral cortex defines the limits of intellectual capacity, and the formation of appropriate synapses is the ultimate step in establishing these functional limits. Since the mid-1970s, developmental neurobiologists whose work focuses on the cerebral cortex have been dedicated to understanding the principles of neuronal production and migration and the rules growing axons follow as they extend to their appropriate postsynaptic targets prior to the formation of synapses (reviewed in Levitt, 1994; Rakic, 1988,1995). Research on the final step in the establishment of cortical circuitry has been neglected, and our understanding of the relationship between synaptic maturation and function is relatively poor. Among the many questions relevant to cognitive development that must be answered are the following: Does the course of synaptogenesis in the sensory areas precede that in the frontal association cortex? Are there more synapses in some cortical areas than in others? Are there gender differences in synaptic density, and are synapses lost with age? If synapses decline with age, what is the timing and rate of this dissolution? Is there a relationship between synaptic density and functional capacity? Are synapses added as we learn, as many researchers have argued? Finally, does the maturation of the human cerebral cortex follow the same principles as does that of nonhuman primates? Although opinions on these matters are often expressed, hard data, in the form of rigorous quantitative analysis at the ultrastructural level, are rare.

The findings described in this chapter, which were collected in our laboratories beginning in the mid-1980s, begin to address some of these issues, occasionally with counterintuitive results. We have performed quantitative electron microscopic analyses for six major cortical areas in the nonhuman primate brain (Figure

2.1). More than 1 million synapses have been individually identified and quantified, beginning in the first third of gestation and continuing beyond the 20th year of postnatal age. The cerebral cortex of the rhesus monkey is a highly suitable model for such analytical study because of its size, slow gestational incubation, and extended postnatal development. Data can be gathered under strictly controlled conditions, and the brain can be processed for optimal preservation of ultrastructure. These features have enabled us to estimate 1) the density of synapses per unit volume of cortex and unit volume of neuropil at different ages; 2) the change in sizes of synapses during development; 3) the relative distribution of synapses on the soma, dendritic shafts, and spines of target neurons; and, finally, 4) the emergence of the various types of synaptic specializations—for example, symmetric versus asymmetric or axospine versus axoshaft. The study of six major subdivisions of the cortex over the prolonged primate life span offers a particularly comprehensive view of synapse formation. Knowledge of the principles and limits of synaptic plasticity during childhood and adolescence has important implications for educational theory and practice as well as for understanding the pathogenesis and treatment of childhood mental disorders.

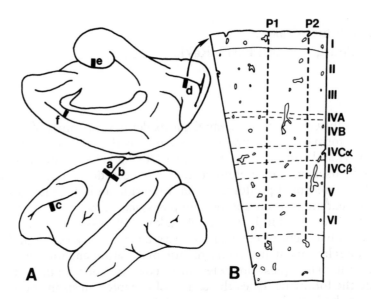

Figure 2.1.   (A) The lateral surface of the left cerebral hemisphere (bottom) and the medial surface, inverted (top), show the six cortical areas examined: a, motor cortex (Brodmann's area 4) in precentral gyrus; b, somatosensory cortex (Brodmann's area 1) in the postcentral gyrus; c, prefrontal cortex (Brodmann's area 9) in the upper bank of the principal sulcus; d, visual cortex (Brodmann's area 17) in the upper bank of the calcarine fissure; e, molecular layer in the dentate gyrus (Brodmann's area 34); and f, anterior cingulate (Brodmann's area 24). The blocks were postfixed in osmium and embedded in Epon-Araldite, and 750-Å sections were cut across the entire width of the cortex. (B) An outline of an ultrathin section across the visual cortex (shown for d from Panel A). The two vertical lines (P1 and P2) indicate the localization of two probes, each of which yields approximately 100 electron micrographs that were printed at a final magnification of ×14,000. Similar probes were prepared for other cortical areas, except the dentate gyrus in which probes were taken only across the width of the molecular layer of the suprapyramidal and infrapyramidal limbs. (Adapted from Rakic, Bourgeois, Eckenhoff, Zecevic, & Goldman-Rakic [1986].)

Herein, the detailed course and kinetics of synaptogenesis are illustrated primarily in the frontal granular cortex of the macaque monkey. This prefrontal area of association cortex is essential for executive functions in both humans and non-human primates (Fuster, 1989; Goldman-Rakic, 1987a; Luria, 1973; Milner, 1964; Stuss & Benson, 1986). The dorsolateral portion of the prefrontal cortex is involved in guiding behavior by transient memory traces, which bridge the temporal distance between past sensory stimuli and prospective responses (Funahashi, Bruce, & Goldman-Rakic, 1989; Fuster, 1989; Goldman-Rakic, 1987a). These integrative functions are subserved by a complex, richly interconnected system of association cortical areas and subcortical nuclei (Goldman-Rakic, 1988a, 1988b; Selemon & Goldman-Rakic, 1988). Neuropsychological investigations indicate that full functional maturation of the prefrontal dorsolateral cortex in macaques is achieved slowly, with at least 3 years being required to reach full maturity (Diamond & Goldman-Rakic, 1989; Goldman, 1971; Goldman & Alexander, 1977; Goldman-Rakic & Brown, 1982). Behavioral analysis alone cannot provide a direct reflection of the differentiation of the neural system underlying prefrontal function. In this respect, anatomical descriptions of the organization and maturation of neuronal assemblies and the elaboration of their connectivity are necessary to understand the construction of a neural system that subserves cognitive functions.

MAJOR PHASES OF SYNAPSE PRODUCTION

Synapse formation in the primate cerebral cortex is a prolonged process that begins well before birth, soon after the genesis of neurons at the embryonic ventricular surface. Synapse formation begins as soon as neurons complete their migration across the intermediate zone to settle in the cortical plate and form the cortical layers (Rakic, 1972, 1974, 1988). In the prefrontal cortex, the first synapses are observed at embryonic day (E)60, about 2 months after conception and more than 3 months before birth, which occurs on E165 (Bourgeois, Goldman-Rakic, & Rakic, 1994). Knowledge of the origin of all of these early presynaptic terminals is incomplete, but it is clear that many early afferents arise from the dopamine-, serotonin-, and norepinephrine-containing cell groups in the brain stem. Monoaminergic fibers are present in the marginal zone, subplate layer, and white matter as early as E47 (Berger, Verney, & Goldman-Rakic, 1993; Marin-Padilla & Marin-Padilla, 1982). Some thalamic and cortical fibers innervate the fetal prefrontal cortex by midgestation (Goldman & Galkin, 1978; Schwartz & Goldman-Rakic, 1991; Schwartz, Rakic, & Goldman-Rakic, 1991), and local intrinsic connections have also been observed (Kostovic & Rakic, 1990; Marin-Padilla, 1988). All of these afferents contribute some of the initial synaptic contacts observed in the embryonic cortex.

At midgestation (i.e., E90–E100), synapse production enters an exponential, or rapid, phase that terminates about 2–3 months after birth (Bourgeois et al., 1994). As evident from Figure 2.2, the major accumulation of synapses in the prefrontal cortex occurs around birth (Bourgeois et al., 1994). During this perinatal period, the adult pattern of sulci and gyri is apparent on the surface of the macaque brain (Goldman & Galkin, 1978), perhaps reflecting the growth and differentiation of cellular morphology. The rapid phase coincides with the major wave of corticocortical and thalamocortical afferent penetration into the cortical plate (Schwartz & Goldman-Rakic, 1991). Callosal axons achieve the columnar architecture characteristic of adult prefrontal cortex between E133 and E155 (Goldman-Rakic, 1981).

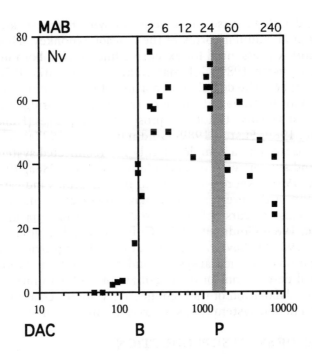

Figure 2.2.   Density of synaptic contacts per 100 μm³ of neuropil in each of the cortical layers during development and maturation. The density was obtained by using Anker and Cragg's (1974) stereological correction. (■ = axospines synaptic contacts; + = axoshaft synaptic contacts.) The number of days after conception is represented in the abcissae (x-axes) by a semilogarithmic plot. (MAB, months after birth; B, birth; P, puberty [shaded line].) (From Bourgeois, J.-P., Goldman-Rakic, P.S., & Rakic, P. [1994]. Synaptogenesis in the prefrontal cortex of rhesus monkey. *Cerebral Cortex, 4,* 87; reprinted by permission.)

The dramatic increase in synaptic density that occurs in the perinatal period shortly before and after birth is predominantly associated with the overproduction of synapses on spines, which proliferate on the dendrites of pyramidal neurons during this time period (Figure 2.3). The density of spine synapses reaches a plateau of 30–60 contacts per 100 μm³ of neuropil 2 months after birth; this value is maintained throughout infancy and childhood, until the onset of puberty (Napier & Napier, 1967; Plant, 1988). There is no comparable overproduction of symmetric synaptic contacts. As a rule, asymmetric synapses in the cerebral cortex are predominantly associated with the excitatory neurotransmitter glutamate, whereas symmetric synapses are associated with the neurotransmitter γ-aminobutyric acid (GABA) and a variety of neuropeptides and monoaminergic synapses, almost all of which have been shown to have inhibitory influences. Asymmetric synapses stabilize earlier than do asymmetric terminals, and the ratio of excitatory to inhibitory synapses increases changes throughout development before reaching the adult profile of 80% asymmetric and 20% symmetric synapses in prefrontal and other cortical areas (Figure 2.4). The changing ratio of synaptic profiles in development was not appreciated previously, and, as of 1997, its functional significance remains to be elucidated.

The rapid phase of synapse formation in the prefrontal area subsides at approximately 3 months of postnatal age, as it does in all other areas of macaque cerebral

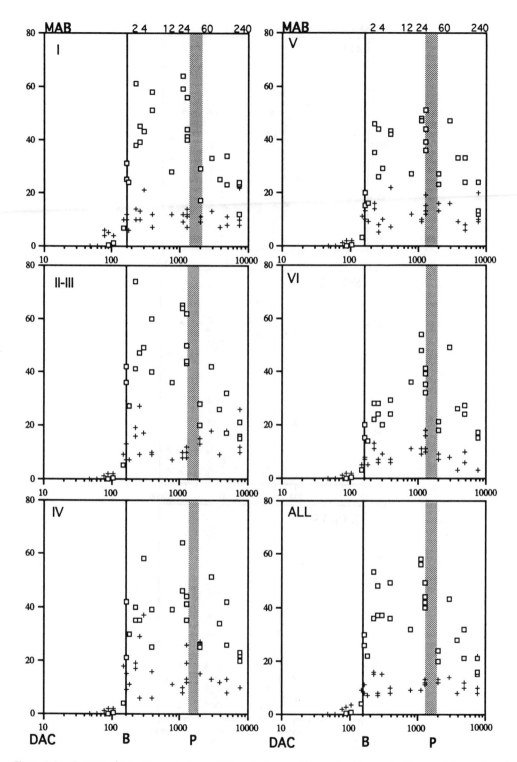

Figure 2.3. Density of synaptic contacts per 100 μm³ of neuropil in each of the cortical layers of the prefrontal cortex during development and maturation. The density was obtained using Anker and Cragg's (1974) stereological correction. (□ = axospine synaptic contacts; + = axoshaft synaptic contacts.) The number of days after conception (DAC) is represented in the abcissae (x-axes) by a semilogarithmic plot. (MAB, months after birth; B, birth; P, puberty [shaded line].) (From Bourgeois, J.-P., Goldman-Rakic, P.S., & Rakic, P. [1994]. Synaptogenesis in the prefrontal cortex of rhesus monkey. *Cerebral Cortex, 4,* 89; reprinted by permission.)

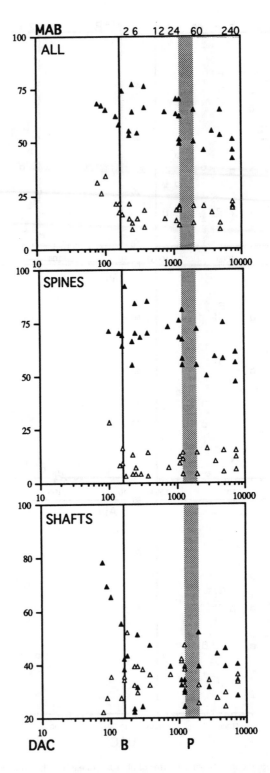

Figure 2.4. Percentages of asymmetric (▲) and symmetric (△) synaptic contacts in the prefrontal cortex (Brodmann's area 46): In the general population of synaptic contacts (top), the population of contacts on dendritic spines (middle), and the population of contacts on dendritic shafts (bottom). The number of days after conception (DAC) is represented in the abcissae (x-axes) by a semilogarithmic plot. (MAB, months after birth; B, birth; P, puberty [shaded lines].) (From Bourgeois, J.-P., Goldman-Rakic, P.S., & Rakic, P. [1994]. Synaptogenesis in the prefrontal cortex of rhesus monkey. *Cerebral Cortex, 4,* 90; reprinted by permission.)

cortex (Bourgeois et al., 1994; Bourgeois & Rakic, 1993; Granger, Tekaia, LeSourd, Rakic, & Bourgeois, 1995; O'Kusky & Colonnier, 1982; Zecevic, Bourgeois, & Rakic, 1989; Zecevic & Rakic, 1991; Zielinski & Hendrickson, 1992). Thereafter, synaptic density in all areas remains at higher-than-adult levels until the approximate time of puberty (see Figure 2.5 on p. xxxiii). We have termed this period of relatively stable synaptic density the plateau period. It is relevant to views of behavioral plasticity that this period of high synaptic density occurs during adolescence, the period in humans that is characterized by intense behavioral change and an enormous capacity for learning coincident with intellectual growth and the achievement of adult-level competence in language and logical thought (e.g., Gelman & Gallistal, 1978; Karmiloff-Smith, 1992; Yates, 1991).

During the third year of life, the density of synapses in prefrontal cortex enters a declining phase, which is defined by a slow but steady decrease (Figure 2.2). This decline parallels changes that have been observed in other cortical areas (Bourgeois et al., 1994). For example, in the prefrontal cortex, the axospine synaptic density declines approximately 50%, a value close to the 40% decrease in density observed in the primary visual cortex from the same hemispheres (Bourgeois & Rakic, 1993). In the prefrontal cortex, the loss of synapses appears to be evenly distributed throughout the entire life span up to 20 years of age (Bourgeois et al., 1994), whereas, in Brodmann's area 17, there appears to be no further decline after 4 years of age (Bourgeois & Rakic, 1993). Whether these differences are genuine or reflect a sampling problem (i.e., fewer points in prefrontal analysis), all evidence indicates that the decreases in synaptic density represent a genuine attrition of synaptic contacts and are not due to enlargement of the volume of the cortex or neuropil (Bourgeois & Rakic, 1993; Rakic, Bourgeois, Eckenhoff, Zecevic, & Goldman-Rakic, 1986; Zecevic et al., 1989; Zecevic & Rakic, 1991). The attrition is primarily due to a selective elimination of asymmetric junctions situated on dendritic spines (Figure 2.4). Again, symmetric synapses situated on shafts remain relatively constant. An age-related decline in excitatory synapses may, to some extent, explain age-related decreases in information-processing capacity that are generally associated with the aging process.

CONCURRENT SYNAPTOGENESIS AND BIOCHEMICAL MATURATION IN DIVERSE CORTICAL AREAS IN MONKEYS AND HUMANS

A commonly held principle of brain development is that it proceeds in a hierarchical temporal sequence, with phylogenetically older structures maturing before newer regions (e.g., see Flechsig, 1920; Greenfield, 1991; Yakovlev & LeCours, 1967). The hierarchical scheme holds true when examining the "vertical" axis of brain maturation, which proceeds in a caudal to rostral sequence, or from spinal cord to brain stem, brain stem to thalamus, and thalamus to cortex. The hierarchical scheme for development of cortical regions is appealing because of the seemingly early development of sensory capacity and the later development of human rational thought and cognitive abilities. Again, quantitative analysis of synaptogenesis in nonhuman primate cortex has caused us to question this assumption and take a new view of the cerebral cortex as an integrated and unified structure that develops as "whole cloth" (Goldman-Rakic, 1987b). The whole-cloth view of the cortex as a woven tapestry in which the entire piece emerges by progressive addition of threads to all portions simultaneously derives from consideration of the comparative time course of synapse formation and synaptic density in diverse regions of the primate cortex. A comparison of findings in the prefrontal (Bourgeois et al., 1994); visual (Bourgeois & Rakic, 1993); cingulate (Granger et al., 1995); motor (Zecevic et al., 1989); and somatosensory (Zecevic & Rakic, 1991) cortices in macaque monkey indicates that a basic course of synaptogenesis, the ascending phase, occurs concurrently in all neocortical areas examined (see Figure 2.5 on p. xxxiii). The strictly linear portion of the rapid phase of synaptogenesis in the six cortical areas that were examined spans a perinatal time window of only 40 days (Granger et al., 1995). This time window is much shorter than the 3-year minimum required for full functional maturation of these cortical areas. The kinetics and changes in one area are paralleled by similar changes in other areas during both the ascending phase and the rapid phase of synaptogenesis.

Similarities among areas extend to later phases of synaptogenesis. For example, the subsequent decrease in synaptic density caused by the elimination of asymmetric junctions situated on dendritic spines occurs contemporaneously in all six areas studied (Rakic et al., 1986). The loss of this class of synapses that support excitatory function during and after puberty is likely to be reflected in decreased excitability of the cerebral hemispheres. Indeed, in studies of individuals between the ages of 10 and 14 years, when substantial synaptic loss occurs in humans (Huttenlocher, 1979), the amplitude of electroencephalograms displays marked decreases in the pattern and duration of the spike activity, which are reflective of cortical excitability associated with sleep during the rapid eye movement stage (Feinberg, Korssko, & Heller, 1967). Likewise, the synaptogenesis curve is paralleled by contemporaneous changes in cerebral metabolism in both human and monkey cerebral cortex (Chugani, Phelps, & Mazziotta, 1987; Jacobs et al., 1995). In humans, positron emission tomography reveals that metabolic activity also increases concurrently in prefrontal, motor, somatosensory, and visual cortex during the postnatal period (Chugani et al., 1987). Furthermore, the synchrony in synaptogenesis observed in the nonhuman primate is in harmony with biochemical and functional data on cortical maturation in the same species. Biochemical studies (Goldman-Rakic & Brown, 1982; Harris & Lewis, 1990) suggest that concentrations of dopamine, noradrenaline, and serotonin increase rapidly in various regions of the cortex of the macaque over the first 2 months after birth and approach adult levels by the fifth month after birth. Studies of the accumulation of major neurotransmitter receptor sites in different cortical areas (Lidow, Goldman-Rakic, & Rakic, 1991; Lidow & Rakic, 1992) show that their maximum density is also reached between 2 and 4 months after birth (Figure 2.6). These observations from several different studies measuring a variety of parameters of maturation in humans and nonhuman primates support the idea that maturation of diverse cortical areas in both monkeys and humans occurs concurrently rather than in a pronounced sequential order. The observations further suggest that the initial formation and maintenance of synapses, as well as their electrophysiological and biochemical maturation, may be determined by intrinsic signals that are common to the entire cortical mantle.

Concurrent synaptogenesis and the accumulation of neurotransmitter receptors in functionally different areas of the cerebrum appear to be at variance with the presumption that myelination in the cerebral cortex follows a hierarchical sequence from sensory to motor and, finally, from motor to association cortex (Flechsig, 1920; Yakovlev & LeCours, 1967; reviewed in Greenfield, 1991). It should be noted that myelination is not a parameter of circuit formation, per se, and that

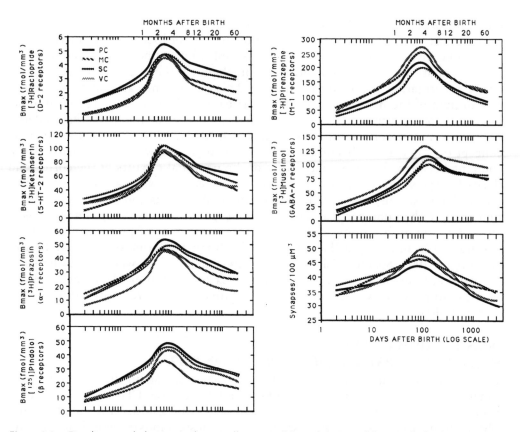

Figure 2.6.   Developmental changes in the overall (across all layers) density of the specific binding of radioligands labeling a representative selection of neurotransmitter receptor subtypes in the prefrontal (PC), primary motor (MC), somatosensory (SC), and primary visual cortical (VC) regions. The figure also includes developmental changes in synaptic density in the same regions (adapted from Rakic et al., 1986). For receptor densities, the curves were obtained by using a locally weighted least squares fit with 50% smoothing (KALEIDA GRAPH, Synergy Software, Reading, Pennsylvania) based on mean (B_{MAX}) values calculated from the measurements of the entire cortical thickness in at least two animals at birth and at 1, 2, 4, 8, 12, 36, and 60 months of age. Age is presented in postnatal days on a logarithmic scale. The original data on synaptogenesis by Rakic et al. (1986) were presented as the number of synapses per unit area of neuropil. We recalculated the data per volume of tissue, which did not alter the timing of events but allowed us to compare the developmental course of cortical synapses with that of neurotransmitter receptors obtained in our present study. The curves representing synaptogenesis per area of neuropil (Rakic et al., 1986) were fitted in the same manner as were those for neurotransmitter receptors. (From Lidow, M.S., Goldman-Rakic, P.S., & Rakic, P. [1991]. Synchronized overproduction of neurotransmitter receptors in diverse regions of the primate cerebral cortex. *Proceedings of the National Academy of Sciences of the United States of America, 88,* 10,219; reprinted by permission.)

hematoxylin staining of sections used to measure the amount of myelin is not a very precise quantitative method. Furthermore, there are clear exceptions to the hierarchical rule of maturation, even in these studies. For example, the corticospinal motor system is among the last to myelinate and becomes stained by hematoxylin only during the second year of life (Yakovlev & LeCours, 1967). The principal sulcus, a major region of association cortex that was thought to be among the last cortical regions to develop mature function, never becomes heavily myelinated, even in the adult monkey (Preuss & Goldman-Rakic, 1991). Furthermore, the callosal axons that connect frontal association areas are either unmyelinated or much less myelinated than are callosal axons of the parietal and occipital lobes (LaMantia & Rakic, 1990). Although myelination is important because it changes the speed and efficiency of conduction and is important to neural transmission, it does not necessarily reflect synaptic maturation, circuit formation, or hierarchical functional organization. Instead, the quantitative data assembled in numerous studies argue for concurrent structural (i.e., synaptic) and biochemical (i.e., neurotransmitters, receptors) maturation of the cortical mantle. This concurrence appears to be reasonable in light of the intricate network of cortical connections that are essential for integration of the sensory, motor, limbic, and associative components that underlie even the simplest cortical functions (Goldman-Rakic, 1987a, 1988a, 1988b). This concept of concurrence becomes even more compelling when one considers the coupling between the early maturation of the neuronal circuits of the cortex and the early expressions of cognitive capacity; it is clear that such a coupling requires integration of sensory, mnemonic, and motor subfunctions and consequent activation of more than one cortical area. The concept of concurrent synaptogenesis is also, therefore, in harmony with contemporary evidence of precocious cognitive maturation in infants (Baillargeon, 1995; Gelman & Gallistal, 1978; Mehler & Christophe, 1995; Spelke, Vishton, & von Hofsten, 1995), as well as with Jerison's evolutionary perspective on prefrontal cortex (see Chapter 1), which stresses, as does our perspective, the integrative nature of distributed cortical networks (Goldman-Rakic, 1988b).

DOES THE HUMAN CORTEX MATURE
SEQUENTIALLY RATHER THAN CONCURRENTLY?

The overall ascending–descending course of synaptogenesis in the human brain is remarkably similar to that in the monkey brain (Anderson, Classey, Conde, Lund, & Lewis 1995; Huttenlocher, 1979; Rakic et al., 1986; Zielinski & Hendrickson, 1992). On the basis of the detailed studies in the rhesus monkey described both previously in this chapter and in the literature, the acceleration, overproduction, and subsequent small but genuine reduction of synaptic contacts to a relatively stable state in adulthood appears to represent a general rule governing the acquisition, maintenance, and reduction of synapses in the mammalian cortex. Although there is little question of the inverted-U shape of the synaptogenesis curve across primate species, a major unsettled issue concerns whether synaptogenesis in all primate species is concurrent across cortical regions. Data on macaque monkeys suggest that, within the time window of 40 days, the timing and sequence of synaptogenesis is very similar for all areas of the neocortex studied. Huttenlocher and colleagues have, however, provided data that suggest that rapid synaptogenesis in primary visual cortex precedes that in prefrontal cortex (Huttenlocher, 1979; Huttenlocher & de Courten, 1987; see also Chapter 4). The implication of this finding is that there may be a basic difference in cortical synaptogenesis between humans and nonhuman primates. Although, we cannot exclude such a difference a priori, to be convincing, a difference between species should be demonstrated by using exactly the same methods in both species. Technical and procedural factors could explain the apparent discrepancy in synaptogenesis curves for humans and monkeys (Rakic, Bourgeois, & Goldman-Rakic, 1994). The phosphotungstic acid method used in human postmortem tissue exposes only the postsynaptic thickening, and stereological corrections cannot be readily applied. Moreover, in the study of monkeys, all neocortical areas (i.e., prefrontal, motor, visual, somatosensory) examined were dissected from the corresponding site and virtually always from the same set of animals fixed and processed by using the same protocol, whereas, in the studies of humans, the visual and prefrontal areas were obtained from different samples of subjects under different conditions, possibly introducing intersubject sampling error.

In our view, it is unlikely that a process as fundamental as circuit formation would differ substantially across mammalian species and even less likely that it would do so between closely related primates. Accordingly, we reexamined the reported human data and expressed them in a manner that is more comparable with the manner in which monkey data are expressed (Rakic et al., 1994). In particular, when the data on synaptogenesis obtained from the human prefrontal (Huttenlocher, 1979) and human visual cortices (Huttenlocher & de Courten, 1987) were normalized to the means of their respective distributions and replotted to the maximum value of the curve on a semilogarithmic scale, both curves (frontal and visual) were found to overlap, as they do in the monkey (Figure 2.7). Moreover, by means of linear regression analysis, the two sets of values were fitted to a straight line (correlation coefficients: .90, $n = 5$, $p < .05$, for striate cortex; and .92, $n = 7$, $p < .05$ for prefrontal cortex). A statistical comparison between the two regression lines failed to reveal a significant difference in their slopes. It seems possible, therefore, that synaptogenesis in both humans and monkeys proceeds concurrently rather than sequentially in visual and prefrontal cortex. Knowledge of how our brains develop and how best to promote their optimal maturation requires such knowledge as can be gained from coordinated life-span developmental studies in both humans and closely related nonhuman primates. Furthermore, the issue of human-nonhuman differences with respect to the sequence of regional maturation in the cortex will continue to be debated until more data are available in both species.

SOME IMPLICATIONS FOR LEARNING AND MEMORY

A common assumption in psychology and neuroscience is that new learning is supported by the acquisition of new synapses (Bailey & Chen, 1988; Greenough & Black, 1992). A different point of view is that maturity and learning result in a net loss of already-formed synaptic connections (Changeux, 1993; Changeux & Danchin, 1976). Although both mechanisms undoubtedly play an important role in functional maturation of some systems, the findings in both humans and nonhuman primates reviewed herein indicate that neither synapse formation nor synapse elimination is the dominant mechanism for storing new information in the adult cerebral cortex. Our view is that learning is associated with the strengthening of existing synapses. The finding that, from sexual maturity (at approximately 3 years) to senescence (older than 25 years), the density of synapses per unit volume of neuropil in the rhesus monkey cortex remains relatively steady or shows only a small decline is in contrast with research in rodents, in which learning, acquisition of new memories, and even exposure to one or more tasks were found to significantly increase the number of synapses; volume of cortex; and number and size of spines, glial cells, and endothelial cells (Greenough & Black, 1992). Extrapolating these findings to primates, whose acquisition of new knowledge increases continuously throughout their much longer life span, one would expect significant increases in both the number of synapses and total brain weight. The evidence, however, of a steady state of synaptic density throughout adolescence and of a subsequent decline throughout adult life does not offer much support for this expectation. Rather, it appears that humans and nonhuman primates store new information within an

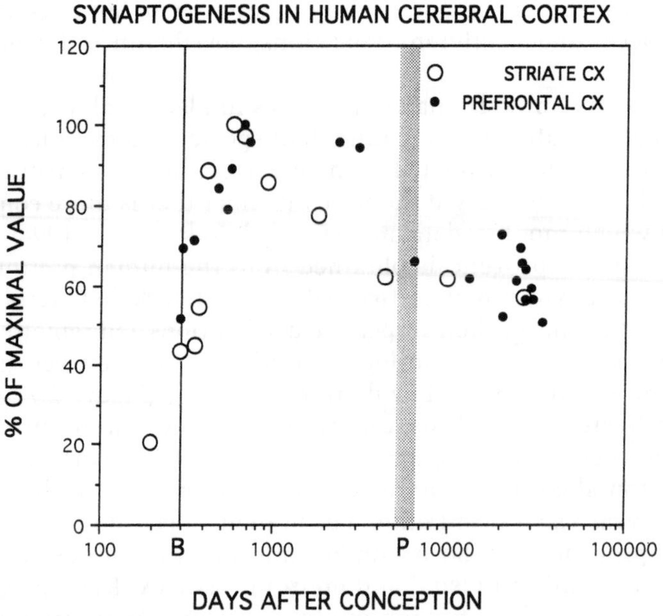

SYNAPTOGENESIS IN HUMAN CEREBRAL CORTEX

Figure 2.7. Synaptic density in the human striate area (○) and prefrontal cortex (•) determined on the basis of studies by Huttenlocher and de Courten (1987) and Huttenlocher (1979), respectively. We replotted each point from the published data on a semilogarithmic scale as a function of conceptual age and normalized them to the maximum value of the curve. Under these conditions, both curves overlap, as they do in monkeys. (From Rakic, P., Bourgeois, J.-P., & Goldman-Rakic, P.S. [1994]. Synaptic development of the cerebral cortex: Implications for learning, memory, and mental illness. *Progress in Brain Research, 102,* 232; reprinted by permission.)

existing set of neurons and their synaptic connections. Perhaps the type of neuronal plasticity that underlies the capacity to learn resides more in a stable circuitry that is capable of changing its functional weights through molecular adjustments at pre- and postsynaptic levels of communication (e.g., Rumelhart, McClelland, & the PDP Research Group, 1988).

In regard to the general issue of synaptic stability, we note the remarkable fact that the *developmental* accumulation of synapses, as studied quantitatively in macaque monkeys, is altered much less by environmental stimulation than has been appreciated or would be expected by conventional wisdom. The primate visual system has been the best model for manipulating these influences, and the data gathered on the normal course of synapse formation in this cortex have provided the normative background for studying them experimentally. On the one hand, monocular enucleation or even brief periods of visual deprivation can cause a dramatic alteration in the size of ocular dominance columns in the primate visual cortex (Hubel, Wiesel, & LeVay, 1977; Rakic, 1981). On the other hand, certain features of cortical connectivity develop quite normally in the absence of normal visual input. A striking example of this unexpected normal development is the finding that ocular dominance columns develop even when monkeys are raised in total darkness (Horton & Hocking, 1996). Similarly, the distribution of cytochrome oxidase patches and major neurotransmitter receptors in the macaque primary visual cortex develops according to the normal adult pattern even when both retinas are ablated in the third month of gestation (Kuljis & Rakic, 1990; Rakic & Lidow, 1995). A number of basic features of cortical architecture, therefore, are found to be surprisingly resistant to degradation by severe deprivation, which indicates that these features likely develop under endogenous and genetic regulation.

Most studies of environmental influence can be categorized as deprivation studies. In contrast, we have performed studies in which fetuses were exposed to sensory input and have evaluated the impact of excessive or precocious stimulation on parameters of synaptic development. In one experiment, fetal monkeys were delivered 3 weeks before their full-term delivery date and were exposed to 3 weeks of visual stimulation to determine whether the growth of synapses in the visual cortex would be accelerated (Bourgeois, Jastreboff, & Rakic, 1989). Contrary to expectations, an analysis of synaptic density in pairs of monkeys that were conceived at the same time but were delivered at different times after conception failed to reveal any difference in synaptic density in any layers of the visual cortex (Bourgeois et al., 1989). In a second experiment, the visual cortex of monkeys that had been enucleated binocularly in utero was examined for possible changes in synaptic density relative to age-matched controls (Bourgeois & Rakic, 1987, 1996). Again, there were no significant differences in synaptic density in the visual cortex between experimental and control subjects. In the binocularly enucleated animal, the visual cortex is drastically reduced in size, but the portion that remains is normal in cytoarchitectonic appearance and maintains connections with the spared relay cells of the lateral geniculate nucleus (Rakic, 1988). Furthermore, synaptic density is not altered in the visual cortex despite the fact that the animal was *totally deprived* of visual stimulation (Bourgeois & Rakic, 1996). The findings of these two studies that experimentally altered cortical activation in immature animals indicate that the timing and rate of synaptic production may be preprogrammed rather than induced by stimulation from the environment, as is commonly assumed. Given that an increasing number of children are born prematurely in the United States, this is an encouraging finding about cortical development in unfavorable circumstances.

The finding that the course of synaptic formation proceeds at the normal pace in the face of bilateral visual deprivation does not negate the possibility that certain synaptic changes could occur after more drastic environmental perturbations and viral, nutritional, and/or other serious afflictions of normal brain development. It is well established that sustained deprivation, abnormal sensory stimulation, and other sustained deleterious influences after birth alter synaptic distribution, efficacy, and viability (Hubel et al., 1977; Lund, Holbach, & Chung, 1991). Our data suggest only that these influences probably act predominantly on synapses that have already been formed rather than on the initiation and establishment of new synapses (Bourgeois et al., 1989). It is, however, notable that even as severe a postnatal deprivation as castration during adolescence does not appear to have an impact on postnatal changes in relative spine density, which is an indirect measure of synaptic density (Anderson et al., 1995). Anderson et al. (1995) reported no change in relative spine density, total dendritic length, or number of immunoreactive terminals (of parvalbumin positive axons, a subset of GABAergic fibers) on the soma of Layer III pyramidal cells in the prefrontal cortex of male monkeys undergoing castration at 14 months of age. Synaptic density, even in the mature cortex, may, therefore, be relatively impervious to change concomitant with an expanded adult life span.

FUNCTIONAL COMPETENCE,
INDIVIDUAL VARIABILITY, AND SYNAPTOGENESIS

The size of the cortex and its cytoarchitectonic areas in the macaque monkey, like that in the human, display considerable individual differences that are presumably related to variations in capacity. In the monkey, individual variability in the density of synaptic contacts is relatively small during the rapid phase of synaptogenesis (Figure 2.2, and Figure 2.5 on p. xxxiii) but considerably larger during the phase of synaptic elimination (Bourgeois & Rakic, 1993). It is possible that the rapid phase of synaptogenesis yields more homogeneity because it is regulated by a unitary intrinsic developmental mechanism (Rakic et al., 1986). In contrast, the phases of synaptic elimination may display higher individual variability because of the diverse epigenetic events and various environmental factors that become more pronounced postnatally (Bourgeois et al., 1989).

A high degree of variability, similar to the one reported herein, has also been observed during the development of axodendritic spines (Boothe, Greenough, Lund, & Wrege, 1979; Lund et al., 1991) and axosomatic contacts in layer IVC in area 17 of macaque monkeys (Lund & Harper, 1991; Mates & Lund, 1983). High variability has also been found in the number of neurons in the macaque neocortex (Vincent, Peters, & Tigges, 1989; Williams & Rakic, 1985); the size of cytoarchitectonic areas (Loftus et al., 1993; Rajkowska & Goldman-Rakic, 1995); and the concentrations of several neurotransmitters (Wenk, Pierce, Struble, Price, & Cork, 1989) and neurotransmitter receptors (Rakic, Gallager, & Goldman-Rakic, 1988). There is little doubt, therefore, that there are considerable quantitative differences among synaptic densities in the cerebral cortex of individual macaque monkeys at any age, as well as pronounced differences in the rate of their elimination. The functional significance of these differences encountered during the elimination phase remains to be determined. Variability of a similar magnitude is expected in the developing human brain. Samples based on a small number of specimens and/or on uneven numbers of males and females may, therefore, give misleading results. Even gross morphological features, such as the gyral pattern and the size of areas, differ considerably from individual to individual (Rajkowska & Goldman-Rakic, 1995). Again, the functional significance of these individual variations is not clear.

The balance between overproduction and elimination of neurons, axons, and synapses ultimately determines the size of a given pathway or the extent of territories devoted to a given terminal field in the mature cortex (O'Leary & Koester, 1993; Rakic, 1988). Although a number of mechanisms have been proposed to regulate the specificity and therefore the selection of specific synaptic connections in the brain, this problem has not been resolved at the level of cellular and molecular processes. In fact, many processes studied by developmental neurobiologists could all be engaged in the development and subsequent maintenance of the synaptic neuropil. Studies in a variety of species, including humans, support the hypothesis that competitive interactions among two or more populations of neurons play a significant role in the selective elimination of excess synapses during development, before the adult level is reached. The coincidence of the period of synaptic loss with the period of sexual maturation points logically toward a possible major role of steroid hormones, which have been reported to influence synaptogenesis both in vivo and in vitro (Arai & Matsumoto, 1987; Toran-Allerand, 1984). Experience is another crucial factor, in particular in the primate cortex, where synaptic loss occurs postnatally during adolescence and young adulthood (when the broadest of interactive experiences take place).

We assume that the main lines of cortical circuitry are connected during the rapid phase of synaptogenesis. The plateau phase of synaptic density (i.e., between birth and puberty), however, covers the period of intense behavioral plasticity during which synapses might be strengthened, weakened, or repositioned by turnover without a net gain or loss in number. A close correspondence has been demonstrated between the maturation of working memory capacity (Diamond & Goldman-Rakic, 1989) and the point of peak synaptic density in the prefrontal cortex of rhesus monkey (Bourgeois et al., 1994). Strong parallels between the developmental course of delayed-response performance and that of Piaget's AB Object Permanence Test (Piaget, 1954) have been shown in both humans (Diamond & Doar, 1989) and monkeys (Diamond & Goldman-Rakic, 1989). As monkeys and humans develop, so does the length of the delay period over which they are able to hold sensations or memories "in mind"; this presumably occurs as a consequence of the fine tuning developing in the prefrontal circuitry that mediates this important capacity. The emergence and evolution of working memory capacity from the end of the rapid phase through the plateau period of synaptogenesis in the monkey, therefore, provide a valuable animal model for investigating postnatal structure–function relationships relevant to cognition (Goldman-Rakic, 1987a).

Longitudinal experimental studies in cats and monkeys have revealed that periods of cortical plasticity can extend well beyond the rapid phase of synaptogenesis. For example, in macaque monkeys, Vernier hyperacuity, which depends critically on the circuitry of the striate cortex, does not develop fully until 2 years of age (Harwerth, Smith, Duncan, Crawford, & von Noorden, 1986). Likewise, the development of spatial resolution and contrast sensitivity in the foveal representation requires at least 1 year to reach adult-level competence (Blakemore, Garey, & Vital-Durand, 1978; Blakemore, Vital-Durand, & Garey, 1981; Vital-Durand & Blakemore, 1983). Studies in the cat suggest that there is also a period of cortical plasticity in response to monocular deprivation, which ends only at the onset of puberty; that is, at 1 year of age in this species (Daw, Fox, Sato, & Czepita, 1992). Similar critical periods may exist for the specific cognitive functions subserved by the prefrontal cortex, although these have not been characterized. During the 3-year period between birth and puberty, young macaques learn survival skills, the complexities of social relations, and their ranking within their troops. Sensory, motor, and social deprivation at different points in this plateau phase may have different effects, and there is little doubt that adequate sensory and motor experience; training; and, in the case of humans, education are essential for the proper *maintenance* of cortical structure and function.

A logical strategy for understanding the basic mechanisms of synaptogenesis would be to determine which connections and synapses are lost and whether the type of loss and retention can be influenced by training. The studies conducted to date have revealed only the basic course of developing synapses, their morphological types, and the sites of their termination; their origin has not been determined. As a result, we have only preliminary ideas about the basis for the temporal correlation of various developmental events and the functions of the neural systems involved. Many modifications in the morphofunctional maturation of the cerebral cortex have, however, been proposed to explain the dramatic behavior change during adolescence; these possible modifications include reorganization and turnover of synaptic circuitry (Purves, 1988), synaptic vesicle proliferation (Miller, 1988), axonal myelination (Gibson, 1970), and biochemical differentiation (Goldman-Rakic & Brown, 1982). Any or all of these parameters could contribute to the functional maturation of the cerebral cortex because most of these cellular events occur during the plateau phase of synaptogenesis. Nevertheless, this period of intense and highly efficient learning and rapid behavior modification does not appear to be paralleled by either significant net accretion or net loss of synapses. In humans, the plateau phase for prefrontal cortex would correspond to the entire period of childhood through puberty, which is roughly 13 years (Figure 2.7; Chugani et al., 1987; Huttenlocher, 1979). The findings obtained in nonhuman primates seem to indicate that the systemic/experiential factors that improve synaptic efficiency may be more critical than shifts in synaptic density as a neural basis for behavioral maturation and plasticity during this prolonged postnatal period.

As argued elsewhere, "a prolonged period of interaction with the environment, as pronounced as it is in all primates, especially humans, requires a stable set of neurons to retain acquired experiences in the pattern of their synaptic connectivity" (Rakic, 1985, p. 155). This stability is in contrast with the continuing turnover and addition of neurons in some nonmammalian vertebrates (Nottebohm & Alvarez-Buylla,1993) and possibly in rodents, which continue to acquire some new neurons in the hippocampus (Altman & Bayer, 1993) and perhaps in the neocortex (Kaplan, 1985). The stability of neurons in primates may be an evolutionary adaptation (Rakic, 1985; Rakic & Kornack, 1993). Humans can remember events that occurred 70–80 years earlier, perhaps because their experiences and memories are imprinted in stable neuronal assemblies that are equally old or even older. The existence of newly generated neurons and axons to replace older sets would conceivably render us eternal infants who would be incapable of retaining learned behavior. Neurogenesis in the primate cerebral cortex neither occurs after sexual maturity (Rakic, 1985) nor contributes to the recovery of function following trauma sustained after the normal production of neurons has ceased (reviewed in Rakic & Kornack, 1993). Prolonged maintenance of the same set of neurons and connections throughout a lifetime, therefore, has the evolutionary advantage of permitting the retention and updating of acquired information that is essential for survival and transmission of culture (Rakic, 1985; Rakic & Kornack, 1993).

REFERENCES

Altman, J., & Bayer, S.A. (1993). Are new neurons formed in the brain of adult mammals? In C. Cuello (Ed.), *Restorative neurology: Vol. 6. Neuronal cell death and repair* (pp. 203–225). Amsterdam: Elsevier.

Anderson, S.A., Classey, J.D., Conde, F., Lund, J.S., & Lewis, D.A. (1995). Synchronous development of pyramidal neuron dendritic spines and parvalbumin-immunoreactive chandelier neuron axon terminals in layer III of monkey prefrontal cortex. *Neuroscience, 67*, 7–22.

Anker, R., & Cragg, B.G. (1974). Estimation of the number of synapses in a volume of nervous tissue from counts in thin sections by electron microscopy. *Journal of Neurocytology, 3*, 725–735.

Arai, Y., & Matsumoto, A. (1987). Gonadal steroid control of synaptogenesis in the neuroendocrine brain. In P.C.K. Leung, D.T. Armstrong, K.B. Ruf, & H.G. Fresen (Eds.), *Endocrinology and physiology of reproduction* (pp. 13–21). New York: Plenum.

Bailey, C.H., & Chen, M. (1988). Long-term sensitization in *Aplysia* modulates the total number of varicosities of single identified sensory neurons. *Proceedings of the National Academy of Science of the United States of America, 85*, 2373–2377.

Baillargeon, R. (1995). Physical reasoning in infancy. In M.S. Gazzaniga (Ed.), *The cognitive neurosciences* (pp. 181–204). Cambridge, MA: MIT Press.

Berger, B., Verney, C., & Goldman-Rakic, P.S. (1993). Prenatal monoaminergic innervation of the cerebral cortex: Differences between rodents and primates. In I. Kostovic, S. Knezevic, H. Wisniewski, & G. Spilich (Eds.), *Neurodevelopment, aging and cognition* (pp. 18–36). Boston: Birkhauser.

Blakemore, C., Garey, L.J., & Vital-Durand, F. (1978). The physiological effects of monocular deprivation and their reversal in the monkey's visual cortex. *Journal of Physiology, 283*, 223–262.

Blakemore, C., Vital-Durand, F., & Garey, L.J. (1981). Recovery from monocular deprivation in the monkey. I. Reversal of physiological effects in the visual cortex. *Proceedings of the Royal Society of London (B), 213*, 399–423.

Boothe, R.G., Greenough, W.T., Lund, J.S., & Wrege, K. (1979). A quantitative investigation of spine and dendrite development of neurons in visual cortex (area 17) of *Macaca nemestrina* monkeys. *Journal of Comparative Neurology, 186*, 473–489.

Bourgeois, J.-P., Goldman-Rakic, P.S., & Rakic, P. (1994). Synaptogenesis in the prefrontal cortex of rhesus monkey. *Cerebral Cortex, 4*, 78–96.

Bourgeois, J.-P., Jastreboff, P.J., & Rakic, P. (1989). Synaptogenesis in visual cortex of normal and preterm monkeys: Evidence for intrinsic regulation of synaptic overproduction. *Proceedings of the National Academy of Science of the United States of America, 86*, 4297–4301.

Bourgeois, J.-P., & Rakic, P. (1987). Distribution, density and ultrastructure of synapses in the visual cortex in monkeys devoid of retinal input from early embryonic stages. *Abstract Society for Neuroscience, 13*, 1044.

Bourgeois, J.-P., & Rakic, P. (1993). Changes of synaptic density in the primary visual cortex of the macaque monkey from fetal to adult stage. *Journal of Neuroscience, 13*, 2801–2820.

Bourgeois, J.-P., & Rakic, P. (1996). Synaptogenesis in the occipital cortex of macaque monkey devoid of retinal input from early embryonic stages. *European Journal of Neuroscience, 8*, 942–950.

Changeux, J.-P. (1993). A critical view of neuronal models of learning and memory. In P. Anderson (Ed.), *Memory concepts* (pp. 413–433). Amsterdam: Elsevier.

Changeux, J.-P., & Danchin, A. (1976). Selective stabilization of developing synapses as a mechanism for the specification of neural networks. *Nature, 264*, 705–712.

Chugani, H.T., Phelps, M.E., & Mazziotta, J.C. (1987). Positron emission tomography study of human brain functional development. *Annals of Neurology, 22*, 487–497.

Daw, N.W., Fox, K., Sato, H., & Czepita, D. (1992). Critical period for monocular deprivation in the cat visual cortex. *Journal of Neurophysiology, 67*, 197–202.

Diamond, A., & Doar, B. (1989). The performance of human infants on a measure of frontal cortex function, the delayed-response task. *Developmental Psychobiology, 22*, 271–294.

Diamond, A., & Goldman-Rakic, P.S. (1989). Comparison of human infants and rhesus monkeys on Piaget's AB task: Evidence for dependence on dorsolateral prefrontal cortex. *Experimental Brain Research, 74*, 24–40.

Eckenhoff, M.E., & Rakic, P. (1991). A quantitative analysis of synaptogenesis in the molecular layer of the dentate gyrus in the rhesus monkey. *Developmental Brain Research, 564*, 129–135.

Feinberg, I., Korssko, R.L., & Heller, N. (1967). EEG sleep patterns as a function of normal and pathological aging in man. *Journal of Psychiatric Research, 5*, 107–144.

Flechsig, P. (1920). *Anatomie des menschlichen gehirns und ruckenmarks auf myelogenetischer grundlage* [Anatomy of the human brain and spinal cord on the basis of myelogenetics]. Leipzig, Germany: Thieme.

Funahashi, S., Bruce, C.J., & Goldman-Rakic, P.S. (1989). Mnemonic coding of visual space in the monkey's dorsolateral prefrontal cortex. *Journal of Neurophysiology, 61*, 1–19.

Fuster, J.M. (1989). *The prefrontal cortex: Anatomy, physiology, and neuropsychology of the frontal lobe*. New York: Raven Press.

Gelman, R., & Gallistal, C. (1978). *The child's understanding of numbers*. Cambridge, MA: Harvard University Press.

Gibson, K.R. (1970). *Sequence of myelinization in the brain of Macaca mulatta*. Unpublished doctoral dissertation, University of California, Berkeley.

Goldman, P.S. (1971). Functional development of the prefrontal cortex in early life and the problem of neuronal plasticity. *Experimental Neurology, 32*, 366–387.

Goldman, P.S., & Alexander, G.E. (1977). Maturation of prefrontal cortex in the monkey revealed by local reversible cryogenic depression. *Nature, 267,* 613–615.

Goldman P.S., & Galkin, T.W. (1978). Prenatal removal of frontal association cortex in the fetal rhesus monkey: Anatomical and functional consequences in postnatal life. *Brain Research, 152,* 451–485.

Goldman-Rakic, P.S. (1981). Development and plasticity of primate frontal association cortex. In F.O. Schmidt, F.G. Worden, S.G. Dennis, & G. Edelman (Eds.), *The organization of cerebral cortex* (pp. 69–97). Cambridge, MA: MIT Press.

Goldman-Rakic, P.S. (1987a). Circuitry of primate prefrontal cortex and regulation of behavior by representational memory. In V.B. Mountcastle, F. Plum, & S.R. Geiger (Eds.), *Handbook of physiology* (Vol. 5, Part 1, pp. 373–417). Bethesda, MD: American Physiological Society.

Goldman-Rakic, P.S. (1987b). Development of cortical circuitry and cognitive functions. *Child Development, 58,* 642–691.

Goldman-Rakic, P.S. (1988a). Changing concepts of cortical connectivity: Parallel distributed cortical networks. In P. Rakic & W. Singer (Eds.), *Neurobiology of the neocortex* (pp. 177–202). New York: John Wiley & Sons.

Goldman-Rakic, P.S. (1988b). Topography of cognition: Parallel distributed networks in primate association cortex. *Annual Review of Neuroscience, 11,* 137–156.

Goldman-Rakic P.S., & Brown, R.M. (1982). Postnatal development of monoamine content and synthesis in the cerebral cortex of rhesus monkeys. *Developmental Brain Research, 4,* 339–349.

Granger, B., Tekaia, F., LeSourd, A.M., Rakic, P., & Bourgeois, J.-P. (1995). Tempo of neurogenesis and synaptogenesis in the primate cingulate mesocortex: Comparison with the neocortex. *Journal of Comparative Neurology, 360,* 363–376.

Greenfield, P.M. (1991). Language, tools and brain: The ontogeny and phylogeny of hierarchically organized sequential behavior. *Behavior and Brain Sciences, 14,* 531–595.

Greenough, W.T., & Black, J.E. (1992). Induction of brain structure by experience: Substrates for cognitive development. In M.R. Gunnar & C.A. Nelson (Eds.), *Developmental behavioral neuroscience* (Minnesota Symposia on Child Psychology, Vol. 24, pp. 155–200). Hillsdale, NJ: Lawrence Erlbaum Associates.

Harris, H.W., & Lewis, D.A. (1990). Postnatal changes in the dopaminergic innervation of monkey prefrontal cortex: A tyrosine hydroxylase immunohistochemical study. *Society for Neuroscience Abstracts, 16,* 1094.

Harwerth, R.S., Smith, E.L., III, Duncan, G.C., Crawford, M.L., & von Noorden, G.K. (1986). Multiple sensitive periods in the development of the primate visual system. *Science, 232,* 235–238.

Horton, J.C., & Hocking, D.R. (1996). An adult-like pattern of ocular dominance columns in striate cortex of newborn monkeys prior to visual experience. *Journal of Neuroscience, 16,* 1791–1807.

Hubel, D.H., Wiesel, T.N., & LeVay, S. (1977). Plasticity of ocular dominance columns in monkey striate cortex. *Philosophical Transactions of the Royal Society of London (B), 278,* 377–409.

Huttenlocher, P.R. (1979). Synaptic density in human frontal cortex-developmental changes and effects of aging. *Brain Research, 163,* 195–205.

Huttenlocher, P.R., & de Courten, C. (1987). The development of synapses in striate cortex of man. *Human Neurobiology, 6,* 1–9.

Jacobs, B., Chugani, H.T., Allada, V., Chen, S., Phelps, M.E., Pollack, D.B., & Raleigh, M.J. (1995). Developmental changes in brain metabolism in sedated rhesus macaques and vervet monkeys revealed by positron emission tomography, *Cerebral Cortex, 5,* 222–233.

Kaplan, M.S. (1985). Formation and turnover of neurons in young and senescent animals: An electronmicroscopic and morphometric analysis. *Annals of the New York Academy of Science, 457,* 173–192.

Karmiloff-Smith, A. (1992). *Beyond modularity.* Cambridge, MA: MIT Press.

Kostovic, I., & Rakic, P. (1990). Developmental history of transient subplate zone in the visual and somatosensory cortex of the macaque monkey and human brain. *Journal of Comparative Neurology, 297,* 441–470.

Kuljis, R.O., & Rakic, P. (1990). Hypercolumns in primate visual cortex develop in the absence of cues from photoreceptors. *Proceedings of the National Academy of Science of the United States of America, 87,* 5303–5306.

LaMantia, A.S., & Rakic, P. (1990). Cytological and quantitative characteristics of four cerebral commissures in the rhesus monkey. *Journal of Comparative Neurology, 291,* 520–537.

Levitt, P. (1994). Experimental approaches that reveal principles of cerebral cortical development. In M.S. Gazzaniga (Ed.), *The cognitive neurosciences* (pp. 147–163). Cambridge, MA: MIT Press.

Lidow, M.S., Goldman-Rakic, P.S., & Rakic, P. (1991). Synchronized overproduction of neurotransmitter receptors in diverse regions of the primate cerebral cortex. *Proceedings of the National Academy of Science of the United States of America, 88,* 10218–10221.

Lidow, M.S., & Rakic, P. (1992). Scheduling of monoaminergic neurotransmitter receptor expression in the primate neocortex during postnatal development. *Cerebral Cortex, 2,* 401–416.

Loftus, W.C., Tramo, M.J., Thomas, C.E., Green, R.L., Nordgren, R.A., & Gazzaniga, M.S. (1993). Three-dimensional quantitative analysis of hemispheric asymmetry in the human superior temporal region. *Cerebral Cortex, 3,* 348–355.

Lund, J.S., & Harper, T.R. (1991). Postnatal development of thalamic recipient neurons in the monkey striate cortex. III. Somatic inhibitory synapse acquisition by spiny stellate neurons of layer 4C. *Journal of Comparative Neurology, 309,* 141–149.

Lund, J.S., Holbach, S.M., & Chung, W.W. (1991). Postnatal development of thalamic recipient neurons in the monkey striate cortex. II. Influence of afferent driving on spine acquisition and dendritic growth of layer 4C spiny stellate neurons. *Journal of Comparative Neurology, 309,* 129–140.

Luria, A.R. (1973). The frontal lobes and the regulation of behavior. In K.H. Pribram & A.R. Luria (Eds.), *Psychophysiology of the frontal lobes* (pp. 3–26). New York: Academic Press.

Marin-Padilla, M. (1988). Early ontogenesis of the human cerebral cortex. In A. Peters & E.G. Jones (Eds.), *Cerebral cortex* (Vol. 7, pp. 1–34). New York: Plenum.

Marin-Padilla, M., & Marin-Padilla, T.M. (1982). Origin, prenatal development and structural organization of layer I of the human cerebral (motor) cortex: A Golgi study. *Anatomy and Embryology, 164,* 161–206.

Mates, S.L., & Lund, J.S. (1983). Developmental changes in the relationship between type 1 synapses and spiny neurons in the monkey visual cortex. *Journal of Comparative Neurology, 221,* 91–97.

Mehler, J., & Christophe, A. (1995). Maturation and learning of language in the first year of life. In M.S. Gazzaniga (Ed.), *The cognitive neurosciences* (pp. 943–958). Cambridge, MA: MIT Press.

Miller, M.W. (1988). Development of projection and local circuit neurons in neocortex. In A. Peters & E.G. Jones (Eds.), *Cerebral cortex* (Vol. 7, pp. 133–175). New York: Plenum.

Milner, B. (1964). Some effects of frontal lobectomy in man. In J.M. Warren & K. Akert (Eds.), *The frontal granular cortex and behavior* (pp. 313–334). New York: McGraw-Hill.

Napier, J.R., & Napier, P.H. (1967). *A handbook of living primates.* New York: Academic Press.

Nottebohm, F., & Alvarez-Buylla, A. (1993). Neurogenesis and neuronal replacement in adult birds. In A.C. Cuello (Ed.), *Restorative neurology: Vol. 6. Neuronal cell death and repair* (pp. 227–236). Amsterdam: Elsevier.

O'Kusky, J., & Colonnier, M. (1982). A laminar analysis of the number of neurons, glia and synapses in the adult cortex (area 17) of the adult macaque monkey. *Journal of Comparative Neurology, 210,* 278–290.

O'Leary, D.D., & Koester, S.E. (1993). Development of projection neuron types, axon pathways and patterned connections of the mammalian cortex. *Neuron, 10,* 991–1006.

Piaget, J. (1954). *The construction of reality in the child.* New York: Basic Books. (Original work published in 1937)

Plant, T.M. (1988). Neuroendocrine basis of puberty in the monkey (*Macaca mulatta*). In L. Martin & W. Ganong (Eds.), *Frontiers in neuroendocrinology* (Vol. 10, pp. 215–238). New York: Raven Press.

Preuss, T.M., & Goldman-Rakic, P.S. (1991). Myelo- and cytoarchitecture of the granular frontal cortex and surrounding regions in the strepsirhine primate *galago* and the anthropoid primate *macaca*. *Journal of Comparative Neurology, 310,* 429–474.

Purves, D. (1988). *Body and brain: A trophic theory of neural connections.* Cambridge, MA: MIT Press.

Rajkowska, G., & Goldman-Rakic, P.S. (1995). Cytoarchitectonic definition of prefrontal areas in the normal human cortex: Variability in locations of areas 9 and 46 and relationship to the Talairach coordinate system. *Cerebral Cortex, 5,* 307–322.

Rakic, P. (1972). Mode of cell migration to the superficial layers of fetal monkey neocortex. *Journal of Comparative Neurology, 145,* 61–84.

Rakic, P. (1974). Neurons in the monkey visual cortex: Systematic relation between time of origin and eventual disposition. *Science, 183,* 425–427.

Rakic, P. (1981). Development of visual centers in primate brain depends on binocular competition before birth. *Science, 214,* 928–931.

Rakic, P. (1985). Limits of neurogenesis in primates. *Science, 227,* 154–156.

Rakic, P. (1988). Specification of cerebral cortical areas. *Science, 241,* 170–176.

Rakic, P. (1995). Development of cerebral cortex in human and nonhuman primates. In M. Lewis (Ed.), *Child and adolescent psychiatry* (2nd ed., pp. 9–29). Baltimore: Williams & Wilkins.

Rakic, P., Bourgeois, J.-P., Eckenhoff, M.F., Zecevic, N., & Goldman-Rakic, P.S. (1986). Concurrent overproduction of synapses in diverse regions of the primate cerebral cortex. *Science, 232,* 232–235.

Rakic, P., Bourgeois, J.-P., & Goldman-Rakic, P.S. (1994). Synaptic development of the cerebral cortex: Implications for learning, memory, and mental illness. *Progress in Brain Research, 102,* 227–243.

Rakic, P., Gallager, D., & Goldman-Rakic, P.S. (1988). Areal and laminar distribution of major neurotransmitter receptors in the monkey visual cortex. *Journal of Neuroscience, 8,* 3670–3690.

Rakic, P., & Kornack, D.R. (1993). Constraints on neurogenesis in adult primate brain: An evolutionary advantage? In A.C. Cuello (Ed.), *Neuronal death and regeneration: Vol. 6. Restorative neurology* (pp. 257–266). Amsterdam: Elsevier.

Rakic, P., & Lidow, M.S. (1995). Distribution and density of neurotransmitter receptors in the absence of retinal input from early embryonic stages. *Journal of Neuroscience, 15,* 2561–2574.

Rumelhart, D.E., McClelland, J.L., & the PDP Research Group. (1988). *Parallel distributed processing: Explorations in the microstructure of cognition: Vol. 1. Foundations.* Cambridge, MA: MIT Press.

Schwartz, M.L., & Goldman-Rakic, P.S. (1991). Prenatal specification of callosal connections in rhesus monkey. *Journal of Comparative Neurology, 307,* 144–162.

Schwartz, M.L., Rakic, P., & Goldman-Rakic, P.S. (1991). Early phenotype expression of cortical neurons: Evidence that a subclass of migrating neurons have callosal axons. *Proceedings of the National Academy of Science of the United States of America, 88,* 1354–1358.

Selemon, L.D., & Goldman-Rakic, P.S. (1988). Common cortical and subcortical targets of the dorsolateral prefrontal and posterior parietal cortices in the rhesus monkey: Evidence for a distributed neural network subserving spatially guided behavior. *Journal of Neuroscience, 8,* 4049–4068.

Spelke, E., Vishton, P., & von Hofsten, C. (1995). Object perception, object-directed action, and physical knowledge in infancy. In M. Gazzaniga (Ed.), *The cognitive neurosciences* (pp. 165–180). Cambridge, MA: MIT Press.

Stuss, D.T., & Benson, D.F. (1986). *The frontal lobes.* New York: Raven Press.

Toran-Allerand, C.D. (1984). On the genesis of sexual differentiation of the central nervous system: Morphogenetic consequences of steroidal exposure and possible role of α-fetoprotein. *Progress in Brain Research, 61,* 63–98.

Vincent, S.L., Peters, A., & Tigges, J. (1989). Effects of aging on the neurons within area 17 of rhesus monkey cerebral cortex. *Anatomical Record, 223,* 329–341.

Vital-Durand, F., & Blakemore, C. (1983). The first few weeks in monkey's visual cortex. *Behavioral Brain Research, 8,* 283.

Wenk, G.L., Pierce, D.J., Struble, R.G., Price, D.L., & Cork, L.C. (1989). Age-related changes in multiple neurotransmitter systems in the monkey brain. *Neurobiology of Aging, 10,* 11–19.

Williams, R.W., & Rakic, P. (1985). Deployment of growth cones in the retina and optic pathway of rhesus monkeys. *Investigative Ophthalmology and Visual Sciences, 26*(Suppl.), 286.

Yakovlev, P.I., & LeCours, A.R. (1967). The myelogenetic cycles of regional maturation of the brain. In A. Minkowsky (Ed.), *Regional development of the brain in early life* (pp. 3–70). Oxford, England: Blackwell Scientific.

Yates, T. (1991). Theories of cognitive development. In M. Lewis (Ed.), *Child and adolescent psychiatry* (pp. 109–129). Baltimore: Williams & Wilkins.

Zecevic, N., Bourgeois, J.-P., & Rakic, P. (1989). Changes in synaptic density in motor cortex of rhesus monkey during fetal and postnatal life. *Developmental Brain Research, 50,* 11–32.

Zecevic, N., & Rakic, P. (1991). Synaptogenesis in monkey somatosensory cortex. *Cerebral Cortex, 1,* 510–523.

Zielinski, B.S., & Hendrickson, A.E. (1992). Development of synapses in macaque monkey striate cortex. *Visual Neuroscience, 8,* 491–504.

Development of the Prefrontal Cortex: Evolution, Neurobiology, and Behavior
edited by Norman A. Krasnegor, Ph.D., G. Reid Lyon, Ph.D.,
and Patricia S. Goldman-Rakic, Ph.D.
copyright © 1997   Paul H. Brookes Publishing Co., Inc.
Baltimore • London • Toronto • Sydney

3

Organization and Development of Callosal Connectivity in Prefrontal Cortex

Michael L. Schwartz

The corpus callosum is the principal pathway for the communication of sensory and cognitive information between cortical areas of the two cerebral hemispheres (Gazzaniga, 1985; Sperry, 1974, 1982) and has been the subject of considerable clinical interest because of its role as the primary substrate for the interhemispheric spread of discharges in generalized epileptic seizures (Reeves & O'Leary, 1985; Wilson, Culver, Waddington, & Gazzaniga, 1975). Studies of callosal connections within sensory and motor regions of the cerebral cortex since the 1960s have provided important insight into the functional, organizational, and developmental features of these pathways. In contrast, the study of callosal connections for association regions of the cerebral mantle has not kept pace. This chapter presents data from ongoing studies of corticocortical connectivity in which the focus has been on the organization and development of interhemispheric connections between areas of the monkey prefrontal association cortex. The chapter describes general features of the topographic, laminar, and columnar organization of these connections in the mature monkey and concludes with results of studies examining the prenatal development and maturation of these connections.

The prefrontal cortex (PFC) is of particular interest because of its prominence both anatomically and functionally in primates. In humans, this region of the frontal lobes comprises 24%–29% of the entire surface of the cerebral cortex (Brodmann, 1912; Rakic, 1982) and is involved in many aspects of cognitive activity that are considered to be distinctively human (Goldman-Rakic, 1987; Goldman-Rakic, Isseroff, Schwartz, & Bugbee, 1983). We have used the rhesus monkey as a model for understanding the functional organization and development of this region because the cytoarchitectonic differentiation and proportion of cortical surface occupied by the PFC in the monkey are greater than those found in any nonprimate

This chapter was supported by grants from the National Science Foundation (BNS-8617585) and the National Institutes of Health (NS22807).

species. Moreover, damage to this area in mature monkeys produces a pattern of cognitive and behavior deficits that are in many ways analogous to those seen in human infants and in adults with frontal lobe damage (Diamond & Goldman-Rakic, 1989; Goldman-Rakic, 1987).

The prefrontal cortex in humans and in monkeys can be divided into a number of distinctive cytoarchitectonic areas that are characterized by unique connectional and functional features (Barbas, 1992; Brodmann, 1909; Goldman-Rakic, 1987; Walker, 1940). This chapter focuses on Walker's area 46 (Walker, 1940), a subdivision of the PFC in monkeys that occupies the dorsolateral surface of the frontal lobes, including the cortex lining the banks of the principal sulcus. This area is characterized by a well-demarcated granular Layer IV, a distinctive feature of the dorsolateral PFC in primates that is not present in any region of the PFC in nonprimate species (Akert, 1964). In addition, clinical studies of humans with damage encompassing this portion of the PFC (Freedman & Oscar-Berman, 1986; Guitton, Buchtel, & Douglas, 1985; Milner, 1982) and behavior studies of monkeys with experimental lesions of this region (for review, see Goldman-Rakic, 1987) reveal striking parallels in the resulting constellation of cognitive deficits.

CALLOSAL CONNECTIONS IN THE
PREFRONTAL CORTEX OF MATURE MONKEYS

Areal Topography

Fibers connecting areas of the PFC of the two hemispheres are found within the genu and rostral portions of the body of the corpus callosum (Barbas & Pandya, 1984; Pandya, Karol, & Heilbronn, 1971). The axons within these regions are topographically distributed. However, their topography is not purely a reflection of the relative tangential positions of their cells of origin; it is also determined by the degree of architectonic differentiation of the cytoarchitectonic area from which they originate. Axons from areas with similar patterns of architectonic differentiation therefore tend to occupy adjacent positions in the callosum, although they may occupy nonadjacent regions on the cortical surface (Barbas & Pandya, 1984).

Since the mid-1970s, a number of studies have applied sensitive tract-tracing techniques to map both the targets and the sources of callosal axons connecting prefrontal area 46 with regions of the contralateral hemisphere. Two principles of callosal organization have emerged from these studies: 1) connections between area 46 and cytoarchitectonic areas of the contralateral hemisphere are reciprocal, and 2) all cortical areas that have a callosal connection with area 46 also maintain an ipsilateral associational projection with area 46 of the same hemisphere. The majority of callosal connections with area 46 are restricted to cytoarchitectonic areas of the contralateral PFC. These include the homotopic area 46 as well as heterotopic areas 8a, 8b, 9, 10, and 45 on the dorsolateral surface; orbital areas 11 and 12; and cingulate area 24 on the medial surface of the hemisphere (Jacobson & Trojanowski, 1977b; McGuire, Bates, & Goldman-Rakic, 1991; Schwartz & Goldman-Rakic, 1984). The density of these connections is greatest between area 46 of the two hemispheres (McGuire et al., 1991; Schwartz & Goldman-Rakic, 1984); is somewhat diminished for areas 8A, 8B, 24, and 45; and is relatively modest for areas 9, 10, 11, and 12. Only a small subset of prefrontal areas lacks callosal connections with area 46 of the opposite hemisphere. These include areas 13 and 14 on the orbital surface and medial area 25. Callosal connections between area 46 and regions of the contralateral hemisphere outside the PFC are sparse and are limited to premotor area 6 and to the supplementary motor area (SMA) (Jacobson & Trojanowski, 1977a; McGuire et al., 1991; Schwartz & Goldman-Rakic, 1984).

Columnar and Laminar Organization
Studies of the microarchitecture of the dorsolateral PFC in monkeys indicate that the afferent, efferent, and local circuit elements of this area are organized in a modular pattern in both the radial and the tangential domains (Goldman & Nauta, 1977; Goldman-Rakic & Schwartz, 1982; Schwartz & Goldman-Rakic, 1984; Schwartz, Zheng, & Goldman-Rakic, 1988). This modularity was first appreciated in an autoradiographic study of the callosal and associational projections of area 46 by Goldman and Nauta (1977). Following injection of ^{3}H-leucine and ^{3}H-proline into the dorsolateral PFC of one hemisphere, they observed that the pattern of terminal and axonal labeling in the homotopic area of the opposite hemisphere appeared as a series of vertically oriented stripes or columns. These stripes were roughly .5 mm in width, extended through all six cortical layers, and alternated with unlabeled regions of approximately the same dimensions. Subsequent studies focusing on the topography of projections to area 46 from areas of the ipsilateral PFC, the posterior parietal cortex, and the SMA have reported a similar modularity in the pattern of afferent terminations (Goldman-Rakic & Schwartz, 1982; Leichnetz, 1980; McGuire et al., 1991; Schwartz & Goldman-Rakic, 1984; Selemon & Goldman-Rakic, 1988). Thus, the columnar distribution and regular periodicity of callosal terminations within the dorsolateral PFC appears to be a general feature that characterizes all corticocortical afferent terminations within prefrontal areas of the association cortex.

Consistent with the disjunctive organization of afferent terminations within the PFC, corticocortical projection neurons of area 46 are also unevenly distributed. For example, the tangential distribution of area 46 neurons that project to the homotopic region of the opposite hemisphere wax and wane in density across the cortical surface. However, few regions of the PFC are truly devoid of labeled neurons. For this reason, the true modularity and periodicity of efferent neuronal populations is not fully appreciated in the absence of careful quantitative examination of the density of labeled cells across the cortical surface. For example, generating a histogram of variations in the density of identified efferent populations across the cortical surface readily reveals that projection neurons also have a repeating modular distribution (Figure 3.1). This distribution shares the cyclical dimensions of the more sharply defined afferent territories. This is best demonstrated by the results of our horseradish peroxidase (HRP) tracing studies, in which areas containing the highest density of retrogradely labeled callosal projection neurons were also found to correspond with anterogradely labeled columns of callosal terminations (Figure 3.2) (Goldman-Rakic & Schwartz, 1982; Schwartz & Goldman-Rakic, 1984). A similar registration in the periodicities of projection neuron density and afferent termination zones is evident for corticocortical connections of the PFC with other areas of the same and the opposite hemisphere.

Similarities in the periodicity of afferent and efferent modules interconnecting area 46 with cortical areas of the ipsilateral and contralateral hemispheres raise the issue of how these different modules might be related. For example, what sources of input and which projection neuron populations occupy cortical regions between callosal projection columns? Do different corticocortical connections occupy unique or overlapping modular territories within the PFC? We initially addressed these questions using an anterograde double-labeling paradigm to simultaneously

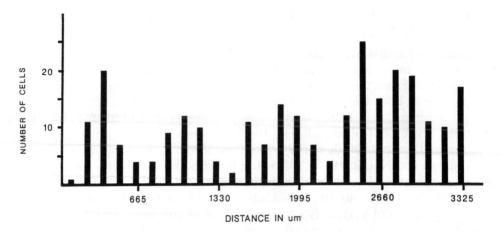

Figure 3.1. Histogram representing the tangential distribution of retrogradely labeled callosal neurons in the dorsal bank of the principal sulcus (PS) from a representative 40-μm coronal section. The injection of the fluorescent tracer fast blue was made into homotopic area 46 of the opposite hemisphere. The dorsal bank of the PS was divided into a series of adjacent 133-μm-wide bins extending from the pial surface to the Layer VI–white matter border. The number of retrogradely labeled callosal projection neurons in each bin was determined and is indicated by the height of each black bar in the histogram. Adjacent bars represent adjacent cortical bins. Note the regularly repeating waxing and waning in callosal neuron number across the surface of the cortex.

identify the terminal territories of two sources of corticocortical input that converge in the dorsolateral PFC. For this purpose, rhesus monkeys were unilaterally injected with ^{3}H-leucine and ^{3}H-proline into the dorsal bank of the principal sulcus (i.e., area 46) to label columns of callosal axons and terminals in the cortex of the principal sulcus of the contralateral hemisphere. Horseradish peroxidase was then injected into the posterior bank of the intraparietal sulcus of the opposite hemisphere to identify the termination zones of this associational projection within the PFC (Figure 3.3). Alternate sections through the principal sulcus of the PFC were processed autoradiographically or for HRP visualization, and the distributions of labeled afferents were reconstructed. The principal finding of this study was that callosal and associational terminals from these two sources occupy unique and interdigitated columnar territories within the PFC (Figure 3.3).

Using a similar double-labeling strategy with retrogradely transported fluorescent dyes, we have also examined the relationship between efferent neuron populations within area 46. In these studies, the tracer fast blue was injected into the cortex lining the principal sulcus of one hemisphere and diamidino-yellow was injected into the posterior bank of the intraparietal sulcus of the opposite hemisphere. The distributions of labeled neurons containing either fast blue, diamidino-yellow, or both tracers were then charted in area 46 of the PFC that was not injected. An example of the pattern of labeling found in these studies is illustrated in Figure 3.4. As was expected from the results of previous single-labeling studies, the tangential distributions of callosal and associational projection neuron populations showed considerable overlap and were not separated by sharp boundaries. Despite the intermixing of these efferent populations, both had periodic variations in neuron density across the cortical surface that were inversely related. That is, areas of peak callosal neuron density corresponded to areas containing relatively few associ-

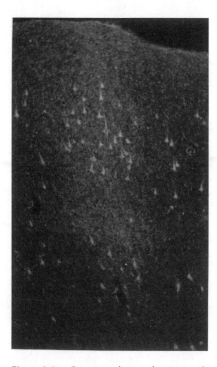

Figure 3.2.   Correspondence of anterograde and retrograde HRP labeling in the dorsal bank of the PFC following an injection in area 46 of the opposite hemisphere. Note that the fine, dustlike anterograde labeling of terminals and axons is coincident with the region of densest retrograde labeling of callosal projection neurons.

ational neurons, whereas areas of low callosal neuron density were coincident with regions containing the highest densities of associational projection neurons. Taken together with our results concerning the modularity of afferent terminations, these data indicate that information carried over callosal and associational pathways is topographically segregated at the stages of initial input and final output in prefrontal cortical areas. Therefore, the ultimate integration of information between these modules must rely heavily upon the local circuit connections of the PFC.

In addition to the spatially disjunctive distribution of corticocortical efferents and afferents in the tangential domain, these connections also exhibit a very distinctive pattern of laminar or radial termination and origin. For example, retrograde tracing studies using either HRP or fluorescent dyes indicate that callosal and associational neurons within area 46 have a bilaminar distribution. Approximately 80% of all callosal and 70% of associational corticocortical projection neurons are distributed within Layer III (Schwartz & Goldman-Rakic, 1984). The bulk of the remaining neurons of each class are distributed within Layer V (19% and 14%, respectively). Although, as noted, callosal and associational projection neurons have similar patterns of laminar origin and are often intermixed across the cortical surface, our studies using multiple fluorescent tracers indicate that less than 1% of these neurons project simultaneously to areas of both hemispheres. The low inci-

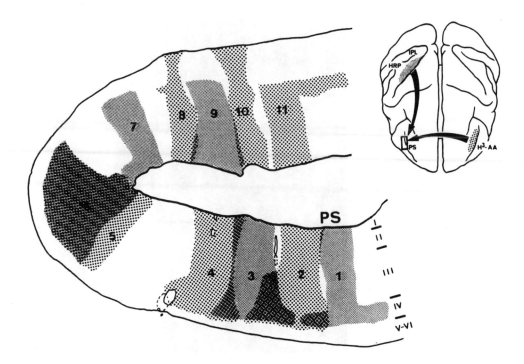

Figure 3.3.   Composite diagram of two adjacent 50-μm coronal sections cut through the convergence zone in the principal sulcus (PS; see inset). Autoradiographically labeled (³H-AA) callosal fiber columns (2, 4, 5, 8, 10, and 11) are indicated by coarse stipple; associational fiber columns arising from neurons in the posterior bank of the intraparietal sulcus (IPL) labeled by anterograde transport of HRP (1, 3, 6, 7, and 9) are indicated by fine stipple. Blood vessels in HRP-reacted sections are indicated by dashed lines; those from autoradiograms are indicated by continuous lines. Several blood vessels penetrating Layers I and II orthogonally were used to align adjacent sections. (Adapted from Goldman-Rakic & Schwartz [1982].)

dence of neurons with bilateral projections to areas of the two hemispheres in mature monkeys underscores the independence and segregation of information communicated by callosal and associational pathways to and from the dorsolateral PFC.

Callosal Neuron Morphology

Consistent with the results of previous studies in the PFC (Jacobson & Trojanowski, 1977b) and other areas of the monkey cerebral cortex (Jones & Wise, 1977; Rockland & Pandya, 1979), our studies using retrograde tracers have generally confirmed that the vast majority of callosal projections of area 46 arise from neurons with a pyramidal morphology (Schwartz & Goldman-Rakic, 1984). These data are in agreement with the long-standing view that callosal projections exert an excitatory influence on target neurons of the contralateral hemisphere (Toyama & Matsunami, 1976; Toyama, Matsunami, Ohno, & Tokashiki, 1974). However, careful analyses of the morphological features of callosal projection neurons in our studies have suggested that a small population of these projections may originate from nonpyramidal neurons found predominately within Layers V and VI. In these studies, we examined the morphological features of HRP-labeled neurons with reaction product extending into proximal portions of the dendritic tree following an injection of tracer into the homotopic area of the opposite hemisphere. Neurons of uncertain morphology as a result of insufficient dendritic labeling were considered

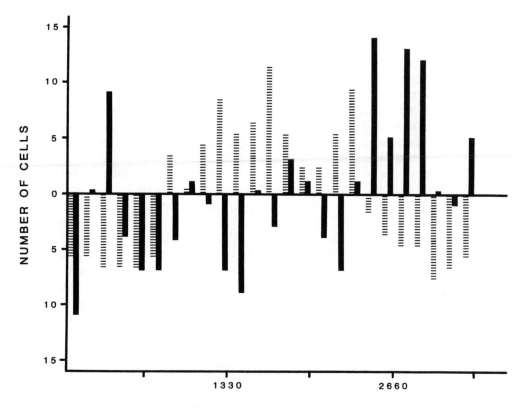

Figure 3.4.   Relative distributions of callosal and associational projection neurons in the principal sulcus of the PFC. The number of neurons labeled by each fluorescent tracer was determined for adjacent 133-μm-wide cortical slabs (bins) extending from the pial surface to the border of Layer VI with the underlying white matter. Adjacent hatched and solid bars in the histogram represent the values for each cell class in a single bin or unit area of cortex. The value for each bin represents the number of callosal neurons (solid bars) and ipsilateral neurons (hatched bars) represented as deviations from their respective means. The line at zero denotes the mean; downward deviations signify values below the mean, and upward deviations signify density values greater than the mean. (From Schwartz, M.L., & Goldman-Rakic, P.S. [1984]. Callosal and intrahemispheric connectivity of the prefrontal association cortex in rhesus monkey: Relation between intraparietal and principal sulcal cortex. *Journal of Comparative Neurology, 226,* 419; reprinted by permission.)

as pyramids. Thus, our analysis was conservatively biased toward the pyramidal phenotype. Despite this bias, we classified approximately 15% of all labeled Layer V neurons and 60% of labeled Layer VI neurons as having a nonpyramidal morphology (Schwartz & Goldman-Rakic, 1984). We have pursued this issue by using a double-labeling strategy in the ferret PFC. Cholera toxin conjugated to colloidal gold was used to retrogradely label callosal projection neurons and was combined with immunocytochemistry to simultaneously label γ-aminobutyric acid (GABA)-containing neurons. The major finding of these studies was that a small population of infragranular callosal projection neurons were also immunocytochemically identified as GABA-containing neurons (Figure 3.5). These data suggest that a limited population of callosal projections has a direct inhibitory influence on neurons of the opposite hemisphere and may explain the results of physiological studies demonstrating inhibitory interactions related to callosal connections (Asanuma & Okuda, 1962).

DEVELOPMENT OF CALLOSAL CONNECTIONS
IN THE PREFRONTAL CORTEX OF FETAL MONKEYS

Many of the important milestones in the development of cortical organization and connectivity take place prior to birth in both humans and monkeys. The timing of these events has made them inaccessible to experimental examination until the development of prenatal surgical techniques (Rakic & Goldman-Rakic, 1984). With the perfection of these surgical methods, it has now become feasible to design studies that incorporate surgical interventions to perturb normal development and to apply modern tract-tracing methodologies to the study of connectional organization at different stages of fetal development. This section describes the results of studies that have combined sensitive retrograde tract-tracing techniques and prenatal neurosurgery to explore the timing and specificity of developing callosal projections of the dorsolateral PFC of the monkey.

An important issue that must be addressed in developmental studies of corticocortical connections is how one defines the target and source of a projection. In the retrograde tracing studies described here, our goal has been to characterize the distribution of callosal projection neurons whose axons have entered the dorsolateral cortex of the opposite hemisphere and could therefore be said to project to this cortical area (cortex-specific callosal neurons). To address this point, we confined our tracer injections to the layers of the emerging cortical plate and were careful not to allow their encroachment into the prospective white matter and transient development zones that are present below the cortex during early stages of cortical development. Previous studies have demonstrated that these subcortical areas con-

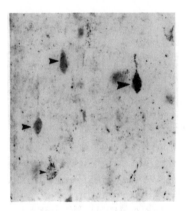

Figure 3.5. Photomicrograph of callosal and GABA-containing neurons in infragranular cortical layers of the ferret PFC. Callosal neurons are retrogradely labeled by a conjugate of cholera toxin–colloidal gold (CT–gold), which was injected into the prefrontal cortex of the opposite hemisphere (small arrowhead). GABA-immunoreactive neurons are indicated by medium-size arrowheads. Double-labeled neuron containing both CT–gold and GABA is indicated by the large arrowhead.

tain growing axons—fibers of passage passing to and from other cortical areas—and form a waiting compartment for axonal populations prior to their growth into appropriate cortical targets (Goldman-Rakic, 1981; Kostovic & Rakic, 1990; Shatz, Chun, & Luskin, 1988; Wise & Jones, 1978). Thus, the restriction of our injections to the cortical plate was essential because the objective of our studies was to characterize the distribution and development of callosal projections that actually innervate rather than those approaching or waiting under prefrontal area 46.

We began these studies by examining the distribution of callosal projections to the dorsolateral PFC in fetal monkeys at midgestation, Embryonic Day 82 (E82) of the 165-day gestational period. By this age, most neurons of Layers III through VI that will give rise to the callosal connections of area 46 have been generated and have migrated or are in the process of migrating to their final resting positions within the cortical layers (Schwartz, Rakic, & Goldman-Rakic, 1991). Animals in our earliest fetal group received injections of retrogradely transported fluorescent dyes or HRP into the cortical layers of the dorsolateral PFC between E82 and E89. We confirmed that the lateral spread of tracer within the cortex did not extend into areas outside the dorsolateral PFC by examining the pattern of retrograde thalamic labeling in each case. Thalamocortical axons are already within their cortical targets at these early fetal ages, and the restriction of retrogradely labeled neurons to lateral portions of the mediodorsal thalamic nucleus in these cases was consistent with the pattern of thalamic projections to area 46 in mature monkeys (Giguere & Goldman-Rakic, 1988; Goldman-Rakic & Porrino, 1985). Fetuses with injections of tracer that were restricted to the cortical layers had only a small number of retrogradely labeled neurons in the opposite hemisphere (usually only 1–5 per 40-μm section). The few labeled neurons were generally confined to the cortical layers of the dorsolateral cortex homotopic to the injection sites and to regions of the prospective cingulate cortex on the medial surface of the hemisphere. Both are regions that maintain projections to the dorsolateral PFC of the opposite hemisphere in mature monkeys. Although we consistently identified labeled neurons in these cases, the extremely small number indicated that these fetal ages are near the very beginning of callosal axon ingrowth into the PFC. In contrast to the paucity of neurons labeled by cortically restricted injections, even small injections placed below the cortical plate at these ages labeled a substantial population of neurons. Although most of these labeled neurons were restricted to the cortical layers, many were also present within the developmentally transient subplate and intermediate zones lying below the cortical plate. The greater density of labeled neurons in cases with injections extending below the cortical plate is consistent with the pattern of labeling that would be expected based upon the results of anterograde tracing studies of the monkey PFC (Goldman-Rakic, 1981). These studies indicate that the majority of callosal axons at these ages wait below the cortical plate for a period of weeks or months prior to entering their cortical targets. Therefore, although callosal axons are present within the contralateral hemisphere prior to E90, few have actually innervated their cortical targets.

We had expected that injections of retrograde tracers into the subcortical waiting compartment would label a greater number of neurons in the layers of the cortical plate of the opposite hemisphere than cortically restricted injections. However, we were surprised that many retrogradely labeled cells were also present within the subcortical subplate and intermediate zones of the opposite hemisphere. These data raised the question of whether these cells represent a subpopulation of developmentally transient subplate cells extending axons into the contralateral hemisphere or whether they may be presumptive Layer III callosal neurons extending axons into the opposite hemisphere during their migration into the cortical plate. Although previous studies have suggested that axogenesis is a relatively late event in neuronal development that occurs only after neurons have completed their migration into the cortical plate (Berry & Rogers, 1965; Morest, 1970), several pieces of data favor the possibility that some of these retrogradely labeled cells may indeed be migrating neurons:

1. Many retrogradely labeled callosal neurons in subcortical areas of fetuses injected at E89 or before have a morphology resembling that of migrating cortical neurons (Rakic, 1972; Schwartz et al., 1991).
2. The density of labeled callosal neurons within these subcortical regions is sharply reduced between E84 and E104 coincident with an increasing density of neuronal labeling in Layer III.
3. The reduction in labeled subcortical neurons by E104 coincides with the time at which the majority of neurons in the lower half of Layer III have completed their migration into the cortical plate but when subplate neurons are still at their peak density (Schwartz & Meinecke, 1992; Schwartz et al., 1991).

We directly tested the possibility that these subcortically located neurons may represent a population of cells extending axons toward the contralateral PFC during migration using a double-labeling paradigm combining ^{3}H-thymidine birthdating and retrograde tracing with fluorescent dyes. Briefly, we injected fetuses between E74 and E76 with ^{3}H-thymidine to label prospective Layer III neurons that were being generated at this time. We subsequently injected the PFC of one hemisphere with fluorescent tracers at E84, a time when these neurons would be in the last half of their migration toward the cortical plate. Examination of the cerebral wall contralateral to the tracer injections revealed many neurons singly labeled with either ^{3}H-thymidine or retrograde tracer, which were distributed among all cortical layers, the subplate, and intermediate zones. However, a smaller number of neurons were labeled with both ^{3}H-thymidine and retrograde tracer (Figure 3.6). These neurons were most prominent in Layers III and IV of the cortical plate, but small numbers of double-labeled neurons were also found in Layers V and VI, as well as in the subplate and intermediate zones below the cortex. The presence of double-labeled neurons within the intermediate and subplate zones provided direct evidence that some migrating neurons extend an axon into the opposite hemisphere. These data further suggest that some features of axonal projections may be specified for cortical neurons well in advance of their attainment of their final positions within the laminae of the cerebral cortex.

In contrast to the limited number of neurons innervating the cortical layers of the contralateral PFC in fetuses with cortically restricted injections prior to E90, the results of our analysis of fetuses injected after E90 suggest that the major wave of callosal axon growth into the six layers of the dorsolateral PFC takes place between E100 and E124. For example, injections of HRP restricted to the cortical layers of prospective area 46 at E111 labeled many neurons in both homotopic and heterotopic areas of the opposite hemisphere (Figure 3.7). Although the immaturity of cortical sulcal and lamination patterns at these early ages limits the precision with which one can identify specific cortical areas, comparisons of the topographic dis-

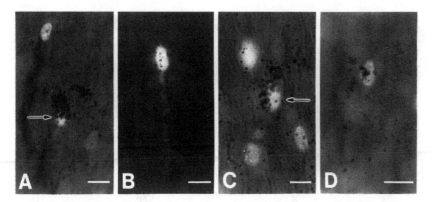

Figure 3.6.   Double-labeled neurons: ³H-thymidine injected at E74 and E76 and retrograde fluorescent tracers injected at E84. (A) Diamidino-yellow (DY)-labeled subplate/intermediate zone neuron heavily labeled with ³H-thymidine. (B) DY- and ³H-thymidine–labeled neuron in the upper subplate zone. (C) DY- and ³H-thymidine–labeled neuron at the border of Layer VI and the subplate. (D) DY- and ³H-thymidine–labeled neuron in Layer III. Arrows in A and C indicate double-labeled neurons. Scale bars equal 10 μm. (From Schwartz, M.L., Rakic, P., & Goldman-Rakic, P.S. [1991]. Early phenotypic expression of cortical neurons: Evidence that a subclass of migrating neurons have callosal axons. *Proceedings of the National Academy of Sciences of the United States of America, 88,* 1357; reprinted by permission.)

tributions of labeled neurons with those in animals at older fetal ages and with the pattern found in mature monkeys reveal very similar distributions (Figure 3.7). At the earliest ages for which we could conclusively identify cytoarchitectonic areas of the PFC (fetuses injected between E124 and E137), the topography of projections was similar to that seen at earlier fetal ages and resulted in retrograde labeling of callosal neurons in all cytoarchitectonic areas of the PFC that have callosal projections to area 46 in mature monkeys. Conversely, we found no ectopic labeled cells in cytoarchitectonic areas of the PFC of the opposite hemisphere, which do not project to area 46 in adults. Thus, the data from these retrograde tracing studies lead us to conclude that 1) the constellation of cytoarchitectonic areas that have callosal projections to the PFC of the opposite hemisphere appears to be stable from E111 through adulthood, 2) the pattern of projections between different areas of the PFC in opposite hemispheres is highly specified at the time of axonal growth into the cortical layers, and 3) callosal axons from divergent areas of the opposite hemisphere innervate the contralateral PFC in unison. Because most of these fibers wait for some period of time below the cortex of the PFC prior to growing in (Goldman-Rakic, 1981), the synchrony of ingrowth for afferents of diverse sources suggests that the waiting compartment may be important for coordinating their entrance into the cortical layers, possibly to ensure competitive interactions between the different afferent populations for the establishment of synaptic and columnar territories.

Another aspect of callosal topography that we have examined is the emergence of the intra-areal columnar organization of callosal projection neurons in area 46 (Schwartz & Goldman-Rakic, 1990, 1991). This analysis of the emergence of modular features for the callosal neuron distribution focused on areas of the greatest and most complete callosal neuron labeling. Thus, we determined the distribution of labeled neurons across the cortex lining the banks and rims of the principal sulcus homotopic to the injection of tracer in the opposite hemisphere. The pattern of

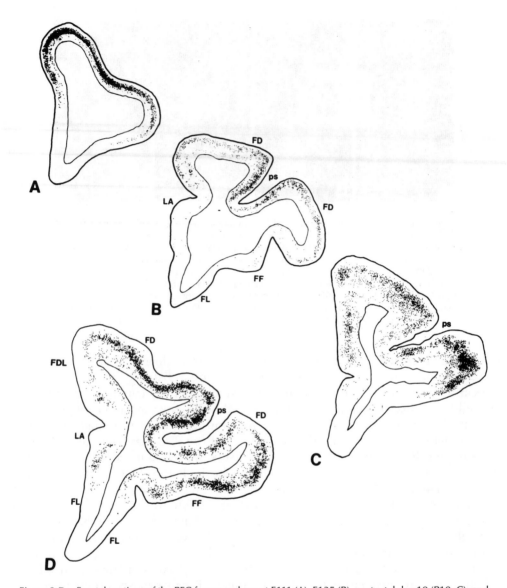

Figure 3.7.   Frontal sections of the PFC from monkeys at E111 (A), E135 (B), postnatal day 10 (P10; C), and adulthood (>3 years of age; D). Anterior–posterior levels represented at the different ages are from areas homotopic to the injection site of the opposite hemisphere and represent roughly equivalent regions of the PFC based upon landmarks such as sulcal location and comparable positions between the frontal pole and the head of the caudate nucleus. All labeled neurons are represented in each plot. Note the similiarities in the distribution and areas of concentration for callosal neurons at the different fetal ages and the similarity with the distribution found in the adult monkey. Letter designations for von Bonin and Bailey's (1941) cytoarchitectonic areas LA, FD, FDL, FF, and FL are shown for the E135 and adult cases. Walker's area 46 and von Bonin and Bailey's area FD are approximately coextensive. (ps, principal sulcus.)

labeling at each age examined between E100 and maturity revealed a band of labeled callosal neurons extending across the entire breadth of the cortex lining the principal sulcus (Figure 3.7). As in mature monkeys, the density of neuronal labeling within this band waxed and waned at each fetal age. Quantitative analyses of these variations were made for each age; representative histograms for fetuses injected at E111, E135, and Postnatal Day 12 (P12) are illustrated in Figure 3.8. Although the distribution of labeled neurons displayed periodic variations in density across the cortical surface at all ages, the tangential dimensions and regularity that characterize this modular organization in mature animals are not apparent until somewhere between E136 and the early postnatal period. These data raise the question of how the inverse relationship between callosal and associational projection fields emerges during this period. We addressed this issue using the same double-labeling paradigm we previously used in mature monkeys. The retrogradely transported fluorescent dye fast blue was injected into the cortex of the principal sulcus of one hemisphere, and a second fluorescent tracer, diamidino-yellow, was injected into the posterior bank of the intraparietal sulcus in the opposite hemisphere (Schwartz & Goldman-Rakic, 1982, 1990). In order to examine the spatial relationship of associational and callosal projection neurons, we generated histograms of their densities across the cortical surface of area 46 (Figure 3.9). These data revealed that, despite the irregularity of the individual distributions of these two efferent populations, there is a tendency for areas of high callosal neuron density to coincide with regions of low associational neuron density, and vice versa. Therefore, although the basic inverse relationship between these efferent projection domains is apparent during the fetal period, the refinement of their periodicities continues into the early postnatal period. These data are consistent with the data of LaMantia and Rakic (1990) demonstrating that the number of axons within the corpus callosum continues to undergo modification and attrition throughout the early postnatal period in monkeys.

A final feature of callosal neuron organization that we have examined is the laminar distribution of these cells at different stages of fetal development. Following injections restricted to the cortex at the earliest fetal ages (E82 through E89), the few labeled neurons were concentrated within prospective Layers V and VI of the cortical plate. These data indicate that some of the earlier generated neurons of the infragranular layers innervate the contralateral PFC at a time when neurons destined for Layer III are still being generated and migrating to their cortical positions. At the time of greatest ingrowth of callosal axons into the cortex of the opposite hemisphere (E100 through E124), the majority of callosal projection neurons are present within Layer III of area 46. Quantitative analysis of the number of labeled neurons within supragranular and infragranular cortical laminae at different fetal and postnatal ages revealed that the proportion of supragranular neurons contributing to the callosal projections of area 46 peaks at approximately E124 (94%) and gradually diminishes to the level found in adults (80%–84%) during the late fetal and early postnatal period (Figure 3.10). It is unlikely that this reduction in the proportion of supragranular callosal neurons is due to an increase in the number of infragranular callosal neurons because these cells are generated prior to the cells of Layer III, and therefore their axons are likely to innervate the opposite cortex prior to or in synchrony with axons of later generated Layer III neurons. Rather, it seems reasonable that this temporally restricted overrepresentation of Layer III neurons is reduced by a selective, and possibly exclusive, susceptibility to cell death or callosal axon loss by the supragranular layers. Similar observations on the selective susceptibility of later generated neurons to attrition by cell death or axonal loss have been made in studies of callosal connections in developing rat sensory cortex (Finlay & Slattery, 1983; Ivy & Killackey, 1981; Olavarria & Van Sluyters, 1985).

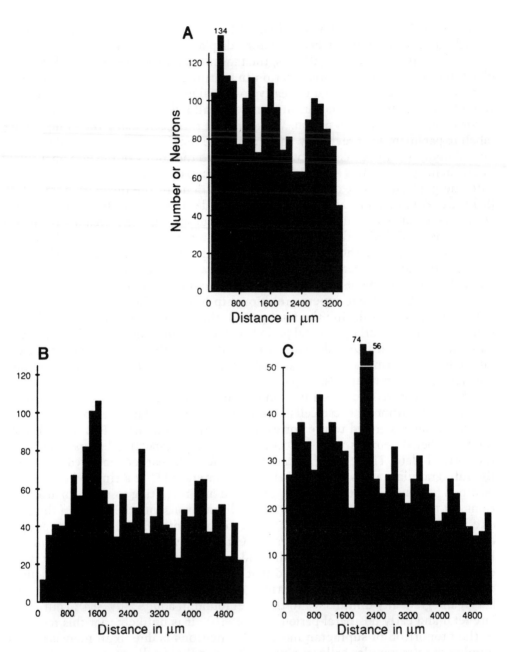

Figure 3.8.   Histograms representing the tangential distribution of callosal neurons at E111 (A), E135 (B), and P12 (C). The bins in each histogram represent the number of labeled callosal neurons in a region of cortex 160-μm wide and spanning the entire cortical depth from the white matter to the pial surface. Although all ages exhibited a somewhat columnar distribution of retrogradely labeled neurons, the regular periodicity and gradual waxing and waning that characterize the adult distribution was well established only in the P12 monkey.

In summary, the conclusion we draw from these studies of the development of cortex-specific callosal projections for prefrontal area 46 is that many features of the areal and intra-areal organization of callosal projections are specified prior to or just after birth. Of these features, the areal topography of connections between

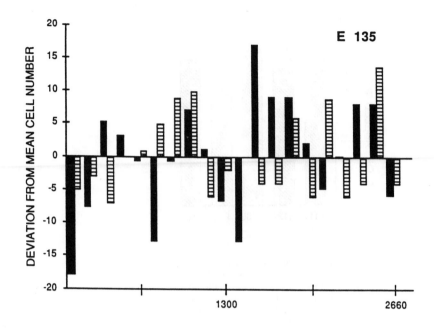

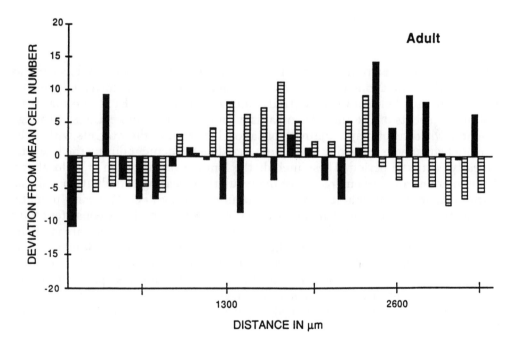

Figure 3.9.   Relative distributions of callosal and associational projection neurons in the principal sulcus of the PFC at E135 (top panel) and in the adult monkey (bottom panel). The relationship between the densities of cells projecting to the posterior bank of the ipsilateral intraparietal sulcus (hatched bars) and those projecting to the cortex of the contralateral principal sulcus (solid bars) are represented in the same graphic conventions as used in Figure 3.4. As before, both populations are plotted as deviations from their mean density across the dorsal bank of the principal sulcus.

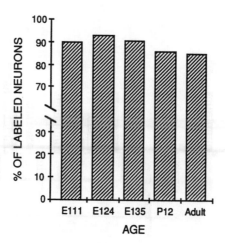

Figure 3.10.   Histogram of the percentages of all labeled callosal neurons that were located in supragranular Layer III from animals injected at E111, E124, E135, and P12, and in an adult monkey. (From Schwartz, M.L., & Goldman-Rakic, P.S. [1991]. Prenatal specification of callosal connections in rhesus monkey. *Journal of Comparative Neurology, 307,* 157; reprinted by permission.)

different cytoarchitectonic regions of the two hemispheres is specified as early as the time when the axons of callosal neurons have entered the cortex of the contralateral hemisphere and is essentially unchanged between E111 and maturity. Still other aspects of the modular organization of callosal connections, although present at the time of major ingrowth of callosal axons into their targets within the opposite hemisphere, continue to undergo a gradual refinement during the late fetal and early postnatal period. These include the laminar organization of callosal projection neurons and the emergence of the regularly repeating periodicity of callosal neuron densities that characterizes the mature monkey PFC. The early prenatal specification of callosal neuron organization in the primate PFC is consistent with the prenatal specification of callosal neuron distributions in other areas of the developing primate cortex, such as the visual (Chalupa, Killackey, Snider, & Lia, 1989; Dehay, Kennedy, Bullier, & Berland, 1988) and somatosensory (Killackey & Chalupa, 1986) cortices. These data also suggest a greater level of specificity in the initial patterning of these corticocortical connections than is present in many nonprimate species (for review, see Kennedy & Dehay, 1993, and Schwartz & Goldman-Rakic, 1990).

REFERENCES

Akert, K. (1964). Comparative anatomy of the frontal cortex and thalamo-cortical connections. In J.M. Warren and K. Akert (Eds.), *The frontal granular cortex and behavior* (pp. 372–396). New York: McGraw-Hill.

Asanuma, A., & Okuda, O. (1962). Effects of transcallosal volleys on pyramidal tract activity of cat. *Journal of Neurophysiology, 25,* 198–208.

Barbas, H. (1992). Architecture and cortical connections of the prefrontal cortex in the rhesus monkey. *Advances in Neurology, 57,* 91–115.

Barbas, H., & Pandya, D.N. (1984). Topography of commissural fibers of the prefrontal cortex in the rhesus monkey. *Experimental Brain Research, 55,* 187–191.

Berry, M., & Rogers, A.W. (1965). The migration of neuroblasts in the developing cerebral cortex. *Journal of Anatomy, 99,* 691–709.

Brodmann, K. (1909). *Vergleichende Lokalisationslehre der Grosshirnrinde.* Leipzig, Germany: Verlag J.A. Barth.

Brodmann, K. (1912). Neue ergebnisse über die vergleichende histologische lokalisation der grosshirnrinde mit besonderer berüksichtigung des stirnhirns. *Anatomischer Anzeiger, 41,* 157–216.

Chalupa, L.M., Killackey, H.P., Snider, C.J., & Lia, B. (1989). Callosal projection neurons in area 17 of the fetal rhesus monkey. *Developmental Brain Research, 46,* 303–308.

Dehay, C., Kennedy, H., Bullier, J., & Berland, M. (1988). Absence of interhemispheric connections of area 17 during development in the monkey. *Nature, 331,* 348–350.

Diamond, A., & Goldman-Rakic, P.S. (1989). Comparison of human infants and rhesus monkeys on Piaget's AB task: Evidence for dependence on dorsolateral prefrontal cortex. *Experimental Brain Research, 74,* 24–40.

Finlay, B.L., & Slattery, M. (1983). Local differences in the amount of early cell death in neocortex predict adult local specializations. *Science, 219,* 1349–1351.

Freedman, M., & Oscar-Berman, M. (1986). Bilateral frontal lobe disease and selective delayed-response deficits in humans. *Behavioral Neuroscience, 100,* 337–342.

Gazzaniga, M.S. (1985). Some contributions of split-brain studies to the study of human cognition. In A.G. Reeves (Ed.), *Epilepsy and the corpus callosum* (pp. 341–348). New York: Plenum.

Giguere, M., & Goldman-Rakic, P.S. (1988). Mediodorsal nucleus: Areal, laminar, and tangential distribution of afferents and efferents in the frontal lobe of rhesus monkeys. *Journal of Comparative Neurology, 277,* 195–213.

Goldman, P.S., & Nauta, W.J.H. (1977). Columnar distribution of cortico-cortical fibers in frontal association, limbic and motor cortex of the developing rhesus monkey. *Brain Research, 122,* 393–414.

Goldman-Rakic, P.S. (1981). Development and plasticity of primate frontal association cortex. In F.O. Schmitt, F.G. Worden, G. Adelman, & S.G. Dennis (Eds.), *The organization of the cerebral cortex* (pp. 69–97). Cambridge, MA: MIT Press.

Goldman-Rakic, P.S. (1987). Circuitry of the prefrontal cortex and the regulation of behavior by representational knowledge. In F. Plum (Vol. Ed.), *Handbook of physiology–revised: Sect. 1. The nervous system: Vol. 5. Higher functions of the brain* (pp. 373–417). Bethesda, MD: American Physiological Society.

Goldman-Rakic, P.S., Isseroff, A., Schwartz, M.L., & Bugbee, N.M. (1983). The neurobiology of cognitive development. In P. Mussen (Ed.), *Handbook of child psychology: Biology and infancy development* (pp. 281–344). New York: John Wiley & Sons.

Goldman-Rakic, P.S., & Porrino, L.J. (1985). The primate mediodorsal (MD) nucleus and its projection to the frontal lobe. *Journal of Comparative Neurology, 242,* 535–560.

Goldman-Rakic, P.S., & Schwartz, M.L. (1982). Interdigitation of contralateral and ipsilateral columnar projections to frontal association cortex in primates. *Science, 216,* 755–757.

Guitton, D., Buchtel, H.A., & Douglas, R.M. (1985). Frontal lobe lesions in man cause difficulties in suppressing reflexive glances and in generating goal-directed saccades. *Experimental Brain Research, 58,* 455–472.

Ivy, G.O., & Killackey, H.P. (1981). The ontogeny of the distribution of callosal projection neurons in the rat parietal cortex. *Journal of Comparative Neurology, 195,* 367–389.

Jacobson, S., & Trojanowski, J.Q. (1977a). Prefrontal granular cortex of the rhesus monkey: I. Intrahemispheric cortical afferents. *Brain Research, 132,* 209–233.

Jacobson, S., & Trojanowski, J.Q. (1977b). Prefrontal granular cortex of the rhesus monkey: II. Interhemispheric cortical afferents. *Brain Research, 132,* 235–246.

Jones, E.G., & Wise, S.P. (1977). Size, laminar and columnar distribution of efferent cells in the sensory-motor cortex of monkeys. *Journal of Comparative Neurology, 175,* 391–438.

Kennedy, H., & Dehay, C. (1993). Cortical specification of mice and men. *Cerebral Cortex, 3,* 171–186.

Killackey, H.P., & Chalupa, L.M. (1986). Ontogenetic change in the distribution of callosal projection neurons in the postcentral gyrus of the fetal rhesus monkey. *Journal of Comparative Neurology, 244,* 331–348.

Kostovic, I., & Rakic, P. (1990). Developmental history of the transient subplate zone in the visual and somatosensory cortex of the macaque monkey and human brain. *Journal of Comparative Neurology, 297*, 441–470.

LaMantia, A.-S., & Rakic, P. (1990). Axon overproduction and elimination in the corpus callosum of the developing rhesus monkey. *Journal of Neuroscience, 10*, 2156–2175.

Leichnetz, G.R. (1980). An intrahemispheric columnar projection between two cortical multisensory convergence areas (inferior parietal lobule and prefrontal cortex): An anterograde study in *macaque* using HRP gel. *Neuroscience Letters, 18*, 119–124.

McGuire, P.K., Bates, J.F., & Goldman-Rakic, P.S. (1991). Interhemispheric integration: I. Symmetry and convergence of the corticocortical connections of the left and right principal sulcus (PS) and the left and the right supplementary motor area (SMA) in the rhesus monkey. *Cerebral Cortex, 1*, 390–407.

Milner, B. (1982). Some cognitive effects of frontal-lobe lesions in man. *Philosophical Transactions of the Royal Society of London, Series B: Biological Sciences, 298*, 211–226.

Morest, D.K. (1970). A study of neurogenesis in the forebrain of opposum pouch young. *Zeitschrift für Anatomie und Entwicklungsgeschichte, 130*, 265–305.

Olavarria, J., & Van Sluyters, R.C. (1985). Organization and postnatal development of callosal connections in the visual cortex of the rat. *Journal of Comparative Neurology, 239*, 1–26.

Pandya, D.N., Karol, E.A., & Heilbronn, D. (1971). The topographic distribution of interhemispheric projections in the corpus callosum of the rhesus monkey. *Brain Research, 32*, 31–43.

Rakic, P. (1972). Mode of cell migration to the superficial layers of fetal monkey neocortex. *Journal of Comparative Neurology, 145*, 61–84.

Rakic, P. (1982). Early developmental events: Cell lineages, acquisition of neuronal positions, and areal and laminar development. *Neurosciences Research Program Bulletin, 20*, 439–451.

Rakic, P., & Goldman-Rakic, P.S. (1984). Use of fetal neurosurgery for experimental studies of structural and functional brain development in nonhuman primates. In R.A. Thompson, J.R. Green, & D. Johnson (Eds.), *Prenatal neurology and neurosurgery* (pp. 1–15). New York: Spectrum Publications.

Reeves, A.G., & O'Leary, P.M. (1985). Total corpus callosotomy for control of medically intractable epilepsy. In A.G. Reeves (Ed.), *Epilepsy and the corpus callosum* (pp. 269–280). New York: Plenum.

Rockland, K.S., & Pandya, D.N. (1979). Laminar origins and terminations of cortical connections of the occipital lobe in the rhesus monkey. *Brain Research, 179*, 3–20.

Schwartz, M.L., & Goldman-Rakic, P.S. (1982). Single cortical neurons have axon collaterals to ipsilateral and contralateral cortex in fetal and adult primates. *Nature, 299*, 154–156.

Schwartz, M.L., & Goldman-Rakic, P.S. (1984). Callosal and intrahemispheric connectivity of the prefrontal association cortex in rhesus monkey: Relation between intraparietal and principal sulcal cortex. *Journal of Comparative Neurology, 226*, 403–420.

Schwartz, M.L., & Goldman-Rakic, P.S. (1990). Development and plasticity of the primate neocortex. *Clinics in Perinatology, 17*, 83–102.

Schwartz, M.L., & Goldman-Rakic, P.S. (1991). Prenatal specification of callosal connections in rhesus monkey. *Journal of Comparative Neurology, 307*, 144–162.

Schwartz, M.L., & Meinecke, D.L. (1992). Early expression of GABA-containing neurons in the prefrontal and visual cortices of rhesus monkeys. *Cerebral Cortex, 2*, 16–37.

Schwartz, M.L., Rakic, P., & Goldman-Rakic, P.S. (1991). Early phenotypic expression of cortical neurons: Evidence that a subclass of migrating neurons have callosal axons. *Proceedings of the National Academy of Sciences of the United States of America, 88*, 1354–1358.

Schwartz, M.L., Zheng, D.-S., & Goldman-Rakic, P.S. (1988). Periodicity of GABA-containing cells in primate prefrontal cortex. *Journal of Neuroscience, 8*, 1962–1970.

Selemon, L.D., & Goldman-Rakic, P.S. (1988). Common cortical and subcortical targets of the dorsolateral prefrontal and posterior parietal cortices in the rhesus monkey: Evidence for a distributed network subserving spatially guided behavior. *Journal of Neuroscience, 8*, 4049–4068.

Shatz, C.J., Chun, J.J.M., & Luskin, M.B. (1988). The role of the subplate in the development of the mammalian telencephalon. In A. Peters & E.G. Jones (Eds.), *Cerebral cortex* (pp. 35–58). New York: Plenum.

Sperry, R.W. (1974). Lateral specialization in the surgically separated hemispheres. In F.O. Schmitt & F.G. Worden (Eds.), *The neurosciences third study program* (pp. 5–19). Cambridge, MA: MIT Press.

Sperry, R. (1982). Some effects of disconnecting the cerebral hemispheres. *Science, 217,* 1223–1226.

Toyama, K., & Matsunami, K. (1976). Convergence of specific visual and commissural impulses upon inhibitory interneurons in cat's visual cortex. *Neuroscience, 1,* 107–112.

Toyama, K., Matsunami, K., Ohno, T., & Tokashiki, S. (1974). An intracellular study of neuronal organization in the visual cortex. *Experimental Brain Research, 21,* 45–66.

von Bonin & Bailey. (1941). *The neocortex of the* macaca mulatta. Urbana: University of Illinois Press.

Walker, A.E. (1940). A cytoarchitectural study of the prefrontal area of the macaque monkey. *Journal of Comparative Neurology, 73,* 59–86.

Wilson, D.H., Culver, C., Waddington, M., & Gazzaniga, M. (1975). Disconnection of the cerebral hemispheres: An alternative to hemispherectomy for the control of intractable seizures. *Neurology, 25,* 1149–1153.

Wise, S.P., & Jones, E.G. (1978). Developmental studies of thalamocortical and commissural connections in the rat somatic sensory cortex. *Journal of Comparative Neurology, 178,* 187–208.

Development of the Prefrontal Cortex: Evolution, Neurobiology, and Behavior
edited by Norman A. Krasnegor, Ph.D., G. Reid Lyon, Ph.D.,
and Patricia S. Goldman-Rakic, Ph.D.
copyright © 1997   Paul H. Brookes Publishing Co., Inc.
Baltimore • London • Toronto • Sydney

4

Developmental Anatomy
of Prefrontal Cortex

Peter R. Huttenlocher
and Arun S. Dabholkar

This chapter considers aspects of the anatomy of prefrontal cortex that are of potential relevance to the function of this cortical region. This is not an easy task, because cortical anatomy per se reveals little concerning cortical function. Areas of cortex with widely different functions have the same basic microstructure, as pointed out by Rockel, Hiorns, and Powell (1980). Exceptions to the basic uniformity of the neocortex are few; they include the calcarine cortex, with its prominent fourth layer and line of Gennari, related to geniculocortical inputs; and the precentral gyrus, with uniquely large pyramidal cells in the fifth layer, related to its specific efferent system, the corticospinal tract. The prefrontal cortex is one of the vast cortical regions without specific anatomical markers, although its prominent granular Layer IV makes it recognizable as a region that is specified for associative or sensory rather than motor functions.

Essentially, all regions of the cerebral cortex consist of vertically arranged repeating units of identical structure. A good example is provided by the ocular dominance columns of the visual cortex (Hubel, Wiesel, & LeVay, 1977). Functional specificity of these units appears to be imparted by differences in connections, including afferent input from sense organs or from other cortical regions, rather than by differences in the intrinsic architecture. Different inputs, in turn, appear to lead to differences in intrinsic synaptic organization that are not visualized by histological methods.

Development represents an exception in that correlations between cortical anatomy and cortical function can be discerned in the immature animal and human. Certain anatomical structures, especially dendritic arbors and synaptic contacts, must be present before functional development can proceed. The timing of

---

This chapter was supported by Grant 5RO1 NS28726 from the U.S. Public Health Service, National Institutes of Health, U.S. Department of Health and Human Services.

these developmental events therefore provides information concerning the minimal age of onset of function in a given neural system. As discussed later, the developmental anatomy of the cerebral cortex may also provide information concerning the age during which the system has increased plasticity or ability to reorganize itself in response to injury or to input from sensory systems or from other cortical regions.

Development of the cerebral cortex proceeds through several temporally distinct stages. The earliest is the migration of postmitotic primitive neurons from the subependymal zone to the cortical plate (Sidman & Rakic, 1973). This is followed by growth of axons and dendrites; myelination of axons; formation of synaptic contacts; and, finally, synaptic reorganization, which includes the loss or pruning of redundant connections.

This chapter focuses on synaptogenesis and synapse elimination in human prefrontal cortex and also summarizes some relevant observations by others on myelination and dendritic development to round out the picture. Findings in humans show important similarities with, but also differences from, the developmental patterns in subhuman primates, which are summarized in Chapter 2.

EARLY OBSERVATIONS ON SYNAPTOGENESIS AND SYNAPSE ELIMINATION IN HUMAN PREFRONTAL CORTEX

Our first observations on synaptogenesis and synapse elimination in developing human cerebral cortex were made in the 1970s in Layer III of the middle frontal gyrus (MFG), a gyrus in the prefrontal cortex (Huttenlocher, 1979). This study was carried out to obtain normative data on synaptogenesis to be used for comparison with brains from people with mental retardation. The expectation was that, with growth of the cerebral cortex, there would be an increase in synaptic contacts and that synapse number and density would be highest in the mature (adult) state. Surprisingly, a plot of synaptic density versus age showed a complex biphasic curve: net synaptogenesis during infancy, up to about age 1 year; followed by a plateau between the ages of 1 and at least 7 years, during which synaptic density is significantly above the adult level; followed by a decrease in synaptic density some time between late childhood and adolescence (Figure 4.1). Adult synaptic density is about 60% of that of the peak in early childhood.

The study also included measurement of neuronal density in the same cortical region. From the synaptic and neuronal density values, it was possible to calculate the approximate mean number of synapses per neuron in Layer III of the MFG. This value reaches a maximum of about 100,000 synapses per neuron at about 1 year of age, which is maintained between ages 1 and 7 years. The mean number of synapses per neuron subsequently decreases to about 80,000 in the young adult, indicating significant pruning of synapses on individual neurons.

The findings were unexpected in two ways: 1) they suggested rather massive synaptic loss during normal development of the cerebral cortex, and 2) they showed that major changes in the anatomy of the cerebral cortex occur remarkably late, at ages when its anatomical development had been thought to be complete, with the exception of myelination, which was known to continue in some systems even in the young adult (Yakovlev & LeCours, 1967).

The importance of regressive events during nervous system development has been demonstrated in many systems. It has been found that synapse elimination

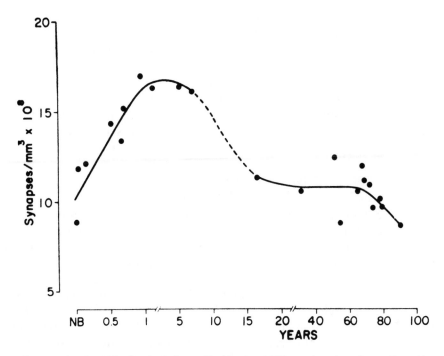

Figure 4.1.   Synaptic density in Layer III of human MFG as a function of age. (From Hutten-locher, P.R. [1979]. Synaptic density in human frontal cortex: Developmental changes and effects of aging. *Brain Research, 163,* 199; reprinted by permission.)

occurs universally during development, including in simple systems such as the neuromuscular junction (Brown, Jansen, & Van Essen, 1976). Pruning of dendrites, loss of dendritic spines and axons, and programmed neuronal death have also been described as important aspects of normal development (Cowan, 1973; Innocenti, 1981; LaMantia & Rakic, 1990; Michel & Garey, 1984; Rakic & Riley, 1983). Some information on these aspects of development in human prefrontal cortex is available (Mrzljak, Uylings, Van Eden, & Judas, 1990).

SYNAPTOGENESIS IN SUBHUMAN PRIMATES

Synaptogenesis and synapse elimination have been studied extensively in the cerebral cortex of subhuman primates (Bourgeois, Goldman-Rakic, & Rakic, 1994; O'Kusky & Colonnier, 1982; Rakic, Bourgeois, Eckenhoff, Zecevic, & Goldman-Rakic, 1986; Rakic, Bourgeois, & Goldman-Rakic, 1994; see also Chapter 2). Synapse formation in the rhesus monkey fetus begins at approximately embryonic day 50 (E50), when synapses appear in the marginal zone (later Layer I of the cerebral cortex) and in the region immediately below the cortical plate (the subplate zone). Synapses first appear in the cortical plate itself at about E65. Synaptic density increases until about postnatal age 2 months, stays at a high plateau until puberty, and then declines to an adult value that is about 60% of the maximum. Synapse elimination is of about the same magnitude as in humans.

Multiple cortical regions have been studied by Rakic, Goldman-Rakic, and associates (Rakic et al., 1986, 1994). This work made it possible to compare developmental events in different cortical regions. A novel and interesting finding of theirs is that, in monkey cerebral cortex, synaptogenesis is concurrent in all cortical areas, including the prefrontal area. This finding suggests that all of the cerebral cortex may respond simultaneously to a general signal that promotes synaptogenesis.

Concurrent synaptogenesis has a startling implication. It has long been assumed that the development of synaptic contacts is linked to the onset of function in a neural system. If so, concurrent synaptogenesis implies that, in the rhesus monkey, all cortical systems become functional approximately simultaneously. Previously, a hierarchical pattern of development, with sensory and motor areas preceding association areas, had generally been assumed (Greenfield, 1991).

SYNAPTOGENESIS AND DEVELOPMENT
OF CORTICAL FUNCTION IN THE HUMAN INFANT

In humans, the demonstration of concurrent synaptogenesis would imply discordance between synaptogenesis and functional development because the functions subserved by some cortical regions are known to develop at different times than those subserved by other cortical regions and at very different rates. For example, basic functions of the visual cortex emerge rapidly between ages 2 and 4 months, as determined by the appearance of binocular interactions such as stereopsis and stereoacuity (Held, Birch, & Gwiazda, 1980; Teller, 1983; Wilson, 1988). Fairly extensive data have been gathered on synaptogenesis in the human visual cortex, for correlation with functional development (Huttenlocher & de Courten, 1987; Huttenlocher, de Courten, Garey, & Van der Loos, 1982). In the visual cortex, emergence of basic functions appears to coincide with the age at which synaptic density increases very rapidly and approaches the maximum value. Synaptic development in this cortical region, as elsewhere, has its onset in the fetus but accelerates markedly between ages 2½ and 4 months. Wilson (1988) found an almost perfect superimposition of this burst of synaptogenesis on the time course of development of stereopsis, which is known to depend on the integrative function of the visual cortex.

The visual cortex is unusual in that its basic functions develop very rapidly over a short period of time, during the first few postnatal months. Functions of the motor cortex develop more slowly, maximally between ages 3 and 12 months, when basic voluntary motor functions such as reaching, sitting, and walking emerge. Emergence of language is slower still, as well as later in occurrence (late in the first and in the second year of life). If synaptogenesis and functional development were linked, one would see maximum synaptogenesis in language areas late in the first year or early in the second. Some data relevant to this point are presented later in this section.

Less is known about the onset of function in the human prefrontal cortex. Performance on delayed response tasks, thought to represent one of the most basic functions mediated by the prefrontal cortex in nonhuman primates, emerges near the end of the first year of life in humans, with progressively increasing competence between ages 7½ and 12 months (Diamond, 1985; Diamond & Goldman-Rakic, 1989). If we assume that these delayed response tasks have a similar cortical representation in humans as in nonhuman primates, then it follows that the human prefrontal cortex develops some functional capacity during the latter part of the first year of life. Other functions thought to be mediated by the prefrontal cortex—often referred to as *executive functions*, which include abstract reasoning, achievement motivation, and judgment—appear to develop slowly during child-hood and into adolescence (Sternberg & Powell, 1983). The complexity of these functions, disagreement about definitions and testing, and large individual differ-ences make it difficult to assign specific ages to their development. If synaptogene-sis and functional development were linked, one would expect later and more grad-ual synaptogenesis in the prefrontal cortex than, for example, in the calcarine cortex.

Data from our laboratory suggest that this may be the case and that synaptic development in the human neocortex may not be totally concurrent, as has been found in subhuman primates. We are presently engaged in a study of synaptic de-velopment in multiple cortical regions in the human brain. Sufficient areas have been analyzed at sufficient ages for some comparisons between cortical regions. Figure 4.2 compares synaptic density data in Layer II of the anterior MFG, Broca's motor speech area, and the visual and primary auditory cortices (Heschl's gyrus) at different ages. At 28 weeks' gestational age, synaptic density is low in all four corti-cal regions and lowest in the prefrontal cortex, where it is less than 20% of that in the auditory cortex. Synaptic density continues to be lower in the MFG at term and at ages 3 and 14 months. By 3 years of age, the prefrontal cortex has caught up to the primary sensory regions. Broca's motor speech area, usually considered part of the prefrontal cortex, appears to follow a developmental time course similar to that of the MFG. Table 4.1 shows data on synaptic density in the auditory cortex, the MFG, and Broca's motor speech area in tabular form, including the standard error of the mean of four counts in the same cortical region. All counts were carried out

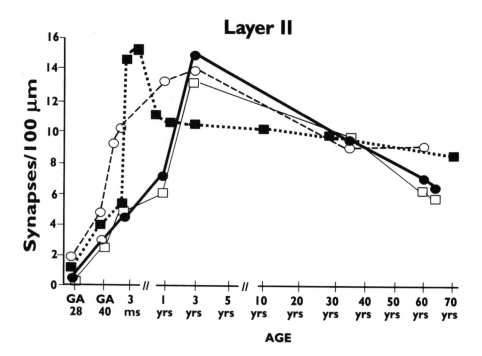

Figure 4.2.   Comparison of synaptic development in four regions of human neocortex: Primary vi-sual, auditory, motor speech, and MFG. (GA, gestational age; O- - -O, Heschl's gyrus; ■- - - -■, cal-carine cortex; □——□, middle frontal gyrus; ●——●, Broca's area.)

Table 4.1. Synaptic density in three areas of Layer II[a]

Area		Age at sampling					
	GA 26 weeks	GA 40 weeks	3 months	14 months	3 years	32 years	59 years
Left Heschl	2.3 (0.1)[b]	5.2 (0.9)	10.0 (0.5)	13.3 (1.2)	13.9 (1.6)	8.5 (0.3)	8.2 (0.4)
Left MFG	0.4 (0.2)	3.2 (0.4)	7.0 (0.5)	6.4 (0.5)	12.8 (1.5)	5.8 (1.0)	5.8 (1.0)
Left Broca	1.0 (0.5)	3.2 (0.3)	5.0 (0.5)	7.7 (1.0)	16.1 (1.0)	7.2 (0.5)	7.2 (0.5)

[a]Synaptic density, in synapses per 100 μm^2, in sections approximately 0.075 μm in thickness.
[b]Numbers in parentheses indicate 1 standard error of the mean of four determinations in the same cortical area.

blind as to the age and cortical location of the samples. They were made on electron microscopy prints from tissue prepared by the phosphotungstic acid method of Bloom and Aghajanian (1968), which stains synaptic profiles selectively (Figure 4.3). This method lends itself well to studies of human postmortem brain tissue because it stains perisynaptic proteins that are very resistant to autolysis. The method does, however, require fresh (unfixed) tissue; and availability of tissue, especially for the age span from late infancy to the adult, is very limited.

We do not have data for the later childhood years in this study. Some data in later childhood are available from our earlier work on Layer III of the MFG and on the visual cortex (Figure 4.4). The figure shows that maximum synaptic density is reached later in the MFG than in area 17, similar to our more recent data, and that synapse elimination also occurs later in the MFG.

In general, both acquisition of synapses and synapse elimination seem to proceed more slowly in the prefrontal cortex and in the motor speech area than in the primary sensory cortex. In other words, synaptogenesis in these cortical regions differs in the direction that would have been predicted if synaptic development and functional development were linked. Function appears to emerge at the time when synaptic density approaches the maximum, at about age 4 months in the visual cortex and at about age 12 months in the frontal cortex. However, it is also clear that functional development progresses long after maximum synaptic density has been reached. These later phases of development probably depend on utilization and rearrangement of existing synaptic contacts rather than on net increase in synapse number. The decline in synaptic density and number that occurs late in childhood may also be of functional significance. It may improve the efficiency of cortical information processing by elimination of synapses that are of no functional significance (Changeux & Danchin, 1976; Changeux, Heidmann, & Patte, 1984).

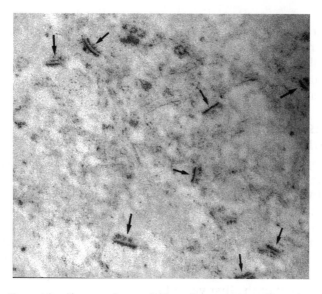

Figure 4.3.   Electron micrograph illustrating synaptic profiles in human cerebral cortex as demonstrated by the phosphotungstic acid method. (Bloom & Aghajanian, 1968; →, synaptic profiles; magnification = ×30,000.)

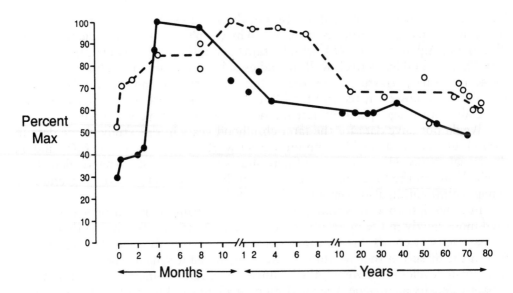

Figure 4.4. Plot of synaptic density as percentage of maximum in visual cortex (solid line) and in MFG (dashed line). (The higher synaptic density in the MFG at birth is related to differences in the mode of data expression in the two studies. The data in the MFG represent synaptic density in neuropil that excludes cell bodies, empty spaces, and blood vessels, whereas the density values in the visual cortex refer to the cortex as a whole. Results of these two methods are most discrepant in the immature brain, where cell bodies, empty spaces, and blood vessels are very numerous, leading to significantly larger differences between the volume of neuropil and that of the cortex as a whole than in the mature state, and to considerably higher synaptic density values for neuropil than for whole cortex.) (From Huttenlocher, P.R. [1994]. Synaptogenesis, synapse elimination, and neural plasticity in human cerebral cortex. In C.A. Nelson [Ed.], *Threats to optimal development: Integrating biological, psychological, and social risk factors* [Minnesota Symposia on Child Psychology, Vol. 27, p. 40]. Hillsdale, NJ: Lawrence Erlbaum Associates; reprinted by permission.)

Although there are regional differences, as outlined, similarities in synaptic development over cortical regions are observed as well. Overproduction of synapses occurs in all cortical areas examined. Layer-specific differences in synaptic density are similar in all cortical regions, as also found in monkey cortex by Bourgeois et al. (1994). Synaptic density is lowest in Layer I and highest in Layers II and III. These differences are already present at term.

REGIONAL DIFFERENCES IN
DENDRITIC DEVELOPMENT AND IN MYELINATION

Data on developmental events other than synaptogenesis confirm that the prefrontal cortex in humans is a late-developing system. With regard to myelination of the subcortical white matter, the earlier observational data on myelination in postmortem brain tissue by Yakovlev and LeCours (1967) have more recently been supplemented with data from imaging studies, especially magnetic resonance imaging (MRI). Myelination of the subcortical white matter as demonstrated by light microscopy begins near term in central regions. It spreads from there posteriorly, most rapidly in the visual radiations, and later anteriorly, reaching prefrontal regions latest, in the second half of the first year of life.

Modern imaging techniques now allow us to view these events in the clinic on an almost routine basis. Several monographs provide data on myelination of the subcortical white matter (Barkovich, 1990; Salamon, 1990; Wolpar & Barnes, 1992).

Magnetic resonance imaging shows the same progression of myelination as the histological method. Myelination of the prefrontal white matter occurs last and appears to be complete around age 1 year at the level of resolution provided by routine MRI. However, subtle differences between cortical regions, persisting beyond this age, would not be demonstrable by this method. Myelination in some fiber tracts, such as the corpus callosum, has been reported to continue into the adult years (Pujol, Vendrell, Junque, Marti-Vilalta, & Capdvila, 1993). Although the relationship of myelination to function remains controversial, evidence from the study of infants with delayed myelination shows an excellent correlation between myelination delay and neurodevelopmental lag (Van der Knaap et al., 1991). It is likely that delayed myelination is a marker for more global developmental delay, involving cortical maturation, that is not demonstrable by presently available imaging techniques.

Dendritic development, as determined by the Golgi method, also occurs later in the prefrontal cortex than in other cortical regions. The most extensive data comparing cortical regions in humans have been published by Conel (1939–1963). They show later development of dendritic branches on cortical pyramidal neurons in the prefrontal cortex than in more posterior neocortical areas (Figure 4.5). The left-hand panels of the figure present drawings from Golgi-Cox–stained sections in the anterior MFG. The right-hand panels present such drawings from sections in the superior temporal gyrus in the region of the primary auditory cortex. At birth (Figure 4.5A), dendritic development of cortical neurons in the MFG is quite immature, especially in the smaller pyramidal cells, which as yet have only a few, very short basal dendritic branches and no branches arising from apical dendrites. There

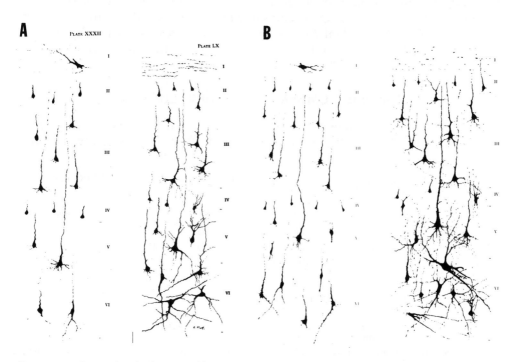

Figure 4.5.   Camera lucida drawings of human cerebral cortex: (A) at birth; (B) at age 1 month. (Left panel, MFG; right panel, superior temporal gyrus.) (From THE POSTNATAL DEVELOPMENT OF THE HUMAN CEREBRAL CORTEX Vols. I & II, by J.L. Conel. Copyright © 1939, 1941 by the President and Fellows of Harvard College, © 1967, 1969 by Jesse LeRoy Conel. Reprinted by permission of Harvard University Press.)

is as yet a very limited substrate for synapse formation. The superior temporal gyrus near the auditory cortex appears more mature. These differences persist at age 1 month (Figure 4.5B) but are no longer evident at 3 months (not shown). In general, dendritic development advances quite remarkably between 1 and 3 months in all cortical regions. Beyond age 3 months, it is difficult to detect much change on mere inspection of Golgi-stained sections.

However, quantitative studies have shown dendritic growth to continue beyond this age and to maintain regional differences into late infancy. A quantitative study of dendritic development in human MFG by Schade and van Groenigen (1961) showed considerable further elongation of dendritic branches, even after age 2 years. This has been confirmed more recently by Mrzljak et al. (1990), who reported maturational changes in neurons of the prefrontal cortex until puberty. These changes include growth of dendrites, especially on Layer III pyramidal cells, and regressive changes, with loss of dendritic spines, especially on nonpyramidal cells (interneurons). Quantitative data on the primary visual cortex have been published by Becker, Armstrong, Chan, and Wood (1984). Data on the mean dendritic length of pyramidal neurons in Layers III and V for the two cortical areas are summarized in Table 4.2 for comparison. They show earlier dendritic growth in visual cortex pyramidal neurons, especially in Layer III, than in pyramidal neurons of the MFG. Differences between the MFG and the calcarine cortex are most marked at birth. Dendritic development appears to progress more rapidly in Layer V than in Layer III, especially in the MFG.

Anatomical data on the development of the cerebral cortex have been supplemented by data on the onset of cortical function as determined by positron emission tomography. The tomographic data show remarkable similarity to the anatomical findings. Regional cerebral glucose metabolism increases postnatally, and this increase occurs last in the prefrontal cortex, toward the end of the first year (Chugani & Phelps, 1986, 1990).

CHANGES IN NEURONAL NUMBER DURING DEVELOPMENT

Possible changes in the number of cortical neurons must be considered during the period of synaptogenesis, dendritic growth, and synapse elimination. In the MFG,

Table 4.2.   Mean dendritic length of cortical pyramidal neurons as measured in Golgi-stained sections at various ages

Area	Birth	6 months	24 months	7 years	Adult
MFG, Layer III[a]	203 (3)[c]	2,369 (35)	3,259 (48)	—[d]	6,836 (100)
Calc, Layer III[b]	950 (33)	1,150 (40)	2,900 (100)	2,400 (83)	—[d]
MFG, Layer V[a]	858 (11)	4,246 (56)	4,669 (62)	—	7,558 (100)
Calc, Layer V[b]	1,250 (42)	2,100 (70)	2,800 (93)	3,000 (100)	—

[a]Data for the MFG are from Schade and van Groenigen (1961).

[b]Data for the calcarine cortex (Calc) are from Becker et al. (1984, Figure 3A–3D). Approximate values for apical dendrites (Becker et al., 1984, Figure 3A, 3B) have been added to values for basal dendrites (Becker et al., 1984, Figure 3C, 3D) for estimates of total dendritic length.

[c]Dendritic length values are in micrometers. Numbers in parentheses indicate percentage of dendritic length at maximum.

[d]Age 7 years was the oldest age examined, and adult data were not available in the study of Becker et al. (1984).

there are no data on such changes. An estimate of total cell number in the MFG is not possible because the anatomical boundaries of this gyrus are indefinite and highly variable from one brain to another. It is unlikely that neuronal number increases past 28 weeks' gestational age because neuronal migration in the neocortex appears to be completed considerably before that age (Sidman & Rakic, 1973). The other possibility that must be considered is the occurrence of neuronal loss through programmed cell death. However, as of 1997, there is no convincing evidence that programmed neuronal death occurs during the development of human neocortex after 26 weeks' embryonic age. Data necessary for calculation of total cell number at various ages are available for the human visual cortex (area 17). Cell counts from Leuba and Garey (1987) were combined with data on volume of the calcarine cortex from Huttenlocher and de Courten (1987), from the same brains that were also analyzed for synaptic density (Huttenlocher, 1990). The estimates of total neuronal number in the calcarine cortex derived from these data fail to show loss of visual cortical neurons between the fetus of 28 weeks' gestational age and the adult. In a more recent publication that includes a larger number of cases, Leuba and Krafsik (1994) found considerable variability in total neuronal number in area 17, but this variability does not appear to be age related. Because of this large normal variability in neuron number, significant programmed cell death could go undetected in the relatively small sample of cases studied. The question of the occurrence and extent of programmed cell death in the human cerebral cortex therefore is unresolved at present.

Available data suggest that programmed cell death may be most significant in simple systems, such as spinal motor neurons, where specific targets for innervation (i.e. myocytes) must be found. Failure to find a target may lead to neuronal death. Target finding may not be a problem in the cerebral cortex, where innumerable targets on neighboring neurons and their dendrites are available. Synapse elimination, in contrast, appears to become more important with increasing complexity of the system (Huttenlocher, 1990).

FUNCTIONAL SIGNIFICANCE OF EXUBERANT SYNAPTOGENESIS

Exuberant synaptogenesis appears to occur widely during development of neural structures. Its functional significance is unknown but invites speculation. A coherent hypothesis has been proposed by Changeux (Changeux & Danchin, 1976; Changeux et al., 1984): Synapse formation may to a large extent be a random process, with synaptic contacts made wherever there is a point of contact of neurites. Random formation of synapses appears likely because the immense number of contacts that are made tends to exclude genetic determination of individual synapses. It is now known that the intrinsic programs for generation of synapses are already present in the cell membranes of developing neurites prior to cell–cell contact. This includes the mechanism for secretion of specific neurotransmitters and the presence of neurotransmitter receptors. Contact between neurites may lead to formation of functional synapses within minutes (Haydon & Drapeau, 1995). Synaptogenesis therefore appears to be closely linked to the growth of axons and dendrites and to random contacts between neurites that share secretory machinery and receptors for the same neurotransmitters.

What evidence is available suggests that the initial burst of synapse formation is determined by intrinsic developmental programs not under environmental influence. Preterm exposure to light, for example, has no effect on the time course of synaptogenesis in the visual cortex (Bourgeois, Jastreboff, & Rakic, 1989). The presence of numerous synaptic contacts, in turn, forms the substrate for the development of functioning neuronal circuits. Changeux and Danchin (1976) postulated that synapses that become incorporated into functioning systems persist, whereas those that are not utilized disappear. This process is referred to as functional validation or functional stabilization. According to this concept, functional development should promote synapse elimination, and we should see a decline in synaptic density of a cortical area as functional circuits form.

Contrary to synapse formation, which is likely to be to a large extent a random process and not environmentally determined, the development of functionally significant neural circuits is likely to depend on input to the system—sensory stimulation and input from other cortical areas. The shaping of connections that occurs during the emergence of function is thought to be dependent on environmental input. An elegant example of these general principles is provided in the development of geniculocalcarine connections in the visual cortex. Initial synaptic connections are diffuse from both eyes. These connections are formed prior to light exposure. Subsequently, after the visual experience that occurs after birth, there is selective elimination of synapses such that areas of input from one eye alternate with those of input from the other eye, the so-called ocular dominance columns. Formation of the ocular dominance columns in turn can be modified by alterations in visual input such as is provided by exclusion of formed images from one eye (Goodman & Shatz, 1993; Wiesel, 1982). Much less is known about environmental influences in synapse formation in other systems. However, it seems likely that developmental events in other cortical regions resemble those in the visual cortex. For example, by age 1 or 2 years, the synaptic substrate for language development is likely to be present in the speech areas of the brain, to an approximately equal extent in all normal brains. The specific type of language that develops and its complexity—and, presumably, the specific synapses that become stabilized and those that are resorbed—are in turn influenced by environmental input during the subsequent years.

The capacity of the system for molding in response to environmental input is often referred to as plasticity. The anatomical data provide some indication as to the ages at which plasticity is apt to be greatest. The brain is likely to be most malleable during the years when synaptic density is highest, that is, when large numbers of synapses not yet specified for functions are available. This period is likely to extend at least into late childhood in the prefrontal cortex. In the visual cortex, the period of plasticity appears to be shorter, ending near age 5 years (Huttenlocher & de Courten, 1987). It is at about that age that strabismic amblyopia is no longer preventable by patching of the dominant eye, suggesting loss of plasticity related to visual input (Assaf, 1982; VonNoorden & Crawford, 1979).

CONCLUSIONS

In the human prefrontal cortex, as in other neocortical regions, synaptic development extends over a long period of time, from the fetal period to late childhood. Three stages can be discerned. The first is that of synapse formation, which begins in the fetus and accelerates postnatally. Maximum synaptic density in the MFG is reached at about age 1 year. Dendritic growth and myelination of the subcortical white matter occur at about the same time as rapid synaptogenesis, during the latter part of the first postnatal year. The second stage of synaptic development is one of exuberant synaptic connections, during which synaptic density is about 40% above the adult value. This stage extends from age 1 to at least age 7 years. Finally, net synapse elimination occurs during either late childhood, adolescence, or both.

Correlation of synaptic density data with data on the onset of cortical functions suggests that the first functions of a cortical region appear during the phase of rapid increase in synaptic density and that considerable competence at basic region-specific tasks exists by the time maximum synaptic density is reached. However, more complex functions in the same cortical areas continue to emerge long after synaptic density reaches its maximum. The anatomical data from the prefrontal cortex suggest that onset of function should occur postnatally, probably late in the first year of life. This fits very well with the time course of development of competence at tasks that are thought to depend on the prefrontal cortex, such as Piaget's "A not B" task, which is mastered by the infant by about age 12 months.

The period from age 1 year to adolescence, during which synaptic density is high, is likely to be one of increased functional plasticity. This is the time during which prefrontal lobe functions that are shaped by the environment, often referred to as executive functions, are refined.

Comparison of developmental events in the human prefrontal cortex with those in the primary sensory cortex suggests that the prefrontal cortex develops more slowly than the sensory cortex. Maximum synaptic density is reached at about 12 months in the prefrontal cortex, approximately 8 months later than in the visual and auditory cortices. The data best fit a hierarchical model of development, although there is considerable overlap. At no age examined were synapses totally absent in the MFG and present in primary sensory regions. Differences were quantitative and extended over the period from 27 weeks' embryonic age to 1 year after birth. By age 3½ years, there was no difference between cortical regions. Synapse elimination also appears to begin later in the MFG than in primary sensory (visual) areas. Data on this point are as yet very limited.

Developmental events in the neocortex in humans appear to differ somewhat from those in the rhesus monkey, in which synaptogenesis is concurrent in all cortical regions. The entire time course of synaptogenesis is much more compressed in the monkey, with synapse formation occurring over a period of only about 4 months versus more than 12 months in humans. Synaptogenesis in monkeys also occurs earlier and is already quite advanced at birth. However, differences in developmental timing between monkeys and humans should not obscure the fact that there are remarkable similarities—in the degree of exuberant synaptogenesis, in the absolute synaptic density in the child and in the adult, and in layer-specific differences in synaptic density. The much more extensive studies on synaptogenesis that are possible in monkeys therefore are of great relevance to our understanding of developmental events in the human cerebral cortex and form an important basis for comparison.

REFERENCES

Assaf, A.A. (1982). The sensitive period: Transfer of fixation after occlusion for strabismic amblyopia. *British Journal of Ophthalmology, 66,* 64–70.

Barkovich, A.J. (1990). Normal development of the neonatal and infant brain. In A.J. Barkovich (Ed.), *Pediatric neuroimaging* (pp. 5–34). New York: Raven Press.

Becker, L.E., Armstrong, D.L., Chan, F., & Wood, M.M. (1984). Dendritic development in human occipital cortical neurons. *Developmental Brain Research, 13,* 117–124.

Bloom, F.E., & Aghajanian, G.K. (1968). Fine structural and cytochemical analysis of the staining of synaptic junctions with phosphotungstic acid. *Journal of Ultrastructural Research, 22,* 361–375.

Bourgeois, J.-P., Goldman-Rakic, P.S., & Rakic, P. (1994). Synaptogenesis in the prefrontal cortex of rhesus monkeys. *Cerebral Cortex, 4,* 78–96.

Bourgeois, J.-P., Jastreboff, P., & Rakic, P. (1989). Synaptogenesis in the visual cortex of normal and preterm monkeys: Evidence for intrinsic regulation of synaptic overproduction. *Proceedings of the National Academy of Sciences of the United States of America, 86,* 4297–4301.

Brown, M.C., Jansen, J.K.S., & Van Essen, D. (1976). Polyneuronal innervation of skeletal muscle in new-born rats and its elimination during maturation. *Journal of Physiology, 261,* 387–422.

Changeux, J.-P., & Danchin, A. (1976). Selective stabilization of developing synapses as a mechanism for the specification of neuronal networks. *Nature, 264,* 705–712.

Changeux, J.-P., Heidmann, T., & Patte, P. (1984). Learning by selection. In P. Marler & H.S. Terrace (Eds.), *The biology of learning* (pp. 115–137). New York: Springer-Verlag.

Chugani, H.T., & Phelps, M.E. (1986). Maturational changes in cerebral function in infants determined by 18FDG positron emission tomography. *Science, 231,* 840–843.

Chugani, H.T., & Phelps, M.E. (1990). Imaging human brain development with positron emission tomography. *Journal of Nuclear Medicine, 32,* 23–25.

Conel, J. (1939–1963). *The postnatal development of the human cerebral cortex* (Vols. 1–6). Cambridge, MA: Harvard University Press.

Cowan, W.M. (1973). Neuronal death as a regulative mechanism in the control of cell number in the nervous system. In M. Rockstein (Ed.), *Development and aging in the nervous system* (pp. 19–41). New York: Academic Press.

Diamond, A. (1985). The development of the ability to use recall to guide action, as indicated by infants' performance on AB. *Child Development, 56,* 868–883.

Diamond, A., & Goldman-Rakic, P.S. (1989). Comparison of human infants and rhesus monkeys on Piaget's AB task: Evidence for dependence on dorsolateral prefrontal cortex. *Experimental Brain Research, 74,* 24–40.

Goodman, C.S., & Shatz, C.J. (1993). Developmental mechanisms that generate precise patterns of neural connectivity. *Neuron, 10,* 77–98.

Greenfield, P.M. (1991). Language, tools and brain: The ontogeny and phylogeny of hierarachically organized sequential behavior. *Behavioral Brain Science, 14,* 531–595.

Haydon, P.G., & Drapeau, P. (1995). From contact to connection: Early events during synaptogenesis. *Trends in Neuroscience, 18,* 196–201.

Held, R., Birch, E., & Gwiazda, J. (1980). Stereoacuity of human infants. *Proceedings of the National Academy of Sciences of the United States of America, 77,* 5572–5574.

Hubel, D.H., Wiesel, T.N., & LeVay, S. (1977). Plasticity of ocular dominance columns in the monkey striate cortex. *Philosophical Transactions of the Royal Society of London: Series B, Biological Sciences, 278,* 377–409.

Huttenlocher, P.R. (1979). Synaptic density in human frontal cortex: Developmental changes and effects of aging. *Brain Research, 163,* 195–205.

Huttenlocher, P.R. (1990). Morphometric study of human cerebral cortex development. *Neuropsychologia, 28,* 517–527.

Huttenlocher, P.R. (1994). Synaptogenesis, synapse elimination, and neural plasticity in human cerebral cortex. In C.A. Nelson (Ed.), *Threats to optimal development: Integrating, biological, psychological, and social risk factors* (Minnesota Symposia on Child Psychology, Vol. 27, pp. 35–54). Hillsdale, NJ: Lawrence Erlbaum Associates.

Huttenlocher, P.R., & de Courten, C. (1987). The development of synapses in striate cortex of man. *Human Neurobiology, 6,* 1–9.

Huttenlocher, P.R., de Courten, C., Garey, L.G., & Van der Loos, H. (1982). Synaptogenesis in human visual cortex: Evidence for synapse elimination during normal development. *Neuroscience Letters, 33,* 247–252.

Innocenti, G.M. (1981). Growth and reshaping of axons in the establishment of visual callosal connections. *Science, 212,* 824–827.

LaMantia, A.C., & Rakic, P. (1990). Axon overproduction and elimination in the corpus callosum of the developing rhesus monkey. *Journal of Neuroscience, 10,* 2156–2175.

Leuba, G., & Garey, L.J. (1987). Evolution of neuronal numerical density in the developing and aging human visual cortex. *Human Neurobiology, 6,* 11–18.

Leuba, G., & Krafsik, R. (1994). Changes in volume, surface estimate, three-dimensional shape and total number of neurons of the human primary visual cortex from midgestation until old age. *Anatomy and Embryology, 190,* 351–366.

Michel, A.E., & Garey, L.J. (1984). The development of dendritic spines in the human visual cortex. *Human Neurobiology, 3,* 223–227.

Mrzljak, L., Uylings, H.B.M., Van Eden, C.G., & Judas, M. (1990). Neuronal development in human prefrontal cortex in prenatal and postnatal stages. *Progress in Brain Research, 85,* 185–222.

O'Kusky, J., & Colonnier, M. (1982). Postnatal changes in the number of neurons and synapses in the visual cortex (A17) of the macaque monkey. *Journal of Comparative Neurology, 210,* 291–296.

Pujol, J., Vendrell, P., Junque, C., Marti-Vilalta, J.L., & Capdvila, A. (1993). When does human brain development end? Evidence of corpus callosum growth up to adulthood. *Annals of Neurology, 34,* 71–75.

Rakic, P., Bourgeois, J.-P., Eckenhoff, M.F., Zecevic, N., & Goldman-Rakic, P.S. (1986). Concurrent overproduction of synapses in diverse regions of the primate cerebral cortex. *Science, 232,* 232–235.

Rakic, P., Bourgeois, J.-P., & Goldman-Rakic, P.S. (1994). Synaptic development of the cerebral cortex: Implications for learning, memory and mental illness. *Progress in Brain Research, 102,* 227–243.

Rakic, P., & Riley, K.P. (1983). Overproduction and elimination of retinal axons in fetal rhesus monkey. *Science, 219,* 1441–1444.

Rockel, A.J., Hiorns, R.W., & Powell, T.P.S. (1980). The basic uniformity in structure of the neocortex. *Brain, 103,* 221–244.

Salamon, G. (1990). *Magnetic resonance imaging of the human brain: An anatomical atlas.* New York: Raven Press.

Schade, J.P., & van Groenigen, D.B. (1961). Structural organization of the human cerebral cortex. I. Maturation of the middle frontral gyrus. *Acta Anatomica, 47,* 74–111.

Sidman, R.L., & Rakic, P. (1973). Neuronal migration with special reference to developing human brain. *Brain Research, 62,* 1–35.

Sternberg, R.J., & Powell, J.S. (1983). The development of intelligence. In P.H. Mussen (Ed.), *Handbook of child psychology* (4th ed., pp. 341–419). New York: John Wiley & Sons.

Teller, D.Y. (1983). Scotopic vision, color vision and stereopsis in infants. *Current Eye Research, 2,* 199–210.

Van der Knaap, M.S., Valk, J., Bakker, C.J., Schooneveld, M., Faber, J.A.J., et al. (1991). Myelination as an expression of the functional maturity of the brain. *Developmental Medicine and Child Neurology, 33,* 849–857.

VonNoorden, G.K., & Crawford, M.L.J. (1979). The sensitive period. *Transactions of the Ophthalmological Society of the United Kingdom, 99,* 442–446.

Wiesel, T.N. (1982). Postnatal development of the visual cortex and the influence of environment. *Nature, 299,* 583–591.

Wilson, H.R. (1988). Development of spatiotemporal mechanisms in infant vision. *Vision Research, 28,* 611–628.

Wolpar, S.M., & Barnes, P.D. (1992). *MRI in pediatric neurosurgery.* St. Louis, MO: Mosby–Year Book.

Yakovlev, P.I., & LeCours, A.-R. (1967). The myelogenetic cycles of regional maturation of the brain. In A. Minkowsky (Ed.), *Regional development of the brain in early life* (pp. 3–70). Oxford, England: Blackwell Scientific Publications.

Development of the Prefrontal Cortex: Evolution, Neurobiology, and Behavior
edited by Norman A. Krasnegor, Ph.D., G. Reid Lyon, Ph.D.,
and Patricia S. Goldman-Rakic, Ph.D.
copyright © 1997   Paul H. Brookes Publishing Co., Inc.
Baltimore • London • Toronto • Sydney

5

Human Frontal Lobe Development

A Theory of Cyclical Cortical Reorganization

Robert W. Thatcher

In this chapter, a theory of frontal lobe development is presented in which the role of the human frontal lobes during normal development is explored. The theory is based on analyses of the development of human electroencephalographic (EEG) coherence that indicate that there are oscillations and cyclical growth processes that operate along the mediolateral and anterior–posterior planes of the human brain. The cycles of EEG coherence are interpreted as repetitive sequences of synaptic overproduction followed by synaptic pruning that reflect a convergence process that narrows the disparity between structure and function by slowly sculpting and reshaping the brain's microanatomy. This process is modeled as a developmental spiral staircase in which brain structures are periodically revisited, resulting in stepwise increases in differentiation and integration throughout the postnatal period. The frontal lobes play a crucial role in the theory because they are largely responsible for the selection and pruning of synaptic contacts throughout the postnatal period. From an integrated biological perspective, a mathematical predator–prey model of cycles of synaptic overproduction and pruning is presented in which the frontal lobes behave as gentle synaptic "predators," whereas posterior cortical regions behave as synaptic "prey" in a periodic reorganization process. Some of the neuropsychological consequences of frontal lobe development are discussed in the context of this theory.

This chapter was supported by Grant JFC36285006, from the Henry M. Jackson Foundation, R.W. Thatcher, Principal Investigator.

The author is indebted to Rebecca A. Walker for her assistance in the typing and construction of the chapter.

The cyclical cortical theory of frontal lobe development is also based upon a consideration of shared phylogenetic, embryological, and postnatal spatial gradients that operate on several biological levels. In the sections that follow, these gradients and their neurological representations are reviewed and integrated into a general biological model of human cerebral development.

SPATIOTEMPORAL GRADIENTS IN THE PHYLOGENETIC DEVELOPMENT OF THE FRONTAL LOBES

Human beings are distinguished from nonhuman primates not only by the phylogenetic recency and size of the frontal lobes but also by the temporal sequence and patterning of their development (Carpenter & Sutin, 1983; Sanides, 1971). In fact, among the most intriguing aspects of frontal lobe development are the parallels among its phylogenetic, embryological, and ontogenetic sequences (Thatcher, 1992b, 1994a). An especially intriguing parallel is the presence of mediolateral and anterior–posterior gradients that spatially guide the phylogenetic, embryological, and ontogenetic development of the frontal lobes (Bayer & Altman, 1991; Carpenter & Sutin, 1983; Smart, 1983; Thatcher, 1992b, 1994a). Intrinsic to the spatial gradients is a shared temporal gradient in which the lateral cortex develops before the medial cortex and the frontal cortex develops before the posterior cortex (Bayer & Altman, 1991; Carpenter & Sutin, 1983; Smart, 1983). Although these gradients have been observed in the EEG during the performance of cognitive tasks for many years (Lilly & Cherry, 1954, 1955; Linas & Ribary, 1992; Nunez, 1981; Rogers et al., 1991; Thatcher & John, 1977; Verzeano, 1972; Verzeano & Negishi, 1960, 1961), it is only since the late 1980s and early 1990s that these same spatial gradients have been observed in the ontogenesis of the human EEG (Hudspeth & Pribram, 1991; Thatcher, 1989, 1991, 1992b, 1994a; Thatcher, Walker, & Guidice, 1987).

SPATIOTEMPORAL GRADIENTS DURING PRENATAL BRAIN DEVELOPMENT

One of the wonders of human development is the process by which a few initial germinal cells so quickly develop into the human brain, which consists of more than 100 billion neurons. Given the large number of neurons that compose the infant brain, it has been estimated that, in utero, neurons are developing at a rate of more than 250,000 per minute (Cowan, 1979). This process is made even more remarkable by the fact that each germinal neuron must not only migrate to its terminal destination but also ultimately become connected to approximately 5,000–15,000 other neurons (Cragg, 1975). Research has shown that the development of the cortex in any mammalian species occurs in a distinct sequence (Cowan, 1979; Rakic, 1985): cell proliferation → cell migration → cell differentiation → dendritic and axonal growth → neuronal and synaptic death. Once the germinal cells migrate to their terminal location in the cortex, they next develop the characteristics of the cell type that they are to be (e.g., stellate, pyramidal); then they begin to grow their dendrites and axons and form synapses. Detailed studies of brain development have shown that, in most altricial mammals, such as rat, cat, monkey, and human, the stages of cell proliferation and migration are largely prenatal, and much of the development of the neuropil (i.e., axons and dendrites) and synaptic death occur during the postnatal period (Kolb, 1989).

SPATIAL GRADIENTS OF PRENATAL DEVELOPMENT

The appearance of prenatal spatial gradients of development is also remarkable (Diamond, Scheibel, & Elson, 1985). For example, shortly after conception, a ball of cells grows symmetrically without a clear left or right or an anterior or posterior plane. However, at the first differentiation, spatial polarization occurs in which a disk with an anterior and a posterior end and medial and lateral planes appears. The inner layer (i.e., the endoderm) differentiates to form the skeleton and gut, and the outer layer of the disk (i.e., the ectoderm) differentiates to form the skin and neural plate, from which the entire nervous system develops. Shortly after the formation of the neural plate (e.g., about 16 days postconception), an indentation appears along the midline that grows into a fold that becomes the neural groove. The neural groove becomes a hollow tube, with the inside of the anterior end of the tube eventually becoming the forebrain ventricles and the middle and posterior end becoming the spinal canal. The neural tube begins to close to form a roof in the center of the embryonic disk. Then, like two zippers moving in opposite directions, the roofing process continues in both an anterior and a posterior direction (Diamond et al., 1985). This process represents one of the first examples of the two dominant prenatal spatial gradients; that is, the embryonic anterior–posterior and mediolateral gradients.

CYCLES OF PRENATAL DEVELOPMENT

The emergence of one of the first "cyclical" processes that is embedded in the anterior–posterior and mediolateral gradients begins at approximately 23 days postconception. The cycle is illustrated in Figure 5.1, where the germinal neuroepithelium (A) of the neural tube is seen to lie between the lumen (F) and the outer limiting membrane (E^1). At about 23 days postconception, a cyclical spatial growth process occurs in which the neuroepithelial cells alternate in activity between cell division, or mitosis (A^1), and synthesis of the genetic material DNA (A^2). The spatial cycle is as follows: 1) the neuroepithelial cell near the lumen divides; 2) the nucleus of each newly formed daughter cell then moves laterally away from the lumen of the neural tube toward the outer limiting membrane; 3) the nucleus then undergoes DNA synthesis, or generation; and 4) the nucleus then moves medially back toward the lumen. To repeat the cycle, the cell then becomes mitotic again (Diamond et al., 1985). The cycle time of this spatial process is approximately 4–24 hours per cycle, and the process continues over a period of days until a large complement of neuroepithelial cells is produced, after which differentiation of the neuroepithelial cells to neuroblasts (G) begins. The neuroblasts migrate laterally away from the lumen to form a new, outer mantle layer (C), which becomes the gray matter of the brain and spinal cord. As the neuroblasts differentiate into mature neurons, their axons form the marginal layer (D), which becomes the white matter of the brain and spinal cord. As with the earlier stages of embryogenesis, the precise timing of the development and migration of cells to different cortical regions occurs along mediolateral and anterior–posterior spatial gradients. Figure 5.2 shows the standard neuroanatomy textbook view of early human embryogenesis, in which migration to the frontal and lateral cortical regions occurs before migration to the medial and posterior cortical areas. Detailed analyses of the operation of the anterior–posterior and mediolateral spatial gradients have also been provided for

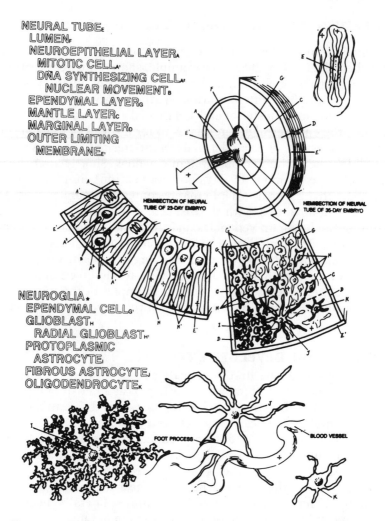

NEURAL TUBE_E
  LUMEN_F
  NEUROEPITHELIAL LAYER_A
    MITOTIC CELL_A'
    DNA SYNTHESIZING CELL_A²
    NUCLEAR MOVEMENT_B
  EPENDYMAL LAYER_G
  MANTLE LAYER_C
  MARGINAL LAYER_D
  OUTER LIMITING
    MEMBRANE_E'

HEMISECTION OF NEURAL
TUBE OF 23-DAY EMBRYO

HEMISECTION OF NEURAL
TUBE OF 35-DAY EMBRYO

NEUROGLIA_*
  EPENDYMAL CELL_G'
  GLIOBLAST_H
    RADIAL GLIOBLAST_H'
  PROTOPLASMIC
    ASTROCYTE_I
  FIBROUS ASTROCYTE_J
  OLIGODENDROCYTE_K

FOOT PROCESS   BLOOD VESSEL

Figure 5.1.   Diagram of a cross-section of the human neural tube of an embryo at 23 days and 35 days. Middle left is a hemisection of the neural tube at 23 days and middle right is a hemisection of the neural tube at 35 days. The emergence of one of the first "cyclical" processes that is embedded in the anterior–posterior and mediolateral gradients is illustrated where the germinal neuroepithelium (A) of the neural tube lies between the lumen (F) and the outer limiting membrane (E¹). At about 23 days postconception, a cyclical spatial growth process occurs in which the neuroepithelial cells alternate in activity between cell division, or mitosis (A¹), and synthesis of the genetic material DNA (A²). In the spatial cycle, the neuroepithelial cell near the lumen divides; then the nucleus of each newly formed daughter cell moves laterally away from the lumen of the neural tube toward the outer limiting membrane; and the nucleus then undergoes DNA synthesis, or generation; and, finally, the nucleus moves medially back toward the lumen. The cycle repeats every 4–24 hours. (From Diamond, M.C., Scheibel, A.B., & Elson, L.M. [1985]. *The human brain coloring book* [p. 3]. New York: HarperCollins; reprinted by permission.)

the embryogenesis of mouse brains (Smart, 1983) and rat brains (Bayer & Altman, 1991). All mammalian species appear to exhibit dominant embryological brain development gradients along the anterior–posterior and mediolateral spatial planes.

Because the embryological sequence of neural development is dependent on cell migration occurring first, it must be the case that the sequence of synapse for-

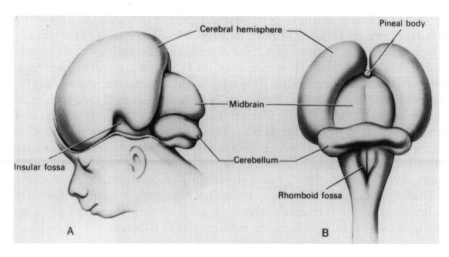

Figure 5.2.   Drawings of the cerebral vesicle and brainstem in a 12-week fetus: (A) lateral view; (B) posterior view. (From Carpenter, M.B., & Sutin, J. [1983]. *Human neuroanatomy* [p. 79]. Baltimore: Williams & Wilkins; reprinted by permission.)

mation followed by synaptic death is also influenced by anterior–posterior and mediolateral spatial gradients. Therefore, it is reasonable to suggest that the findings of a postnatal overproduction of synapses followed by pruning of synapses (Huttenlocher, 1984, 1990; O'Leary, 1987; O'Leary, Stanfield, & Cowan, 1981) also follow anterior–posterior and mediolateral spatial gradients. This is important, given the magnitude of these postnatal processes, in which there is an overproduction of synapses by as much as a factor of 2 (Rakic, Bourgeois, Eckenhoff, Zecevic, & Goldman-Rakic, 1986), with as much as 50% of the early synapses lost by adulthood (Huttenlocher, 1990). The importance of this process is underlined by suggestions that a failure of postnatal cell death or synaptic loss may lead to retardation (Kolb, 1989) or the emergence of other developmental disorders, such as schizophrenia (Feinberg, 1982).

SPATIOTEMPORAL GRADIENTS OF POSTNATAL BRAIN DEVELOPMENT

Because of the expense and difficulty of human anatomical studies, there is a paucity of detailed anatomical information about synaptic overproduction and pruning during human postnatal development. What work has been done has been accomplished largely by Huttenlocher and colleagues (Huttenlocher, 1979; Huttenlocher & deCourten, 1987; Huttenlocher, deCourten, Garey, & Van der Loos, 1982). These workers primarily studied the human visual and frontal cortex, although the age range and the sample sizes are limited. Their data show age-dependent discontinuities in synaptic density in which high synaptic densities are achieved at approximately ages 1 and 7 years for the visual and frontal cortices, respectively. At these ages, synaptic density is about twice that for adults. Unfortunately, the human neuroanatomical data are too sparse to observe mediolateral and anterior–posterior gradients of synaptic development.

In contrast to anatomical experiments, computerized EEG analyses of the development of the human cortex are noninvasive and less expensive, thus allowing for the use of large sample sizes and analyses over the entire human life span (Hudspeth & Pribram, 1990; Matousek & Petersen, 1973; Thatcher et al., 1987). These studies clearly show cyclical patterns of cortical development in which the different regions of the cortex develop at different rates and ages.[1] In the Thatcher et al. (1987) study, there were many examples of rapid and significant increments in EEG coherence that were characterized as growth spurts, and the timing and sequencing of the growth spurts exhibited a striking similarity to the timing and sequencing of power peaks in the Matousek and Petersen (1973) EEG data as analyzed by a number of people, including Epstein (1980), Fischer (1987), Hudspeth and Pribram (1990), and Thatcher (1980). It is important to note, however, that analyses of EEG coherence and phase have an advantage over power analyses because coherence is sensitive to the magnitude and existence of corticocortical connections (Lopez da Silva, Pijn, & Boeijinga, 1989; Nunez, 1981; Pascual-Marqui, Valdes-Sosa, & Alvarez-Amador, 1988; Thatcher, Krause, & Hrybyk, 1986; Tucker, Roth, & Blair, 1986). Although EEG relative power also exhibits spatiotemporal gradients, the next section only discusses the details of the development of human EEG coherence.

CORTICOCORTICAL CONNECTIONS
AND ELECTROENCEPHALOGRAPHIC COHERENCE

The Thatcher (1992b, 1994a) studies used measures of EEG coherence to estimate changes in the maturation of corticocortical connections; accordingly, a brief introduction to the mathematical and neurophysiological foundations of EEG coherence is necessary to provide a basis by which the conclusions of these studies can be understood. Coherence is mathematically analogous to a cross-correlation in the frequency domain. It is a measure of the degree of "phase synchrony" or "shared activity" between spatially separated generators (Bendat & Piersol, 1980; Glaser & Ruchkin, 1976; Otnes & Enochson, 1972). The application of coherence measures to the human scalp EEG have shown that EEG coherence reflects the coupling between neocortical neurons (Lopez da Silva et al., 1989; Nunez, 1981; Thatcher, McAlaster, Lester, Horst, & Cantor, 1983; Tucker et al., 1986). A "two-compartmental" model of EEG coherence was developed (Pascual-Marqui et al., 1988; Thatcher et al., 1986) based upon Braitenberg's (1978) two-compartment analysis of cortical axonal fiber systems in which compartment A is composed of the basal dendrites that receive input primarily from the axon collaterals from neighboring or "short-distance" pyramidal cells, and compartment B is composed of the apical dendrites of cortical pyramidal cells that receive input primarily from "long-distance" intracortical connections. The short-distance A system primarily involves local interactions on the order of millimeters to a few centimeters, whereas the long-distance B system involves long-range interactions on the order of several centimeters, which represent the majority of white matter fibers. These two systems exhibit two different network properties. System B, because of its reciprocal connections and invariant apical dendrite terminations, is involved in long-distance feedback, or loop systems. In contrast, system A, because of the variable depths of the basal dendrites, is in-

---

[1]This position is contrary to the "concurrent development" hypothesis of Rakic et al. (1986). However, that study and subsequent studies by Rakic's group (Bourgeois, Goldman-Rakic, & Rakic, 1994; Zecevic & Rakic, 1991) relied strongly on the assumptions of linear regression, which may have prevented observing oscillations in their own data. For example, significant nonlinear regression fits and strong Fourier components can be obtained by Fourier analysis and nonlinear regression of the published data in Rakic et al. (1986) and the other papers cited. An interesting aspect of the "concurrent" hypothesis is that it is all or none; that is, either cerebral development involves a single event or it involves multiple events, and, therefore, developmental oscillations do not support a concurrent hypothesis.

volved not in reciprocal loop processes, but rather in a diffusion type of transmission process (Braitenberg, 1978; Pascual-Marqui et al., 1988; Thatcher et al., 1986).

The following mathematical equation was developed to describe the magnitude and slope of decline of human EEG coherence with interelectrode distance (Thatcher et al., 1986):

$$\text{Coherence} = A_i e^{-kd} + B_i e^{kd} \sin kd, \tag{Eq. 5.1}$$

where A_i and B_i are amplitude parameters and k and d are parameters of frequency (in hertz) and scalp interelectrode distance (in centimeters), respectively. The first term on the right side of Equation 5.1 corresponds to the operation of the short-distance A system, and the second term corresponds to the operation of the long-distance B system.

Although the moment-to-moment changes in EEG coherence with interelectrode distance can be understood by Equation 5.1, changes in the development of coherence over long spans of time (i.e., months, years) requires additional considerations. One consideration is that developmental changes in EEG coherence in a large group of subjects reflect changes in the mean coupling constants between connected neuronal networks. For example, if we assume that volume conduction has been controlled, then we can postulate a relationship between EEG coherence and two primary factors: 1) the number of corticocortical connections between neural assemblies and 2) the synaptic strength of connections between neural assemblies. (The terms *corticocortical connections* and *intracortical connections* are considered synonymous.) This relationship is described in Equation 5.2:

$$\text{Coherence} = C_{ij} \times S_{ij}, \tag{Eq. 5.2}$$

where C_{ij} is a connection matrix of the number or density of connections between neural systems i and j, and S_{ij} is the synaptic strength of those connections. Equation 5.2 provides a logical means by which developmental changes in EEG coherence can be interpreted in terms of changes in the number and strength of connections between assemblies of neurons (Pascual-Marqui et al., 1988; Thatcher et al., 1986, 1987). For example, increased coherence is due to an increase in the number or strength of connections or both, and, conversely, decreased coherence is due to a decreased number or reduced strength of connections or both. The neurophysiological mechanisms responsible for the changes in the numbers or strengths of connections include axonal sprouting, synaptogenesis, myelination, expansion of existing synaptic terminals, pruning of synaptic connections, presynaptic changes in the amount of neurotransmitter, and changes in the postsynaptic response to a given neurotransmitter (see discussions by Purves, 1988; Huttenlocher, 1984). Currently, measures of EEG coherence cannot distinguish between these various possibilities.

CYCLES OF POSTNATAL DEVELOPMENT

In the Thatcher (1992b, 1994a) and Thatcher et al. (1987) studies, growth spurts were defined by peaks of velocity in mean EEG coherence or those postnatal ages at which there was a maximum increase in mean coherence as measured by the first derivative. The point of maximum increase in EEG coherence (i.e., peak velocity) was considered to reflect an increase in the number or strength or both of connections between two or more intracortical systems. As described by Thatcher (1992b, 1994a), only positive first derivative values were counted as growth spurts. This decision was based upon the fact that postnatal synaptogenesis often involves a sequence of overproduction of synapses followed by a pruning of synapses (Cowan, 1979; Huttenlocher 1984, 1990; O'Leary, 1987; O'Leary et al., 1981; Rakic et al., 1986). Accordingly, the positive first derivative peaks are expected to correspond to the overproduction phase, and the negative peaks are expected to correspond to the pruning phase.

Figure 5.3 shows the first derivatives or velocity curves of mean EEG coherence from subgroupings of electrode pairs from the Thatcher (1991, 1992b, 1994a) studies. The postnatal ages of the positive first derivatives are indicated by the arrows. Figure 5.4 is a summary of the ages and durations of peak first derivatives in mean EEG coherence that were shown in Figure 5.3. An iterative and sequential anatomical pattern of growth spurts was evident. For example, at age 1½ years, growth spurts were relatively localized (e.g., 6-cm interelectrode distances) and confined to the left parietal and left central to left lateral temporal regions. At age 2½ years, there was a lengthening along the anterior–posterior dimension (e.g., 12-cm interelectrode distances), with a lateral-to-medial rotation of parietal–frontal relations to include left parietal to left dorsomedial frontal regions (i.e., electrodes P3–F3 and T3–F1). At age 3 years, there was a further lengthening of intracortical relations along the anterior–posterior dimension (e.g., 18- to 24-cm interelectrode distances), with continued involvement of dorsomedial frontal to posterior cortex. This sequence of lengthening along the anterior–posterior dimension and rotation along the lateral-to-medial dimension between 1.5 and 3 years was repeated again between ages 5½ and 6½ years and finally again between 14½ and 15½ years and is referred to as "microcycles" of cortical development.

ANATOMICAL "GRADIENTS" OF DEVELOPMENT

Anatomical gradients are defined by one or more of the following factors: 1) they involve dominant spatial dimensions or anatomical axes of EEG coherence development, and 2) they exhibit developmental organizing properties. The dominant patterns of the developmental trajectories of EEG coherence over the period from ages 1½ to 16 years indicate three "gradients" of development from which emerge organizational structure. The gradients are 1) anterior–posterior, 2) mediolateral, and 3) left–right hemisphere.

Postnatal Anterior–Posterior Gradients of Development

An anterior–posterior gradient of development was evident by 1) a frontal-to-posterior dominance of corticocortical relations in both the left and the right hemispheres (Thatcher, 1991; Thatcher et al., 1987); and 2) a developmental sequence from short-distance anterior–posterior interelectrode combinations (e.g., P3–T3 or T5–C3) to longer distance anterior–posterior electrode combinations (e.g., P3–F7 or P3–F1) to even longer distance anterior–posterior electrode combinations (e.g., O1–F1). An example of the anterior–posterior gradient of EEG coherence development is shown in Figure 5.5 over ages 4 to 7½ years.

Postnatal Mediolateral Gradients of Development

A lateral-to-medial gradient of development was evident by 1) differential rates of development of the lateral (i.e., F7/8 and T3/4) as opposed to the dorsomedial frontal regions (F3/4 and C3/4) (see Figure 5.3, Factors 1 and 2); 2) a rotational sequence with a direction from lateral to medial in the left hemisphere and a direction from medial to lateral in the right hemisphere; 3) the fact that interhemi-

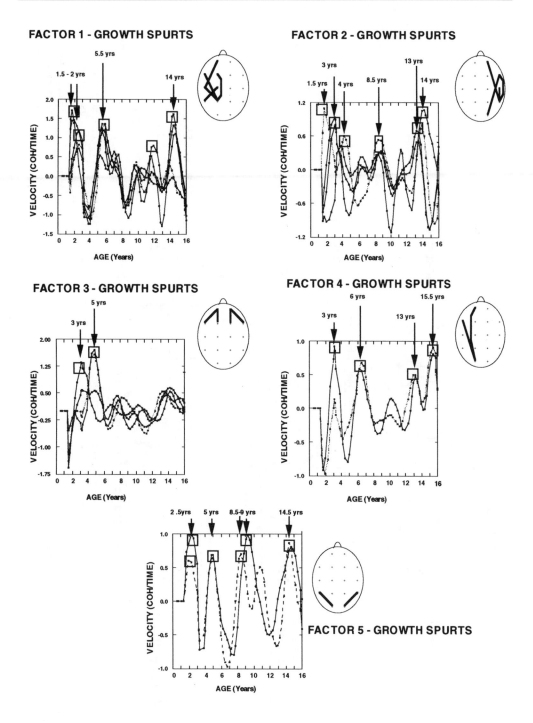

Figure 5.3.   The velocity curves or the first derivatives (change in mean coherence/change in time; Δ COH/Δ TIME) of the developmental trajectories of mean EEG coherence from the subgroupings of electrode pairs that had the highest factor loadings (e.g., > .80) (Thatcher, 1991). Growth spurts were defined by a positive peak in the first derivative (i.e., a postnatal time of maximum growth) in multiple interelectrode combinations. (From Thatcher, R.W. [1994a]. Cyclic cortical reorganization: Origins of cognition. In G. Dawson & K. Fischer [Eds.], *Human behavior and the developing brain* [p. 237]. New York: Guilford Press; reprinted by permission.).

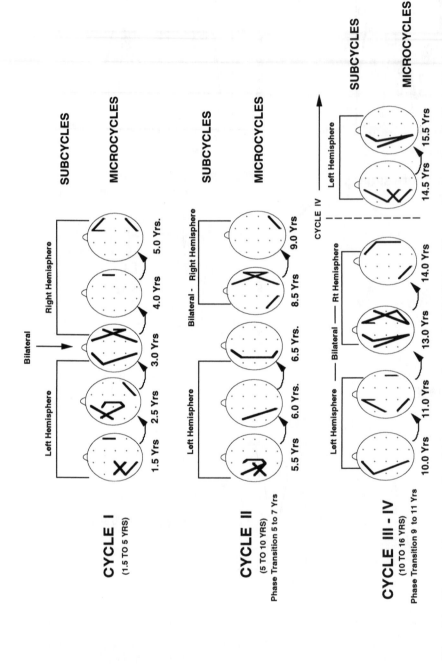

Figure 5.4. Diagrammatic representation of the sequence and anatomical distribution of the growth spurts shown in Figure 5.3. Lines connecting two electrode locations correspond to the electrode locations in Figure 5.3 for the various developmental trajectories that loaded (> .80) on the first five factors (Thatcher, 1991). Microcycles were defined by a developmental sequence involving an anterior–posterior lengthening of interelectrode distances and a mediolateral rotation that cycles from the left hemisphere to bilateral to the right hemisphere in approximately 4-year periods. The microcycles were grouped into subcycles, and the subcycles were grouped into cycles as defined by the age 5–7 and age 9–11 bifurcations. (From Thatcher, R.W. [1994a]. Cyclic cortical reorganization: Origins of cognition. In G. Dawson & K. Fischer [Eds.], *Human behavior and the developing brain* [p. 241]. New York: Guilford Press; reprinted by permission.)

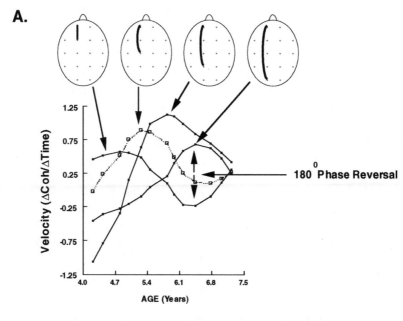

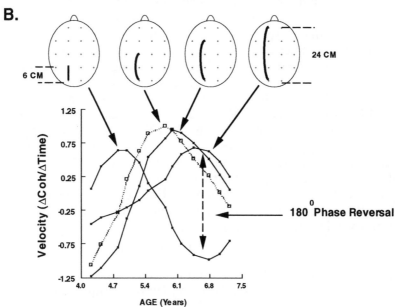

Figure 5.5. Anterior-to-posterior and posterior-to-anterior expansion in the human cortex (approximately 24 cm in 2 years, or 1 cm per month). (A) An expanding sequence of anterior-to-posterior growth spurts that occur in the mediodorsal plane. This process begins at approximately age 4.5 years in the left frontal pole–dorsal frontal region, expands at approximately age 5.3 years to the left frontal pole–central region, then expands again at approximately age 6.0 years to the left frontal pole–parietal region, and, finally, expands at approximately age 6.5 years to the left frontal pole–occipital region. A 180° phase reversal between the short-distance intracortical electrode pair (i.e., F1–F3) and the long-distance intracortical electrode pair (i.e., F1–O1) is evident around age 6.5 years. (B) An expanding sequence complementary to and nearly simultaneous with that observed in (A), but in the posterior-to-anterior direction. This process begins at approximately age 4.5 in the left occipital–parietal region, expands to the left occipital–central region at approximately age 5.75 years, then expands again to the left occipital–dorsal frontal region at approximately age 6.0 years, and, finally, expands to the left occipital–frontal pole at approximately age 6.5 years. A 180° phase reversal between the short-distance intracortical electrode pair (i.e., O1–P3) and the long-distance intracortical electrode pair (i.e., O1–F1) is again evident around age 6.5 years. (Adapted from Thatcher [1992a].)

spheric lateral frontal and lateral temporal regions exhibited 180° phase reversals, whereas interhemispheric dorsomedial frontal regions did not (Thatcher, 1994a); and the fact that 4) dorsomedial interhemispheric trajectories were mostly synchronous, whereas lateral interhemispheric trajectories were mostly asynchronous (see Thatcher, 1994a). Examples of mediolateral gradients of EEG coherence development are shown in Figures 5.4 and 5.6.

Postnatal Left–Right Hemisphere Development
A left-versus-right hemisphere gradient of development was evident by 1) a sequence of predominantly left hemisphere growth spurts followed by predominantly right hemisphere growth spurts, 2) a sequential lengthening of corticocortical connections in the left hemisphere as opposed to a sequential contraction of corticocortical connections in the right hemisphere, and 3) a tendency toward integration of short- to long-distance connections in the left hemisphere, whereas the right hemisphere exhibited a tendency toward differentiation of long-distance connections into shorter-distance connections. Examples of left hemisphere expansion and right hemisphere contraction are shown in Figures 5.4 and 5.7.

NONLINEAR DYNAMICS OF FRONTAL LOBE DEVELOPMENT
The dynamics of the bifurcations or phase transitions observed in the EEG coherence data are similar to those observed in competitive nonlinear oscillator systems in which opposing forces imperceptibly build up until a sudden differentiation or bifurcation occurs (Thom, 1975). The sudden changes in mean EEG coherence observed at ages 3–4, 5–7, and 9–11 years satisfy many of Gilmore's catastrophe flags (Gilmore, 1981) and exhibit characteristics of a "fold" and a "cusp" catastrophe (Thom, 1975; van der Maas & Molenaar, 1992).[2] A clear example of a fold catastrophe is seen in Figure 5.8, in which the P3–F7 EEG coherence trajectory exhibits a change in attractor regimes represented by a rapid change in mean coherence and a frequency shift between ages 5 and 7 years. The Gilmore (1981) catastrophe flags of "modality," "sudden jump," "hysteresis," and "frequency shifts" were present in many of the EEG coherence developmental trajectories. The presence of a bifurcation or catastrophe suggests that the underlying dynamics can be modeled by gradient systems and vector fields of the form

$$\mathbf{x} = -\nabla U(x) \text{ for } \mathbf{x} \text{ in } \mathbb{R}^k \qquad \text{(Eq. 5.3)}$$

in which competition and cooperation between forces are responsible for the dynamics and the stable equilibria (Gilmore, 1981; Thompson & Stewart, 1986).

DOMINANCE OF FRONTAL LOBE CONNECTIONS DURING POSTNATAL CEREBRAL DEVELOPMENT
The developmental trajectories of EEG coherence and phase are dominated by frontal lobe interactions (Thatcher, 1991, 1992b, 1994a; Thatcher et al., 1987). Each postnatal age of development is marked by a different frontal-to-posterior or

---

[2]Mathematically, a catastrophe is defined by a macroscopic vector field **X** on M, where the catastrophe set K is a subset of M. Whenever a point m within the vector field meets K, there will be a discontinuity in the dynamics of the system that is defined as an abrupt change or a "morphogenesis" (Thom, 1975). The "fold" and "cusp" represent two of the elementary geometries of a catastrophe or morphogenesis. A geometric fold in the vector field dynamics of a system occurs when an attractor moves close to an unstable regime and is captured by another stable attractor. A geometric cusp occurs when there are two stable regimes in competition and an attractor either funnels or converges to a stable point or disperses in directions away from a point.

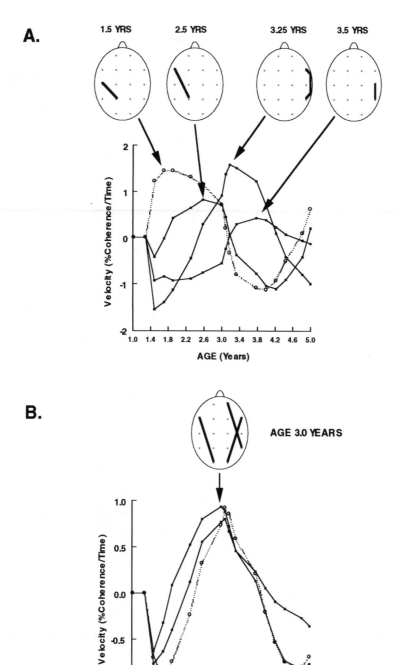

Figure 5.6. Mediolateral clockwise rotation of development of the human cortex. (A) A sequence of expanding and contracting growth spurts that reflect a clockwise anatomical rotation. The process begins at approximately age 1.5 years in the left temporal–parietal region, rotates and extends at approximately age 2.5 years to the left lateral frontal–parietal region, then rotates at approximately age 3.2 years to the right lateral frontal–posterior temporal region, and, finally, rotates and contracts to the right lateral temporal–posterior temporal region at age 3.5–4 years. (B) The long-distance corticocortical growth spurts that are present near the dorsomedial cortex around the age of 3.0 years. Age 3.0 represents the "12 o'clock" or "north pole" of the lateral-to-medial rotational vector and is characterized by a phase lag of about 0.25 years between long-distance left hemisphere frontal connections and long-distance right hemisphere frontal connections. (From Thatcher, R.W. [1992b]. Cyclic cortical reorganization during early childhood development. *Brain and Cognition, 20,* 36; reprinted by permission.)

Left Hemisphere Expansion   Right Hemisphere Contraction

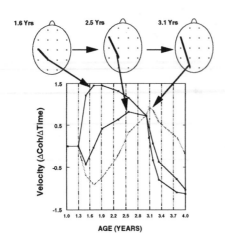

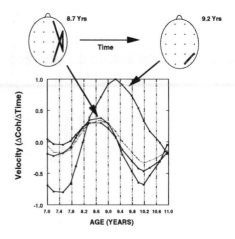

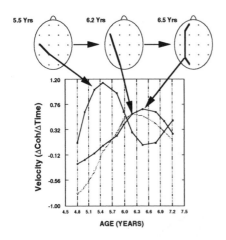

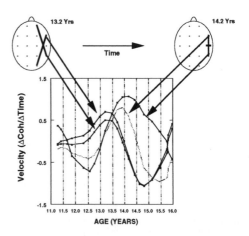

Figure 5.7.   Left panels are examples of left-hemisphere expansion sequences from short-distance intracortical connection systems to longer-distance systems (see Figure 5.4). Right panels are examples of right-hemisphere contraction sequences from long-distance intracortical connection systems to shorter-distance systems. (See Figure 5.4.) (Adapted from Thatcher [1994b].)

frontal-to-temporal or frontal-to-central cortical interaction. Also, the developmental trajectories are different for the left and right hemispheres and different for ventral versus dorsal frontal regions (Thatcher, 1994a; see Figure 5.4). A common finding is the presence of competition between interhemispheric lateral frontal regions but not between interhemispheric medial frontal regions. As suggested elsewhere (Thatcher, 1992b, 1994a), this finding may reflect differences in the anatomy of ventral lateral versus dorsomedial frontal cortex (Abbie, 1940; Dart, 1934; Pandya & Barbas, 1985; Sanides, 1971).

A.

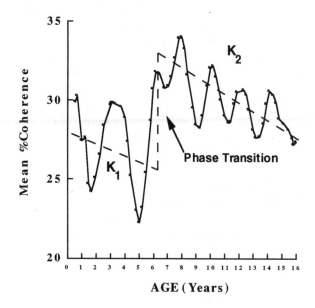

B.

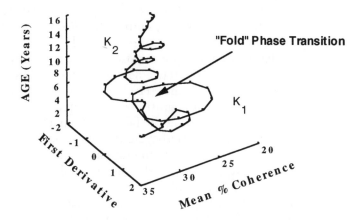

Figure 5.8. (A) Mean percentage EEG coherence (i.e., coherence × 100) in the theta frequency band from left lateral frontal–parietal regions (i.e., F7–P3) from 6 months to 16 years. Two modes of oscillation—mode 1, from birth to approximately age 5, and Mode 2, from approximately age 7 to 16—are fit by regression lines K_1 and K_2. The phase transition between the two developmental states of equilibria or attractor regimes is represented by the line connecting K_1 to K_2. (B) A two-dimensional phase portrait represented in three dimensions by extending the phase space over age. This figure demonstrates that there are two-limit cycles or phase states of EEG coherence oscillation in the left frontal–parietal region (i.e., P3–F7) that are spirals with different radii and frequencies over the life span. (Adapted from Thatcher [1991].)

Finally, some mention should be made about the role of the frontal lobes in the long-distance versus short-distance competition observed in the EEG coherence and phase data (Thatcher, 1991, 1992b, 1994a; Thatcher et al., 1987). Competition as evidenced by 180° phase reversals has been observed in local frontal with respect to long-distance occipital–parietal regions (e.g., F1–F7 versus P3–F7); however, more frequent and larger magnitude competition was noted in local occipital–parietal with respect to long-distance frontal regions (e.g., P3–O1 versus P3–F7). These data indicate that long-distance frontal connections tend to compete with and even displace short-distance posterior cortical connections. As mentioned previously, this process may reflect a dynamic reorganization of increasing differentiation and integration and a developmental progression toward increasing frontal influence and frontal modulatory control of posterior cortical regions.

A CYCLICAL REORGANIZATION THEORY
OF HUMAN FRONTAL LOBE DEVELOPMENT

The essence of the theory of cyclical cortical development is that the iterative growth spurts and patterns of development during the postnatal period reflect a convergence process that narrows the disparity between structure and function by slowly sculpting and reshaping the brain's microanatomy to eventually meet the demands and requirements of an adult world (Thatcher, 1992b, 1994a, 1994b). According to this notion, an individual's gross anatomical structure is established early in development and the postnatal iterative sculpting process is used to fine tune anatomical structure to meet the needs of diverse and unpredictable environments. The sculpting process unlocks or tailors the functional potential of the stable gross anatomy in response to individual needs and environmental demands. According to this theory, the frontal lobes are especially critical in the synaptic sculpting process for the purposes of resource allocation, whereby environmental demands are matched by the cortical resources capable of meeting those demands.

Figure 5.9 is a diagrammatic representation of the structure of cycles and subcycles as observed in the EEG coherence data as they correlate with cognitive development. For continuity, the Fischer (Fischer, 1980; Fischer & Farrar, 1987) and Case (1985, 1987) descriptions of cognitive development are used in Figure 5.9. It should be kept in mind, however, that the labeling of an anatomical organization of growth spurts as a subcycle or a microcycle is somewhat arbitrary. The particular divisions used in Figure 5.9 are meant to emphasize the presence of cyclical patterns of predominantly left, bilateral, and right hemispheric development. The important point, whatever divisions of age one chooses, is that sequential developmental processes are nested within cyclical anatomical patterns.

According to the theory, the oscillations in the mean EEG coherence data are due to delays between the activation and termination of trophic growth factors that are signaled by biochemical mechanisms activated by spatial limits. As shown in Figure 5.10, the engine that drives this process is a traveling wave of nerve growth factor, which is postulated to arise from left hemisphere lateral cortical regions and to rotate clockwise at a rate of approximately 1.0–0.5 cm per month (assuming a 24-cm excursion in the mediolateral direction over a 2- to 4-year period). The leading edge of each cyclical wavefront involves the local production of a surplus of synaptic connections and a periodic reinforcement of existing connections, whereas the trailing edge involves the elimination or pruning of excess connec-

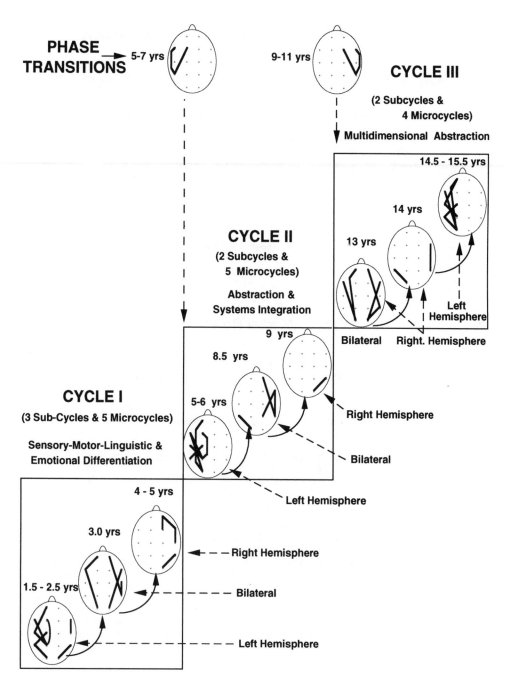

Figure 5.9.   Diagrammatic representation of the predominant developmental cycles and subcycles of neocortical reorganization. Designation of left, bilateral, or right hemisphere is to emphasize the predominant growth spurts during a given age range as shown in Figure 5.4 (e.g., there are six left and two right hemisphere growth spurts between ages 1.5 and 2.5 years as the cycle moves from predominantly left to bilateral). Furthermore, microcycles are not included; instead the microcycles are combined into their respective subcycles from the data in Figure 5.4. This figure illustrates the combination of punctuated equilibria and the presence of a spiral staircase of cyclic reorganization during postnatal cerebral development. The verbal descriptions of the stages of cognitive development are from Fischer (1980), Fischer and Farrar (1987), and Case (1985, 1987). (Adapted from Thatcher [1994a].)

A.   **Anterior - Posterior Expansion and Contraction**

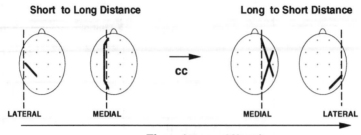

Integration of Differentiation   **Differentiation of Integration**

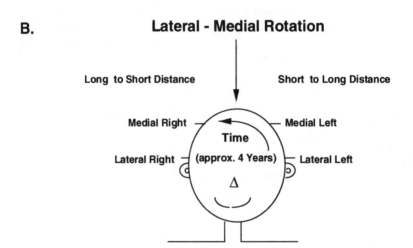

Figure 5.10.   (A) Diagrammatic representation illustrating the anterior–posterior sequence of development in the left and right hemispheres. The left hemisphere exhibits a sequential lengthening of intracortical connection systems, described as a developmental process of integration of differentiation. The right hemisphere exhibits a sequential shortening of the intracortical connection systems, described as a developmental process of differentiation of integration (see Figures 5.4 through 5.6). (B) Diagrammatic representation illustrating the mediolateral sequence of development. The sequence begins at the left lateral cortex, then intrahemispherically expands to the left dorsomedial cortex, then projects through the corpus callosum to the right dorsomedial cortex, and finally intrahemispherically contracts in the right lateral cortex (see Figures 5.1, 5.4, and 5.8). (Adapted from Thatcher [1992a].

tions. It is suggested here that the frontal lobes are largely responsible for selecting and influencing the extent to which environmental factors determine which synaptic connections will survive or be reinforced and which will be pruned or neglected. In the following discussion, an ecological model of synaptogenesis is explored to explain how the frontal lobes operate to cyclically sculpt and select which synaptic influences will be pruned and which will survive.

Let us begin with a search of plausible neural population models that are capable of explaining the presence of oscillations in the development of EEG coherence

(Thatcher, in press). For purposes of simplicity, changes in the number of synapses are emphasized; however, the model will work for modulation of the strength of synapses without a change in the number of synapses. Among the most adaptable population models are those in which two populations are competing for a common food supply (Gause, 1934; Gause & Witt, 1935; Volterra, 1926) and those involving predator–prey relationships (Holling, 1959, 1966; Lotka, 1925; Nicholson & Bailey, 1935; Soloman, 1949; Volterra, 1926). These two models are mathematically related, primarily by the strength of the competitive coupling (Berryman, 1981; Getz, 1984; Real, 1977). In order to adapt these models to cortical development, we must assume 1) a common niche for synapses is the somatodendritic surface area, expressed in squared microns; 2) corticocortical connection systems can compete, cooperate, or both for the available somatodendritic surface area upon which synaptic connections are formed; and 3) competing/cooperating corticocortical connection systems from different brain regions can coexist within a given cortical region, such that displacement of connections or reduced connection strength from Region 1 by connections from Region 2 can occur.

Figure 5.11A is a representation of a competing/cooperating corticocortical connection system representing the lateral frontal–to–parietal corticocortical connections (Fp1–P3, or A), the occipital-to-parietal corticocortical connections (O1–P3, or B), and the somatodendritic domain of the left parietal region (P3) where the corticocortical connections A and B converge (C). Figure 5.11B is a representation of the synaptic populations A and B converging on the somatodendritic area C as depicted in Figure 5.11A. Projections A and B contain multiple synaptic connections, and there are shared spatial locations on the dendrites of C in which the synaptic species from population A cooperate or compete for occupancy, or both, with the synaptic species from population B.

Figure 5.12 is a representation of the mathematical interactions within and between corticocortical synaptic systems as depicted in Figure 5.11. There are three major kinds of interactions between synaptic connection systems: 1) competition, 2) cooperation, and 3) predator–prey. Each of these categories of interaction can be depicted by the sign and magnitude of the interaction coefficients a_{ii}, which are divided into intrasynaptic interaction coefficients (e.g., a_{11} and a_{22}) and intersynaptic interaction coefficients (e.g., a_{12} and a_{21}).

For purposes of examining the fit of the model to the mean EEG coherence developmental data from Thatcher (1992b, 1994a), Equation 5.3 was used. Using the notation of Berryman (1990), we can write one equation for the developmental synaptic dynamics that includes a nonlinear term of coefficient of curvature and terms for carrying capacity:

$$R_i = A_i \left[1 - \left(\frac{N_i}{K_i} \right)^{Q_i} \right] - \frac{a_i N_j}{N_i + E_i} \qquad \text{(Eq. 5.4)}$$

where R_i is the rate of change in the number of synapses, as a function of 1) the maximum per-capita rate of increase of the population in a given environment A_i; 2) the current synaptic density (N_i); and 3) the carrying capacity of the synaptic environment (K_i). The carrying capacity K_i limits the growth of the population because when $N = K$, then $R = 0$. Q_i is the coefficient of curvature to reflect nonlinear properties of the R function; a_i is the intrasynaptic effect of N_i and N_j on themselves as well as the intersynaptic effect between N_i and N_{ji}; and E_i is the con-

A.

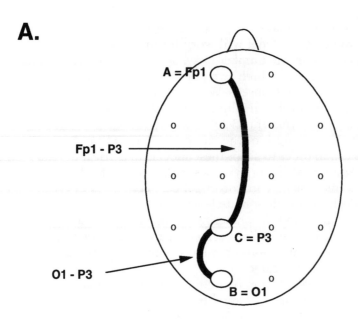

B.

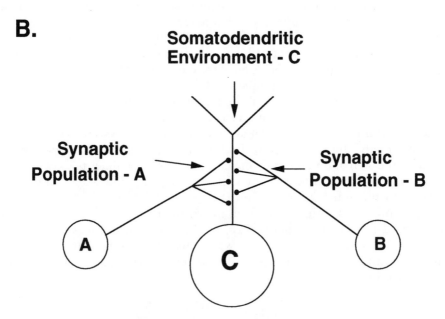

Figure 5.11.   A model of corticocortical connection development. (A) Diagram of left frontal pole regions (e.g., Fp1) that are competing with left occipital regions (e.g., O1) for synaptic influence on the parietal cortex. That is, connections from Fp1 and O1 converge onto P3, where they compete for the available synaptic binding sites on the dentrites or cell body of parietal neurons, or both. (B) An expansion of the synaptic environment for the competing connection systems shown in A. The carrying capacity for synaptic influence is a function of the amount of parietal dendrosomatic area upon which synapses can form and the amount of trophic growth factor. Synapses originating from the frontal and occipital regions converge onto the parietal dendrosomatic surface, where they compete for contact and influence of the parietal neurons. (From Thatcher et al. [1994b]. Psychopathology of early frontal lobe damage: Dependence on cycles of development. *Development and Psychopathology, 6,* 587; reprinted by permission.)

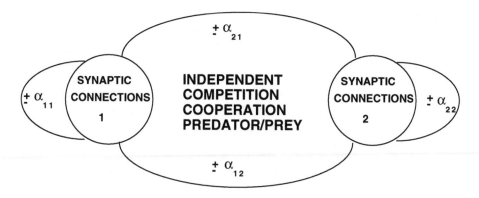

Figure 5.12.   Ecological model in which synapses arising from two different cortical regions interact for influence on a third cortical region. The interaction can be of four types—1) Independent,
2) cooperative, 3) competitive, and 4) predatory–prey—depending upon the sign and magnitude
of the interaction coefficients (α_{ij}), which are divided into intrasynaptic interaction coefficients
(e.g., α_{11} and α_{22}) and intersynaptic interaction coefficients (e.g., α_{12} and α_{21}). (From Thatcher, R.W.
[1994b]. Psychopathology of early frontal lobe damage: Dependence on cycles of development.
Development and Psychopathology, 6, 588; reprinted by permission.)

centration of trophic nerve growth factor that can modulate the number of synapses,
the strength of synapses, or both (see Thatcher, in press, for further details).

Fit of Model to EEG Coherence Development
A stepwise procedure was used to evaluate individual values and combinations of
mean EEG coherence development and to determine the best fit of the data. The
first step was to evaluate the dynamics, stability, and sensitivity of the population
model for single corticocortical connection systems. In these analyses, the EEG coherence trajectories were evaluated for 1) the presence of two or more equilibria
(i.e., the presence of a separatrix and basins of attraction); 2) the magnitude of time
delays; and 3) the magnitude and direction of nonlinearity as measured by the coefficient of curvature of fit (Berryman, 1990). The second step was to evaluate the dynamics of pairs of EEG coherence trajectories using the model of two populations
competing, cooperating, or in a predator–prey mode of interaction. This involved a
least-squares regression analysis to fit the R function, using both the product-
dependent variation and the ratio-dependent variation, followed by simulation of
the best fitting model using deterministic and stochastic simulations. The mode of
interaction as competitive, cooperative, predator–prey, or independent (i.e., no significant interaction) was also determined. The type of two-population interaction
to which each pair of EEG coherence trajectories belonged was determined by the
sign of the coefficients, the squared correlation coefficient (R^2), and the probability
values (i.e., $p < .05$). Once the category of interaction was determined (excluding
the independent interactions), the dynamics of the model were further evaluated by
isocline analyses, in which the structure of the isoclines, the phase space trajectories, and the time-series plots were compared.

Global Characteristics—Limit Cycles and Bifurcations
The fits of all of the EEG developmental trajectories were statistically significant
($p < .05$) using the single-population equations. In 100% of the cases, time delays at
T_3, T_2, or both yielded higher R^2 values than did a time delay of T_1. The highest R^2
values at T_3 or T_2 ranged from 41.78% in F3–C3 to 99.9% in F1–F3. The phase space

trajectories were characterized by 1) sigmoid-type logistic growth, 2) limit cycle behavior, or 3) spiral trajectories that tended to converge toward a limit cycle. Many of the trajectories could be characterized as two or more equilibria separated by an escape threshold or separatrix. From 1.5 to 5 years of age, the separatrix bifurcation occurred primarily in the local right frontal regions (e.g., F2–F8, F2–F4) and in the right frontotemporal regions (F2–T6, F2–T4). Between the ages of 5 and 7 years, the separatrix bifurcation occurred primarily in the left frontotemporal and left frontoparietal regions; a third group of separatrix bifurcations were seen in the right frontotemporal regions around the ages of 9–11 years.

Frontal Cortical Regions as Predators and Posterior Cortical Regions as Prey

The mode of interaction between EEG corticocortical developmental systems could be explained most frequently and with the highest amount of variance accounted for in the predator–prey mode (e.g., 86.7% in the left hemisphere and 48.5% in the right hemisphere). The next most prevalent mode of interaction was of the competitive type, although competitive interactions occurred exclusively in the right hemisphere. The least frequent modes of interaction were the independent and cooperative modes. Clear differences in the anatomical distribution of the various modes were present. In general, the predator–prey modes occurred in the anterior-to-posterior plane, with frontal regions being the predators and posterior cortical regions the prey. The independent and cooperative modes tended to occur in the mediolateral plane, and the competitive modes occurred primarily in right local frontal and right frontotemporal regions.

Figure 5.13 shows an example of actual mean EEG coherence data (a) and simulated data (b) for Fp1–P3 and O1–P3 competitive dynamics. In this case, the least-squares regression fit of the model to the actual mean EEG coherence data had R^2 values of 97.41% for P3–O1 and of 94.97% for Fp1–P3. According to the model, there is a continuous cycling of synaptic abundance followed by synaptic pruning in both frontal and posterior cortical regions. However, the mechanisms of pruning are somewhat different because the frontal regions are directly responsible for the synaptic organization and reorganization in posterior cortical regions. The synaptic sequence, as diagrammed in Figure 5.13(b), is as follows:

Stage 1, at approximately age 1.5 years, is when long-distance frontal–posterior synaptic influences are at a low while short-distance posterior cortical synaptic influences are at a high or surplus. At this age there is minimal frontal cortical reorganization of posterior regions with previously formed frontal connections being influential.

Stage 2, at approximately age 2.5 years, is when short-distance posterior cortical synaptic influences are on the decline while long-distance frontal–posterior synaptic influences are increasing and becoming significantly more influential on posterior cortical neural networks.

Stage 3, at approximately age 3.8 years, appears when long-distance frontal synaptic influence and reorganization is at a maximum; however, there is a diminishing supply of "virgin" local posterior cortical synapses, and therefore frontal influence begins to decline.

Stage 4, at approximately age 5.5 years, is when long-distance frontal–posterior cortical synaptic influences are on the decline and short-distance posterior cortical influences are on the rise; that is, restocking the supply of posterior cortical synapses that the frontal lobes can later "replace" or "reorganize."

EXPERIMENTAL DATA

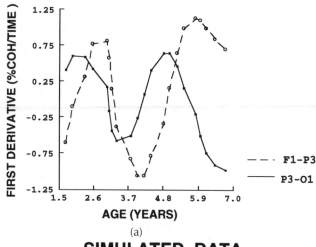

(a)

SIMULATED DATA

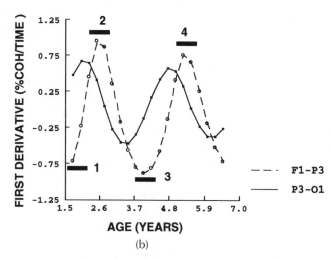

(b)

Figure 5.13.   Comparison of (a) actual first derivatives of mean EEG coherence from the frontal–parietal (F1–P3) and parietal–occipital (P3–O1) regions to (b) simulated first derivative values based upon the predator–prey model described by Equation 5.4. The least-squares regression fit of the model (Equation 5.4) to the actual mean EEG coherence data had an R^2 value for P3–O1 of 97.41% and for Fp1–P3 of 94.97%. (From Thatcher, R.W. [1994b]. Psychopathology of early frontal lobe damage: Dependence on cycles of development. *Development and Psychopathology, 6*, 589; reprinted by permission.)

The adaptation of an ecological predator–prey model to cortical synaptogenesis does not require the exact specification of the predator–prey type, because identical mathematical forms pertain to each of the four different categories of interaction. However, given the long cycle times of cerebral dynamics (e.g., months and years), a somewhat gentle form of predation, similar to that of a herbivore or parasite, would represent a more appropriate ecological analogue.

Functional Interpretation of Frontal Lobe Synaptic Competition and Predation

What is the functional significance of the frontal regions being exclusively the predators and fierce competitors in the dynamic cycle of synaptic surplus followed by synaptic pruning? One interpretation is that the frontal regions control or significantly influence the pruning phase of the synaptic development of posterior cortical regions. That is, frontal synaptic influence significantly determines which synapses will survive and which will be lost during the developmental sculpting process. A hierarchical integration of cortical resources periodically occurs, forming a frontal lobe–mediated spiral of ever-cascading competencies. This process is nonlinear in both space and time and is manifested behaviorally by relatively sudden changes in cognitive competence. The appearance of discontinuous development is often characterized as "sensitive periods" or "growth spurts" (Cicchetti, 1990, 1993; Fischer, 1983). According to the present model, "sensitive periods" reflect the nonlinear manifestation of an underlying and continuous growth process (Thatcher, 1992a, 1992b, 1994a).

Genetic versus Environmental Influences

As defined previously, the positive first derivative of mean EEG coherence change reflects the synaptic surplus phase, and the negative first derivative reflects the synaptic pruning phase (Thatcher, 1992b, 1993, 1994a). One would expect that genetic factors would have a strong influence on the synaptic surplus phase and that environmental factors would have a strong influence on the synaptic pruning phase. Because genetics has the less variable task of turning genes on and off, whereas the environment and the demands placed on the individual are highly variable and complex, it follows that, because the individuals in these studies lived in diverse environments, greater variance in the first derivative of EEG coherence would be expected during the pruning phase than during the surplus phase. Figure 5.14 shows two examples of the relationship between the variance of the first derivative of mean EEG coherence and the actual first derivatives of mean EEG coherence. A 180° phase reversal is strongly present in which variance is greatest during the negative first derivatives, or the synaptic pruning phases, and is small during the positive first derivatives, or the synaptic surplus phases. High EEG coherence variance of the negative first derivative is precisely what is expected if environmental factors dominate the pruning phase while genetic factors dominate the surplus phase.

Figure 5.13(b) illustrates the proposed cycle of synaptic surplus followed by synaptic pruning in which the pruning phase is strongly influenced by the frontal lobes according to the model in Figure 5.11 (i.e., the F1–P3 and O1–P3 model). Both frontal and posterior cortical regions exhibit cycles of synaptic surplus followed by synaptic pruning; however, the frontal regions directly displace or remove posterior cortical synapses, whereas the posterior cortical regions do not displace the frontal synapses. Instead, the growth of frontal synapses is dependent upon the presence of posterior cortical synapses. Therefore, when there is a reduced supply of posterior cortical synapses, frontal synaptic influences decline, and vice versa. The posterior cortical synaptic surplus phase is a type of "restocking" of the supply of posterior cortical synapses that the frontal lobes can subsequently "replace" or "reorganize" based on environmental exigencies.

CONCLUSIONS: NEURAL PLASTICITY AND SENSITIVE PERIODS

The cyclical reorganization model of human brain development explicitly integrates neural plasticity with sensitive periods. That is, each cycle of synaptic sur-

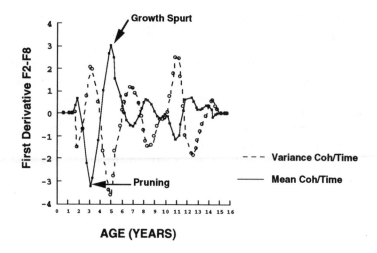

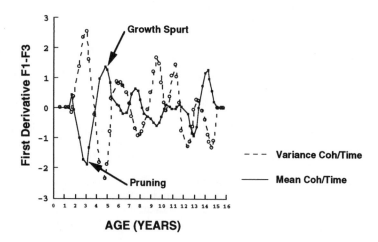

Figure 5.14.   The first derivatives of the mean and variance of EEG coherence from male children for two different cortical regions (top, F2–F8; bottom, F1–F3). A 180° phase reversal is strongly present in which variance is greatest during the negative first derivatives, or synaptic pruning phases, and it is small during the postive first derivatives, or synaptic surplus phases. (From Thatcher, R.W. [1994b]. Psychopathology of early frontal lobe damage: Dependence on cycles of development. *Development and Psychopathology, 6,* 590; reprinted by permission.)

plus followed by pruning represents a "sensitive period" in anatomically localized and interconnected brain regions. Therefore, sensitive periods are continually occurring because they are driven by a diffusion wave of anatomically circulating nerve growth factor. A staging or discontinuous aspect of this process arises because of inherent nonlinearities in both space and time. Spatially, the nonlinearities arise because of the segregation of differentiated function in distributed ensembles of neurons. The functionally differentiated anatomy of the brain guarantees spatial nonlinearities as the wave of growth hormone sweeps across domains of cells. Thus, stages or "sensitive periods" are present because functionally differentiated regions of the brain develop at different ages. A stage–plateau sequence in cognitive development is an outward manifestation of both the continuous and discontinuous aspects of the process. Each stage or period represents rapid synaptic growth within functionally differentiated neural systems, and, as a consequence, neural plasticity involves the genetically driven overproduction of synapses and the environmentally driven maintenance and pruning of synaptic connections. An important point of the theory, whatever divisions of age one chooses, is that sequential developmental processes are nested within cyclical anatomical patterns and that the synaptic drives mediated through frontal corticocortical connections play a crucial role in human development, especially in the process of synaptic pruning and synaptic selection (see Figure 5.9).

REFERENCES

Abbie, A.A. (1940). Cortical lamination in the monotremata. *Journal of Comparative Neurology, 72,* 429–467.

Bayer, S.A., & Altman, J. (1991). *Neocortical development.* New York: Raven Press.

Bendat, J.S., & Piersol, A.G. (1980). *Engineering applications of correlation and spectral analysis.* New York: John Wiley & Sons.

Berryman, A.A. (1981). *Population systems: A general introduction.* New York: Plenum.

Berryman, A.A. (1990). *Population dynamics: A workbook for POPSYS software.* Pullman, WA: Ecological Systems Analysis.

Bourgeois, J., Goldman-Rakic, P.S., and Rakic, P. (1994). Synaptogenesis in the prefrontal cortex of rhesus monkeys. *Cerebral Cortex, 4,* 78–96.

Braitenberg, V. (1978). Cortical architectonics: General and areal. In M.A.B. Brazier & H. Petsche (Eds.), *Architectonics of the cerebral cortex* (pp. 47–63). New York: Academic Press.

Carpenter, M.B., & Sutin, J. (1983). *Human neuroanatomy.* Baltimore: Williams & Wilkins.

Case, R. (1985). *Intellectual development: Birth to adulthood.* New York: Academic Press.

Case, R. (1987). The structure and process of intellectual development. *International Journal of Psychology, 22,* 571–607.

Cicchetti, D. (1990). The organization and coherences of socioemotional, cognitive, and representational development: Illustrations through a developmental psychopathology perspective on Down syndrome and child maltreatment. In R. Thompson (Ed.), *Nebraska symposium on motivation: Socioemotional development* (pp. 259–366). Lincoln: University of Nebraska Press.

Cicchetti, D. (1993). Developmental psychopathology: Reactions, reflections, projections. *Developmental Review, 13,* 471–502.

Cowan, W.M. (1979). The developing brain. In *The brain* (pp. 56–69). San Francisco: W.H. Freeman.

Cragg, B.G. (1975). The development of synapses in the visual system of the cat. *Journal of Comparative Neurology, 160,* 147–166.

Dart, R.A. (1934). The dual structure of the neopallium: Its history and significance. *Journal of Anatomy, 69,* 3–19.

Diamond, M.C., Scheibel, A.B., & Elson, L.M. (1985). *The human brain coloring book.* New York: HarperCollins.

Epstein, H.T. (1980). EEG developmental stages. *Developmental Psychobiology, 13,* 629–631.

Feinberg, I. (1982). Schizophrenia: Caused by a fault in programmed synaptic elimination during adolescence. *Journal of Psychiatric Research, 17,* 319–334.

Fischer, K.W. (1980). A theory of cognitive development: The control and construction of hierarchies of skills. *Psychological Review, 87,* 477–531.

Fischer, K.W. (1983). Developmental levels as periods of discontinuity. In K.W. Fischer (Ed.), *Levels and transitions in children's development* (pp. 23–38). San Francisco: Jossey-Bass.

Fischer, K.W. (1987). Relations between brain and cognitive development. *Child Development, 57,* 623–632.

Fischer, K.W., & Farrar, M.J. (1987). Generalizations about generalization: How a theory of skill development explains both generality and specificity. *International Journal of Psychology, 22,* 643–677.

Gause, G.F. (1934). *The struggle for existence.* Baltimore: Williams & Wilkins.

Gause, G.F., & Witt, A.A. (1935). Behavior of mixed populations and the problem of natural selection. *American Naturalist, 3,* 596–609.

Getz, W.M. (1984). Population dynamics: A per-capita resource approach. *Journal of Theoretical Biology, 108,* 623–643.

Gilmore, R. (1981). *Catastrophe theory for scientists and engineers.* New York: John Wiley & Sons.

Glaser, E.M., & Ruchkin, D.S. (1976). *Principles of neurobiological signal analyses.* New York: Academic Press.

Holling, C.S. (1959). The components of predation as revealed by a study of small mammal predation of the European pine sawfly. *Canadian Entomologist, 91,* 293–320.

Holling, C.S. (1966). The functional response of invertebrate predators to prey density. *Memoirs of the Entomological Society of Canada, 48,* 1–86.

Hudspeth, W.J., & Pribram, K.H. (1990). Stages of brain and cognitive maturation. *Journal of Educational Psychology, 82,* 881–884.

Hudspeth, W.J., & Pribram, K.H. (1991). Physiological indices of cerebral maturation. *International Journal of Psychophysiology, 2,* 19–29.

Huttenlocher, P.R. (1979). Synaptic density in human frontal cortex: Developmental changes and effects of aging. *Brain Research, 163,* 195–205.

Huttenlocher, P.R. (1984). Synapse elimination and plasticity in developing human cerebral cortex. *American Journal of Mental Deficiency, 88,* 488–496.

Huttenlocher, P.R. (1990). Morphometric study of human cerebral cortex development. *Neuropsychologia, 28,* 517–527.

Huttenlocher, P.R., & deCourten, C. (1987). The development of synapses in striate cortex of man. *Human Neurobiology, 6,* 1–9.

Huttenlocher, P.R., deCourten, C., Garey, L., & Van der Loos, H. (1982). Synaptogenesis in human visual cortex: Evidence for synapse elimination during normal development. *Neuroscience Letters, 33,* 247–252.

Kolb, B. (1989). Brain development, plasticity and behavior. *American Psychologist, 44,* 1203–1212.

Lilly, J.C., & Cherry, R. (1954). Surface movements of click responses from the acoustic cerebral cortex of the cat: The leading and the trailing edges of a response figure. *Journal of Neurophysiology, 17,* 521–532.

Lilly, J.C., & Cherry, R. (1955). Surface movements of figures in the spontaneous activity of anesthetized cerebral cortex: The leading and trailing edges. *Journal of Neurophysiology, 18,* 18–32.

Linas, R.R., & Ribary, U. (1992). Rostrocaudal scan in human brain: A global characteristic of the 40-Hz response during sensory input. In E. Basar & T.H. Bullock (Eds.), *Induced rhythms in the brain* (pp. 147–154). Boston: Birkhauser.

Lopez da Silva, F., Pijn, J.P., & Boeijinga, P. (1989). Interdependence of EEG signals: Linear vs. nonlinear associations and the significance of time delays and phase shifts. *Brain Topography, 2,* 9–18.

Lotka, A.J. (1925). *The elements of physical biology.* Baltimore: Williams & Wilkins.

Matousek, M., & Petersen, I. (1973). Frequency analysis of the EEG background activity by means of age dependent EEG quotients. In P. Kellaway & I. Petersen (Eds.), *Automation of clinical electroencephalography* (pp. 32–53). New York: Raven Press.

Nicholson, A.J., & Bailey, V.A. (1935). The balance of animal populations. *Proceedings of the Zoological Society of London, 3,* 551–598.

Nunez, P. (1981). *Electric fields of the brain: The neurophysics of EEG.* New York: Oxford University Press.

O'Leary, D.D.M. (1987). Remodelling of early axonal projections through the selective elimination of neurons and long axon collaterals. In G. Bock & M. O'Connor (Eds.), *Selective neuronal death* (pp. 113–142). New York: John Wiley & Sons.

O'Leary, D.D.M., Stanfield, B.B., & Cowan, W.M. (1981). Evidence that the early postnatal restriction of the cells of origin of the callosal projection is due to the elimination of axon collaterals rather than to the death of neurons. *Developmental Brain Research, 1,* 607–617.

Otnes, R.K., & Enochson, L. (1972). *Digital time series analysis.* New York: John Wiley & Sons.

Pandya, D.N., & Barbas, H. (1985). Supplementary motor area structure and function: Review and hypotheses. *Behavioral and Brain Sciences, 8,* 595–596.

Pascual-Marqui, R.D., Valdes-Sosa, P.A., & Alvarez-Amador, A. (1988). A parametric model for multichannel EEG spectra. *International Journal of Neuroscience, 125,* 73–86.

Purves, D. (1988). *Body and brain: A trophic theory of neural connections.* Cambridge, MA: Harvard University Press.

Rakic, P. (1985). Limits of neurogenesis in primates. *Science, 227,* 1054–1056.

Rakic, P., Bourgeois, J., Eckenhoff, M., Zecevic, N., & Goldman-Rakic, P.S. (1986). Concurrent overproduction of synapses in diverse regions of primate cerebral cortex. *Science, 232,* 232–234.

Real, L. (1977). The kinetics of functional response. *American Naturalist, 111,* 289–300.

Rogers, R.L., Baumann, S.B., Papanicolaou, A.C., Bourbon, T.W., Alagarsamy, S., & Eisenberg, H.M. (1991). Localization of the P3 sources using magnetoencephalography and magnetic resonance imaging. *EEG and Clinical Neurophysiology, 79,* 308–321.

Sanides, F. (1971). Functional architecture of motor and sensory cortices in primates in the light of a new concept of neocortex development. In C.R. Noback & W. Montana (Eds.), *Advances in primatology* (pp. 137–208). New York: Academic Press.

Soloman, M.E. (1949). The natural control of animal population. *Journal of Animal Ecology, 18,* 1–35.

Smart, I.H.M. (1983). Three dimensional growth of the mouse isocortex. *Journal of Anatomy, 137,* 683–694.

Thatcher, R.W. (1980). Neurolinguistics: Theoretical and evolutionary perspectives. *Brain and Language, 11,* 235–260.

Thatcher, R.W. (1989). *Nonlinear dynamics of human cerebral development.* Paper presented at the First International Conference on Mechanisms of Mind. Havana, Cuba.

Thatcher, R.W. (1991). Maturation of the human frontal lobes: Physiological evidence for staging. *Developmental Neuropsychology, 7,* 397–419.

Thatcher, R.W. (1992a). Are rhythms of human cerebral development "traveling waves"? *Behavior and Brain Sciences, 14,* 575.

Thatcher, R.W. (1992b). Cyclic cortical reorganization during early childhood development. *Brain and Cognition, 20,* 24–50.

Thatcher, R.W. (1993). Cyclic cortical morphogenesis: A nonlinear synaptic population model. In *Abstracts of the biennial meeting of the Society for Research in Child Development,* New Orleans.

Thatcher, R.W. (1994a). Cyclic cortical reorganization: Origins of cognition. In G. Dawson & K. Fischer (Eds.), *Human behavior and the developing brain* (pp. 232–268). New York: Guilford Press.

Thatcher, R.W. (1994b). Psychopathology of early frontal lobe damage: Dependence on cycles of development. *Development and Psychopathology, 6,* 565–596.

Thatcher, R.W. (in press). A predator/prey model of human cerebral development. In K. Newell & P. Molennar (Eds.), *Dynamical systems and development.* Hillsdale, NJ: Lawrence Erlbaum Associates.

Thatcher, R.W., & John, E.R. (1977). *Functional neuroscience: Foundations of cognitive processing.* Hillsdale, NJ: Lawrence Erlbaum Associates.

Thatcher, R.W., Krause, P., & Hrybyk, M. (1986). Corticocortical association fibers and EEG coherence: A two compartmental model. *Electroencephalography and Clinical Neurophysiology, 64,* 123–143.

Thatcher, R.W., McAlaster, R., Lester, M.L., Horst, R.L., & Cantor, D.S. (1983). Hemispheric EEG asymmetries related to cognitive functioning in children. In: A. Perecuman (Ed.), *Cognitive processing in the right hemisphere* (pp. 125–145). New York: Academic Press.

Thatcher, R.W., Walker, R.A., & Giudice, S. (1987). Human cerebral hemispheres develop at different rates and ages. *Science, 236,* 1110–1113.

Thom, R. (1975). *Structural stability and morphogenesis.* Reading, MA: W.A. Benjamin.

Thompson, J., & Stewart, H. (1986). *Nonlinear dynamics and chaos.* New York: John Wiley & Sons.

Tucker, D.M., Roth, D.L., & Blair, T.B. (1986). Functional connections among cortical regions: Topography of EEG coherence. *Electroencephalography and Clinical Neurophysiology, 63,* 242–250.

van der Maas, H.L.I., & Molenaar, P.C.M. (1992). A catastrophe theoretical approach to stagewise cognitive development. *Psychological Review, 99,* 395–417.

Verzeano, M. (1972). Pacemakers, synchronization, and epilepsy. In H. Petsche & M.A.B. Brazier (Eds.), *Synchronization of EEG activities in epilepsies* (pp. 154–188). New York: Springer-Verlag.

Verzeano, M., & Negishi, K. (1960). Neuronal activity in cortical and thalamic networks. *Journal of General Physiology, 43*(Suppl.), 177.

Verzeano, M., & Negishi, K. (1961). Neuronal activity in wakefulness and in sleep. In G.E.W. Wolstenholme & M. O'Connor (Eds.), *The nature of sleep* (pp. 108–126). London: Churchill.

Volterra, V. (1926). Variazioni e fluttuaxioni del numero d'individui inspecie animali conviventi. *Memorial R. Academic Lincei Series, 6*(2), 26–43.

Zecevic, N., & Rakic, P. (1991). Synaptogenesis in monkey somatosensory cortex. *Cerebral Cortex, 1,* 5410–5523.

Development of the Prefrontal Cortex: Evolution, Neurobiology, and Behavior
edited by Norman A. Krasnegor, Ph.D., G. Reid Lyon, Ph.D.,
and Patricia S. Goldman-Rakic, Ph.D.
copyright © 1997   Paul H. Brookes Publishing Co., Inc.
Baltimore • London • Toronto • Sydney

II

BRAIN–BEHAVIOR RELATIONSHIPS

6

Competence, Cortex, and Primate Models
A Comparative Primate Perspective

Duane M. Rumbaugh

PREFRONTAL CORTEX AND COMPETENCE

The cortex is held by many scientists to be uniquely involved in our ability to control and shift the topics of our attention and in our capacity to both organize and retrieve information needed for focused learning in schools and productive work. The prefrontal cortex is, of course, but part of the cortex, which, in turn, is only part of the brain. Because the brain generally functions as a whole, we should not expect the functions of the prefrontal cortex to be singularly responsible even for the complex of human behaviors (for reviews, see Armstrong, 1990a, 1990b; Gibson, 1986; Mirsky, 1996). That said, it is to be expected that the prefrontal cortex has primary functions. Because we are so closely related to other primates, it is reasonable that we look to studies of them in our efforts to achieve a better understanding of brain–behavior relationships and, in particular, of cortical function.

The primates most widely used as animal models are chimpanzees and macaque monkeys (*Macaca*). Although the rhesus monkey is not endangered, chimpanzee populations in the wild are increasingly at risk. As primate taxa become rare and endangered, animal model research is being curtailed. Notwithstanding, projected development of *noninvasive* procedures should enable studies of their brain–behavior functions.

This chapter was supported by Grant HD-06016 from the National Institute of Child Health and Human Development, by Grant NAG2-438 from the National Aeronautics and Space Administration, and by additional support from the College of Art and Sciences, Georgia State University, Atlanta.

The author thanks William A. Hillix, David A. Washburn, Rose A. Sevcik, E. Sue Savage-Rumbaugh, and the reviewers of this chapter selected by the editors of this book for critical comments on the manuscript. He also thanks William D. Hopkins, Steve Suomi, Mary P. Williams, and Leslie Burke for data on capuchins and rhesus monkeys that were pooled with other data for their species and included in Figure 6.1; Andrea Clay for the primate figures in Figure 6.1; John Gulledge for assistance with data; Michael Beran, Judith Sizemore, and Tawanna Tookes for manuscript preparation. The views advanced herein are the responsibility of the author. This chapter is dedicated to the memory of Austin H. Riesen—colleague and friend.

Although noninvasive studies of primates have limitations, so do invasive studies. This chapter considers some of the research on intact, healthy primates to obtain a comparative perspective of brain and prefrontal cortical function. All of the tasks herein discussed require the subjects' focused attention, relational learning, memory, and reliable effort in order to do well. How well different kinds of primate species do at various such tasks serves to help us achieve our long-term, primary goal—an improved understanding of the prefrontal cortex and its roles in complex learning and the application of that learning (Armstrong, 1990b; Barkley, 1996; Semendeferi, 1994; Semendeferi, Damasio, & Van Hoesen, 1994). Our general tactic entails assessment of brain complexity in relation to cognition and language in primates. We must await the future and its exciting new, noninvasive technology to achieve the understanding of specific relations between the prefrontal cortex and behavioral competence that we now pursue.

Primates as Models

Behavioral research with primates is basic to our understanding of human behavior, human development, and human competence. The roots of our competence—be it for the complex operations of perceiving relationships between things and events or for the normal acquisition of the ability to understand human speech and language—are now clearly evident in our nearest living relatives of the order Primates. Substantive language skills are now credited to the great apes (*Pongidae*), particularly the larger species of monkeys of the Old World (*Cercopithecidae*) and the New World (*Cebidae*) are now known to have remarkably complex learning and problem-solving skills. More broadly but beyond the scope of this chapter is the recognition that the primates' patterns of perception, anatomy, posture, social development, and so forth have valuable lessons to teach us about ourselves.

This chapter first briefly considers

- Brain evolution and competence
- The human primate
- Homology
- The probable interactive relationships between brain size/complexity and the specific effects of early environment
- The Cartesian and Darwinian perspectives of animals and their mentality

Following that discussion, the merits of nonhuman primates as animal models for language and cognition are reviewed in comparative perspective.

Big Is Better (Generally)   Evolution of the primate brain is noted for increased weight relative to the body (i.e., encephalization [Deacon, 1997; Jerison, 1985; see also Chapter 1]) and for the correlated increase in complexity of the networks within and between the cortex and other structures of the brain (Finlay & Darlington, 1995). Some of the more salient trends of brain evolution within the order Primates include the emergence of color vision; the enhancement of depth perception via binocular disparity; refined motor control of the hands; enhanced cerebral lateralization; and protraction of all critical periods of the life span from gestation to maturity, ages of reproduction, and ages of death (Napier & Napier, 1994). From the perspective of this chapter, no trend is more important than is the enhancement of *learning* and *symbolizing processes*.

These advances are most impressive in the larger primates, among whom lifestyles have become diurnal and social organizational patterns have become both more complex and flexible (Byrne, 1996; Gibson, 1986). Notwithstanding their enhanced behavioral flexibility, the skeletal structures of the larger primates have retained essential arboreal designs (Tuttle, 1986).

Emergence of Human Attributes   *Homo sapiens* is recognized as the most generalized and cognitively competent primate—a form that can exercise dominion over all others and can occupy every climatic region. Le Gros Clark (1959) suggested that the succession from the smallest primates, some of which are not even true monkeys but premonkeys (i.e., *Prosimii*—e.g., galago, lemur, loris), through the taxa of the New and Old World monkeys, and on to the lesser apes (i.e., *Hylobatidae*—gibbon, siamang) and great apes (i.e., *Pongidae*—orangutan, gorilla, chimpanzee) displayed transition points that foreshadowed the emergence of the early hominids. Postural trends toward uprightness and bipedalism were afforded by the translocation of the foramen magnum from the rear to the base of the skull to place it on top of the spinal column. The precision grip became refined as the thumb became opposable and the size and protrusion of the jaw structure were reduced.

Homology   Primates provide a framework of biological and behavioral systems of varying similarity to the human condition. The close genetic relationship between primate forms tends to ensure that structure–function relationships reflect homologous rather than analogous systems. It bears noting, for instance, that the genetic relationship between chimpanzees (*Pan*) and humans is closer than between chimpanzees and gorillas (*Gorilla*) (Andrews & Martin, 1987; Sarich, 1983; Sibley & Ahlquist, 1987).

Importance of Early Environment   Research published since the 1960s has documented the importance of *early* environment in the development of sensory and motor systems (Bryan & Riesen, 1989; Krech, Rosenzweig, & Bennett, 1962; Menzel, Davenport, & Rogers, 1970) as well as learning and memory (Greenough, Withers, & Wallace, 1990; Oden, Thompson, & Premack, 1990). Of special importance here is the evidence that strongly suggests that, as a positive function of species' brain complexity, impoverished rearing during the earliest months and years of life can compromise their social, sexual, and parental competence. Therefore, chimpanzees (Davenport, 1979) but not rhesus monkeys have irreversible deficits in their cognitive and transfer-of-learning abilities if reared as isolates in infancy (Davenport, Rogers, & Rumbaugh, 1973). By contrast, as is discussed later, being reared in a language-structured environment can foster language competencies, including speech comprehension, in chimpanzees in a pattern that parallels that of human children (Nelson, 1985, 1986; Savage-Rumbaugh, 1991; Savage-Rumbaugh et al., 1993).

Cartesian and Darwinian Perspectives of Mentality   The development of animal models for behavioral research has been substantially less than for biomedical and neuroscience research. This disparity is likely a continuing heritage from Descartes (1637/1956), who defined animals as *beast–machines*, void of rationality and feeling, on the premise that they had no souls. Pain was God's punishment, it was believed, for humans who sinned. Having souls, they were accountable for their deeds. Lacking souls, animals should not be held responsible for their actions; hence, they could not sin. Therefore, animals were declared incapable of *ever* experiencing pain because pain was God's retribution for sin, not for bad behavior. Similarities between animals and humans were acknowledged from the perspective of biology but not of psychology. Because a soul was believed necessary for rationality, thought, and cognitive competence and because animals were without souls, the study of their behavior was declared irrelevant to human psychology—a view still advanced by some contemporary authors (e.g., Kennedy, 1992).

The use of the word *mind* is also returning to the parlance of some areas of animal behavioral research. However, rather than spending time arguing about the presence or absence of "mind" in a literal way, we should concentrate on the necessary and indisputably legitimate task of determining the antecedents of complex behaviors and the processes on which they rest. *Mind* is neither a useful explanation nor antecedent; at best, the word references many highly complex behaviors that are *unlikely* to be understood as *reflexive*.

The distinctiveness of humans is now at issue. A basic tenet of this chapter is that Darwin (1871) was correct—*psychological* as well as biological continuities were carried forward as the forces of evolution produced first the hominids and eventually modern humans. For continuity to be advanced in principle, however, it must also be buttressed by evidence. What is the evidence for behavioral continuity? We continue first with a view of complex learning skills in relation to brain size and complexity.

MODE OF LEARNING, DIRECTIONAL TRANSFER, AND BRAIN COMPLEXITY

A *learning set* was initially defined by Harlow (1949) as a generalized form of positive transfer of learning that was a function of *experience*, not of innate intelligence. Learning sets are formed as a function of programmed experience—that is, of training on sets of problems of a given type or class (e.g., two-choice, object-quality visual discrimination problems).

The number of trials (six) on any one problem that Harlow used was initially insufficient for substantial learning by the subject. That notwithstanding, as more problems of a given class were presented, a new problem might be mastered as a result of the very first training trial. Harlow described the subject's change in learning from a mode of gradual improvement, reminiscent of the trial-and-error learning of Thorndike (1911/1970), to one that suggested *insight*—rapid learning of a kind advanced by Koehler (1925) and other Gestalt psychologists. Thus, the subjects' experience changed their learning curve from one that was sigmoidal to one that was discontinuous after the first trial.

The learning-set paradigm was very attractive because it offered a potential explanation of the origins of insight and creativity in terms of the contributions of general experiences, not just of heredity. The learning set proved sensitive to development (Zimmerman & Torrey, 1965) and to variations in human intelligence, particularly for individuals with mental retardation (for a review, see Kintz et al., 1969). Consequently, it was eagerly studied so that primate intelligence might be calibrated from a comparative perspective in terms relative to children's intelligence.

Standardized learning-set testing procedures entailed obvious research risks when applied to diverse primate species, such as the diminutive squirrel monkeys and the substantially larger macaque monkeys and great apes, because these procedures made no allowance among species for differences in size, manual dexterity, temperament, food preferences, sensory systems, and so forth. Accordingly, there was the risk that learning-set capacity might be biased in favor of the species with larger brains, more dexterous hands, and more voracious appetites—the more testable species (e.g., macaques, great apes). There were significant differences among species in learning-set skills that appeared to be related to brain size and complexity. There also were criterion-based training techniques that facilitated use of the learning set in the smaller primate species with relatively simple cortices (Rumbaugh, 1970). These observations encouraged a search for equitable measurements of competence among the diverse species of the order Primates.

Transfer Index

One means of obtaining an improved assay of comparative learning-set potential was defined by the Transfer Index (TI; Rumbaugh, 1970). TI procedures differed from those of the learning set in that subjects had to achieve specific *performance* criteria as a requisite to the administration of test trials, from which the most important measures were obtained. TI procedures assessed not only the subject's ability to transfer but also its ability to transfer operationally defined amounts of learning. Transfer skills are assessed in terms *relative* to the amount of learning to be transferred, not in terms of absolute levels or rates of learning. Accordingly, the TI is intended to serve as a relatively species-fair test of advanced cognitive operations.

Transfer-test trials were trials on which the cue valences of the stimulus objects were exchanged (i.e., reversed). Selection of the object that initially netted food now netted only an empty food well, whereas choosing the initially *incorrect* stimulus was now rewarded. Thus, artifactual differences among species in complex learning and even in differential levels of readiness to attend to and learn a series of two-choice discrimination problems were minimized by requiring that subjects first achieve operationally defined criteria of learning; only then would their ability to transfer that learning be tested.

This tactic worked well. Research affirmed that initial learning-to-criterion provided varying opportunities (i.e., numbers of trials per problem) to learn while fortuitously reserving transfer-test performance to be primarily a function of brain complexity and age, not simply an artifact of trials required to achieve the prior criteria. Two criterion-based training schedules were developed, on both of which the criterion level was only somewhat better than chance and well short of task mastery—the 67% and 84% levels, respectively.

Qualitatively Different Transfer of Learning in Interaction with Brain Complexity

TI testing with several different species (e.g., cat, prosimians, various taxa of New and Old World monkeys, lesser and great apes) affirmed the strong relationship between brain evolution and transfer of learning. Even more important, a qualitative difference emerged between the *direction* of transfer and how much learning had been afforded by the criterion-based training levels employed prior to tests of transfer.

Species with relatively small and simple brains gave evidence of increased *negative* transfer as the amount learned prior to the test trials increased from 67% to 84%! The more they had learned about the reinforcement values of the stimuli that composed a given discrimination problem, the *poorer* they did on transfer-test trials. Conversely, the species with relatively larger and more complex brains frequently manifested *positive transfer*; that is, they did better on the test trials when the criterion-based training level was advanced from 67% to 84% (see Figure 6.1). Therefore, the evolution of brain size and complexity afforded an important shift toward behavioral flexibility rather than rigidity.

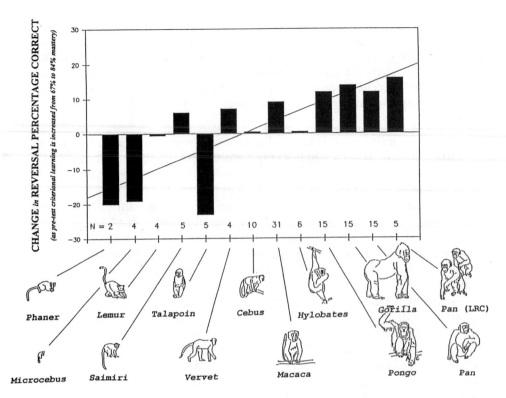

Figure 6.1.   The enhancement of transfer of learning in relation to brain complexity of primates ($N = 121$). The baseline of complexity is essentially a dimension of "extra" brain and neurons (see text). The vertical axis quantifies the *change* in the percentage of correct responses as a result of the pre–transfer test learning criterion being increased from 67% to 84% correct. Each point on the baseline is for a particular species, except for the one at the farthest right, which represents three language-competent chimpanzees and two bonobos at the Language Research Center (LRC). (See Cooper [1980] for data on *Phaner* and *Microcebus* and de Lillo and Visalberghi [1994] for data on capuchin monkeys included here. Also, see footnotes on page 117 for contributions of unpublished data from others.)

The quantitative analysis is based on comparisons of means among species. There was a high and positive correlation (Spearman $\rho = 0.79$) between the rank ordering of brain complexity and ability to transfer. Brain complexity had been adjudged on the basis of a broad reading of a variety of authors' studies of primates' brains. Fortuitously, the ranking of brain complexity subsequently was found to correlate very highly with H. Jerison's (personal communication, February 1995) estimations of the "extra neurons" ($\rho = 0.98$) and of "extra brain volume" ($\rho = 0.96$) afforded by encephalization. In turn, the y-axis values of Figure 6.1 correlated with *extra* brain volume ($r = .82$) and with *extra* neurons $r = .79$). Thus, the reader should basically equate brain complexity with extra brain/neurons afforded species by encephalization.

Emergent Processes

In proposing a schema for the interaction of transfer of learning and brain complexity, we may consider two hypothetical continua—one for brain complexity and a second one for transfer of training—along which increments are quantifiable. We may visualize a pointer that moves gradually from relatively simple to more complex brains as a second pointer moves from strong negative transfer to no transfer and then on to increasingly positive transfer. As these two dimensions are scaled in this manner, a *qualitative shift* has been obtained. Although increments in brain complexity are conceivably unidimensional and simply quantitative in this schema, the transfer of training effects as described is qualitative as well as quantitative: Whereas negative transfer *impedes* performance, positive transfer *facilitates* performance. Therefore, a model is suggested whereby qualitatively different changes in learning and behavior can be associated with or produced by quantitative evolutionary advances in the primate brain.

To be able to use (i.e., transfer) small amounts of learning or knowledge to an advantage can be important. It is evidence of flexibility. By contrast, negative transfer indicates behavioral inflexibility. To date, the best psychometric predictor of ability to master a wide variety of computer-monitored tasks in our research programs is the TI. Hence, within limits, it serves as the species-fair test of advanced and comprehensive cognitive operations for primates that it was designed to be.

I referred earlier to the contributions of rearing to competence and later elaborate on these in connection with the high TI average for the language-competent chimpanzees and bonobos of the Language Research Center (see Figure 6.1). Their performance levels may reflect the effects of rearing and their language skills because they were not selected for our research on the basis of any intuition about their intelligence.

Figure 6.1 corroborates the emergence of a very important *qualitative* advance, of *positive* transfer associated with amount learned in relation to brain size and complexity. It seemingly would have taken this kind of evolutionary advance to provide for the insightfulness, invention, and creativity that provide for human competence and culture. These attributes, generally considered prima facie evidence of high intelligence in humans, are far more common to the great apes than to monkeys and prosimians (Meador, Rumbaugh, Pate, & Bard, 1987) and probably reflect refinements in the cortex and prefrontal cortex.

Modes of Learning in Interaction with Brain Complexity

Was this contrasting outcome in transfer of learning in association with complexity of the primate brain solely a reflection of altered transfer-of-learning mechanisms, or was it also coupled with alteration in mode of learning? I have pursued the answer in part through use of the *mediational paradigm* (Rumbaugh, 1971).

On all problems, subjects were trained to a criterion of 9 of 10 trials correct, a level higher than that used during prior TI testing. Carrying forward the basic principle of the TI reversal test condition (where A+B− during training became A−B+ during transfer tests), I compared this transfer of learning with two other test conditions that entailed the substitution of cues. In one condition, the initially incorrect stimulus, which had just become the correct one on the first reversal test trial, was replaced by a novel stimulus (i.e., A+B− during training became A−C+ on the second and following reversal test trials). The second condition entailed substitution for the stimulus that during criterion-based training had been reinforced (i.e., A+B− during training became C−B+ on the second and following reversal test trials). Table 6.1 presents a summary of the training and three test conditions.

The logic for the substitution was as follows. If the pretest criterion had been achieved through basic stimulus–response habit learning, then transfer of learning should be most difficult in the condition that paralleled the TI test condition (where A+B− becomes and remains A−B+ for all reversal test trials). The subject

Table 6.1. Associative versus mediational learning paradigm

Acquisition	Reversal trial	Reversal trials
Learn to 9/10 correct with	1	2–11
		A–B+ (control)
A+B−	A−B+	C–B+
		A–C+

Note: A, B, and C each refer to different stimuli.

animal would have to extinguish its preference for the initially correct stimulus (A+), which had just become the incorrect one (A−), on the first test trial. It also would have to overcome the inhibition accrued to B− as a result of nonreinforced selection of B during training. Both of these processes take time and trials and would reduce the percentage of correct responses during test.

Just the opposite would be the case for subjects as they encountered the other conditions that entailed replacement of stimuli. If after the first test trial the initially *incorrect* stimulus were replaced (e.g., B, which became + on the first test, is discarded and is replaced with a novel stimulus, C+, resulting in A−C+ on all ensuing test trials), then subjects would not have to overcome their inhibition to selection of B, although they would have to extinguish their preference for A, the initially correct stimulus. Rather, choice of the new and novel stimulus C+ would be uncompromised and reinforced promptly. Conversely, if the initially correct stimulus, A, were discarded and replaced with C− after the first test trial, then the subject would only have to overcome its reticence to select B. Extinction of habit A was obviated because all test trials then consisted of C−B+.

It is important that the reader note, first, that the critical data from this study come from the *relative* performance levels within species on these three kinds of test trials. Second, it should be noted that all of these subjects had extensive histories of discrimination learning research and, therefore, should have been giving their best performances.

On the assumption that brain evolution might avail more of a comprehensive, relational mode of learning rather than only one of stimulus–response habit formation, it was predicted that primates with more complex brains might find all three conditions equivalent in difficulty. After all, adequate information was present for the subject to select the stimulus to be reinforced on all but the first reversal-of-cues test trial (i.e., A−B+), which was unannounced. Hence, the following strategy would support accurate choice: If, on test trials, A were present, then it was to be *avoided*; if B were present, then it was to be *selected* (Rumbaugh & Pate, 1984).

The data supported these expectations. The smaller-brained primates' performances indicated that they were basic stimulus–response habit learners. By contrast, the apes found all test conditions equally easy. Furthermore, as the brains were graded as becoming increasingly complex across an array of species, accuracy levels gradually became higher, although not so high as to define a ceiling effect. The group of bright apes was composed of subjects that had extraordinarily high TI values. Two language-skilled chimpanzees, Sherman and Austin (Savage-Rumbaugh, 1986), did best of all in terms of overall accuracy, a suggestion that language might help mediate the complexities of relational learning (Figure 6.2).

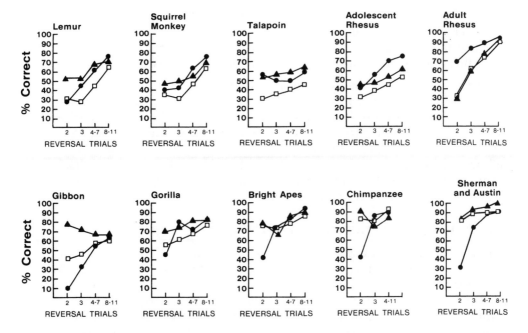

Figure 6.2.   The evolution of mediational learning in relation to brain complexity. (□——□ = A−B+, ●——● = C−B+, ▲——▲ = C+A−.) Here it is the relative difficulty of test conditions within a species and not the absolute levels of accuracy across species that are the most important data. That the three transfer-of-learning conditions were differentially difficult for the species with the relatively less complex or immature brains or both is interpreted to mean that they learned their prior two-choice visual discrimination problems as stimulus–response habits or associations. By contrast, the species with the more complex brains, notably the great apes, tended to learn in a relational manner that served to render all three test conditions equally easy or difficult. The graph on the bottom right is for Sherman and Austin, two language-competent chimpanzees. Their enhanced performance is attributed to their extensive research participation and language competence. The data for "bright apes" are from apes that were superior on their prior TI tests. (Refer to text for details of the training and test conditions.)

If we ask what animals can tell us about cognition and behavior in relation to evolution of the brain and an elaborated cortex, the following points afford at least partial answers:

- Learning becomes more rapid and flexible.
- Transfer of training is more likely to be advantageous, even if only a small amount of knowledge is subject to transfer.
- Learning is more likely to be relational, overarching, and rule based than it is to be of a stimulus–response format.
- The capacity for developing abilities to focus attention and to shift it in a controlled, adaptive manner is markedly enhanced.

With increasing brain complexity and elaboration of the cortex, notably in the great apes and humans, there are important advances in the capacity to break old stimulus–response associations and to supplant them with relational patterns of learning. High TI values clearly rest on the ability of subjects to *shift* their choice of objects subsequent to the first trial of transfer testing, the trial on which the cue values are changed. The same is true for subjects' ability to find all three reversal test conditions equivalent in the mediational paradigm. The ability to shift choice in this manner is held by Mirsky (1996) to be a function relatively specific to the prefrontal cortex, including the anterior cingulate gyrus. Therefore, it is suggested that, as primate brains become larger and more complex, the prefrontal cortex becomes inceasingly proficient in the service of behavioral flexibility.

Protracted Training Can Change Mode of Learning

Other research has affirmed that, given extended learning experience, some species noted primarily for stimulus–response learning, particularly those of the genus *Macaca*, eventually shift to relational learning patterns that otherwise are generally found among the great apes and humans (Washburn & Rumbaugh, 1992b). This finding suggests that the learning modes of children with learning disabilities might similarly be advanced by special regimens of learning that emphasize complex relationships and overarching principles.

SYMBOLIC COMPETENCE, COMPLEXITY, AND PLASTICITY

Cross-Modal Skills and Language

Complex symbolic operations are not unique to *Homo sapiens*. The abilities of great apes to perform accurately on Trial 1 tests of novel cross-modal perceptions (e.g., from touch to vision and vice versa) (Davenport & Rogers, 1970) likely provide an important part of the foundations for symbolism and representational thought more generally. From the perspective developed by Mirsky (1996), these kinds of skills must entail all of the various attentional functions that his factor-analytical studies have defined—the abilities to *focus/execute, sustain, stabilize, shift,* and *encode*. In coordination with the prefrontal cortex, however, a number of other cortical areas and brain structures—including those of the rostral midbrain, the midline–thalamic and brainstem structures, and those of the hippocampus and amygdala—are involved (Mirsky, 1996).

It is important to note that language-competent apes are able to select by touching or feeling the referent objects that are represented only by the word-symbols presented to them visually (Savage-Rumbaugh, Sevcik, & Hopkins, 1988). A related study with the chimpanzee Lana (Rumbaugh, 1977) demonstrated that she did substantially better in declaring whether a palpated, out-of-sight object was or was not the same as the object presented visually if the objects had names. Therefore, symbols extend the dimensions of cross-modal perceptions in the apes to areas germane to language.

Other relevant observations were afforded by the language-trained chimpanzees Sherman and Austin (Savage-Rumbaugh, 1986), who were able to categorize 17 word-lexigrams according to whether they represented a food or a tool item on Trial 1 controlled tests. If those 17 word-lexigrams had not served as symbolic representations of the various foods (e.g., raisin, sweet potatoes) and tools (e.g., lever, wrench, stick) to the chimpanzees, it is difficult to conceive how they could have determined the correct conceptual category for each one. These kinds of findings are but selections of a vast literature that documents ways whereby the formation and conceptual use of symbols can operate richly in the great apes. Because these operations surely provide the basic foundations for the processes of human thinking and reasoning, they merit continued study.

Statements of Imminent Actions

Sherman and Austin also "announced" which of several food items they would retrieve after they had inspected a limited array of randomly selected foods and drinks (Savage-Rumbaugh, Pate, Lawson, Smith, & Rosenbaum, 1983). On their first visit to the array of items, they made a choice that they next identified at their keyboard. If their declared choice was then retrieved on their return visit, the chimpanzees were praised and permitted to consume it. Sherman and Austin did this task with about 90% concurrence between lexigrams used and items retrieved. It bears emphasizing that, as they did this task, they used symbols to declare their *future* courses of action (Rumbaugh, Savage-Rumbaugh, & Washburn, 1994).

Social Learning Enhanced in Language-Competent Apes

Contrary to common belief, neither monkeys nor apes are generally noted by trained observers for acts of imitation. By contrast, the apes with language skills can learn quite readily to attempt replication or emulation of actions demonstrated as models to them. "Educated apes," as they have been called by Tomasello and his colleagues (Tomasello, Savage-Rumbaugh, & Kruger, 1993), are clearly superior in observational learning and modeling behaviors when compared with other chimpanzees reared in standard laboratory conditions. Such competence was impressively manifested by Kanzi (*Pan paniscus*) as he learned, by observation, the principles of stone flaking and fabricating sharp stone chips, which he then used to cut ropes and gain access to incentives (see Figure 6.3; Toth, Shick, Savage-Rumbaugh, Sevcik, & Rumbaugh, 1993). This also was the case for Sherman and Austin (both *Pan troglodytes*) in learning how to use joysticks (Savage-Rumbaugh, 1986).

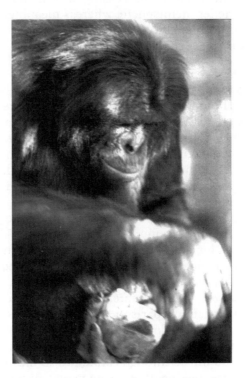

Figure 6.3.   Kanzi (a bonobo) makes flakes from flint and uses them to cut ropes and cables to open puzzle boxes. His skills as a knapper were acquired by observation. (Courtesy of R.A. Sevcik.)

It is important that we achieve a better understanding of social learning, observational learning, and even imitation because, as discussed next, apes garner a great deal of complex knowledge and competence through these processes during infancy—even competence for language.

ANIMALS AND LANGUAGE

Questions pertaining to the requisites for language (Krasnegor, Rumbaugh, Schiefelbusch, & Studdert-Kennedy, 1991) and animal language research (Parker & Gibson, 1990; Roitblat, Herman, & Nachtigall, 1993; Savage-Rumbaugh & Lewin, 1994) are enjoying a productive renaissance. Dolphins have carried out novel requests (Herman, Pack, & Morrel-Samuels, 1993); sea lions have learned the referents for new hand signals apparently on the basis of exclusion (e.g., hand signs, given by the experimenter when new objects are introduced, are learned as their "names") (Schusterman, Gisiner, Grimm, & Hanggi, 1993); a parrot responds to questions regarding multiple characteristics of objects (Pepperberg, 1993); and great apes (*Gorilla, Pan*, and *Pongo*) learn symbol sets (e.g., hand signals, plastic tokens, geometric symbols) for communicating with humans and for problem solving (Fouts & Fouts, 1989; Gardner & Gardner, 1969; Gardner, Gardner, & Van Cantfort, 1989; Matsuzawa, 1990; Miles, 1990; Patterson & Linden, 1981; Premack & Premack, 1983; Rumbaugh, 1977; Terrace, 1979). Although the topic is beyond the scope of this chapter, it should be noted that language-competent chimpanzees show *cerebral lateralization* in the processing of symbols. Meaningful lexigrams are processed best by the left hemisphere, whereas meaningless ones are processed equally well by either hemisphere (Hopkins & Morris, 1989; Hopkins, Morris, Savage-Rumbaugh, & Rumbaugh, 1992).

Language Abilities of the Great Apes

The most recent reports are of chimpanzees and bonobos (both of the genus *Pan*) coming to comprehend human speech—novel sentences of request as well as single words. Of particular significance is the fact that these apes acquired their language competencies *not* by specific teaching or training but naturally and with apparent spontaneity through the course of being reared from shortly after birth in a language-structured environment (Savage-Rumbaugh, Brakke, & Hutchins, 1992). This environment emphasized the use of lexigram keyboards in coordination with human speech to describe things and to organize activities. Thus, language served as an important predictor of future events and narrator of the present for apes much as it does for the human child (Bruner, 1972; Lock, 1980). The apes came to *comprehend* both speech and lexigrams before they *produced* language via lexigrams, a pattern reminiscent of the one whereby normal children acquire language—where comprehension precedes production (i.e., speech).

Sentence Comprehension Kanzi's sentence comprehension at the age of about 8 years was assessed in direct comparison with a 2.5-year-old human child, Alia (Savage-Rumbaugh et al., 1993). Controls for the test trials (415 for Kanzi; 407 for Alia) entailed having the experimenter sit behind a one-way vision mirror with attendants listening to loud music through earphones so they could not hear the test sentences. Throughout the testing, there were varied arrays of objects on the floor in front of the subjects with which they might work.

An important control was that the subjects were asked to fulfill a variety of requests with the items of any given set so that it could not be argued that the subjects were asked only to carry out "obvious" actions (e.g., to hit a nail with a hammer) and thereby be speciously "correct." Generally, there were duplicate items so that, for instance, Kanzi had to get item X from location Y, even though there was another identical item X in front of him.

Seven different sentence types were given. Type 1 entailed asking that object X be placed in or on a transportable versus nontransportable object Y (e.g., "Put the milk in the water," "Put the backpack on the Fourtrax"). Type 2 sentences required subjects to "Give [or Show] object X to animate A" (e.g., "Give Rose a carrot"); "Give object X and object Y to animate A" (e.g., "Give the peas and the beans to Kelly"); "Do action A on animate A" (e.g., "Hide the gorilla"); and "Do action A on animate A with object X" (e.g., "Make the snake bite Linda"). Type 3 sentences required subjects to "Do action A on object X (with object Y)" (e.g. "Bite the picture of the oil," "Stab your ball with the sparklers"). Type 4 sentences announced impending events in which the subjects were to engage, such as "Alia is going to chase Mommy," whereupon she was to do so. Type 5 sentences asked that object X be taken to location Y (e.g., "Take the can opener to the bedroom"); that subjects go to location Y and get object X (e.g., "Go to the microwave and get the tomato"); and that subjects go get object X that is in location Y (e.g., "Get the telephone that's outdoors"). Type 6 sentences asked subjects to pretend that animate A does action B on recipient Y (e.g., "Can you make the bug bite the doggie?"). Type 7 sentences consisted of all other variations on the previous categories (e.g., "Take the potato outdoors and get the apple"). On the controlled trials, Kanzi (age 8 years) was 74% correct (307 of 415 sentences), and Alia (age 2.5 years) was 66% correct (267 of 407 sentences). The overall difference between them was not statistically reliable, although both subjects were well above chance levels in their individual performances.

Other studies addressed the issue of word order directly through the use of three kinds of reversals (e.g., "Take the potato outdoors" versus "Go outdoors and get the potato"; "Put the doggie in the refrigerator" versus "Go get the dog that's in the refrigerator"; "Put the shoe in the raisins" versus "Put the raisins in the shoe"). Overall, Kanzi (71 of 88 responses correct; 81%) was better than Alia (53 of 83 responses correct; 64%) on reversal sentences, although both of them were sensitive to word order as well as to semantic and syntactic cues.

Sentence Production   Greenfield and Savage-Rumbaugh (1991, 1993) found that Kanzi's productive competence (e.g., his use of lexigrams in combination with gestures) was comparable to that of a 1.5-year-old child. Although some of Kanzi's grammatical rules were modeled after those used by his human caregivers, he invented others of his own. For example, Kanzi formed his own rule for combining agent *gesture* with an action *lexigram*: Place *lexigrams* first (e.g., Kanzi would ask a caregiver to go hide by using the lexigram, LIZ, and then gesture HIDE by placing his hand over his eyes).

Methodology accepted for child language studies indicated that Kanzi's two-element combinations (lexigram–lexigram and lexigram–gesture) were classifiable according to their semantic relations, such as agent–action and action–object. Although Kanzi's use of grammar designed to alter meaning was limited, it frequently occurred in social games. When playing "chase," for instance, he would first designate the person to do the chasing by putting his hand on the person. Next, by hand, he would lead the agent selected to do the chasing over to the person to be chased and place the agent's hand on that person; then Kanzi would take a vantage point, as on a tree branch, to observe "the game." Thus Kanzi selected both the agent and the recipient of action, and his choice of persons for these roles changed frequently and unpredictably.

Summary Kanzi's comprehension of spoken English was commensurate with that of a 2.5-year-old child and his production commensurate with that of a 1.5-year-old child—a competence that was instated *without* formal training programs. Bates (1993) assessed the study as "a fair test of the hypothesis that apes are capable of at least some language comprehension, at both the lexical and the structural levels," and concluded that at least one bonobo "is capable of language comprehension that approximates (in level if not in detail) the abilities of a human 2-year-old on the threshold of full-blown sentence processing" (pp. 222–223; see also Bates, Thal, & Marchman, 1991, for an evolutionary perspective of language). Given that the keyboard is, at best, a poor substitute for speech, one wonders how Kanzi's utterances might have been increased in grammar and syntax as well had he been able to speak.

In contrast to Kanzi's spontaneous acquisition of the capacity for speech comprehension, lexigram meaning, and lexigram usage was his mother's *inability* to learn. Matata, his mother, was a wild-born female bonobo who dwelled in the forest until an estimated age of 6 years. Even with protracted training, she failed to use even a small number of lexigrams reliably and gave no evidence that these few served as symbolic representations. Matata's inability to learn language is believed to be the consequence of her feral early rearing. By the time she was given the opportunity to learn language in our laboratory, her cognition had already been structured in ways that pertained to the forest—none of which entailed lexigrams and computers.

A Sensitive Age for Language Acquisition
The accomplishments of Kanzi and his sisters, Panbanisha and Panzee, stand in contrast with those obtained with all other apes in language research where specific instruction cultivated language skills in other apes. Their data strongly suggest that a sensitive period exists during infancy for language acquisition both for children (Greenough, Black, & Wallace, 1987; Greenough et al., 1990) and for apes (Rumbaugh, Hopkins, Washburn, & Savage-Rumbaugh, 1991). Exposure to language, including speech, especially during the first few months of life, is critical if the acquisition of language is to be optimal (Savage-Rumbaugh et al., 1993; Velichkovsky & Rumbaugh, 1996). Opportunity to observe language use and its consequences in the social contexts of everyday life appears to be more effective in the acquisition of language than are event-specific reinforcements of language productions (Lock, 1978, 1980), be they speech or use of a lexigram-embossed keyboard. Through the course of such observations, the apes first came to *comprehend* language—as does the human child long before the speech musculature has matured enough for competent speech (Golinkoff, Hirsh-Pasek, Cauley, & Gordon, 1987).

Animal Models and Child Language Acquisition
Mental retardation, a consequence of brain damage, frequently is reflected in both language acquisition and use. Whether research with ape models might yield new insights into the processes of language acquisition and facilitate both research and remediation of language deficits of people with mental retardation was a question addressed in the Lana Project when first proposed in 1970 (Figure 6.4).

The invention of the highly successful computer-monitored, symbol-embossed keyboard for that project established principles that are reflected in the design of

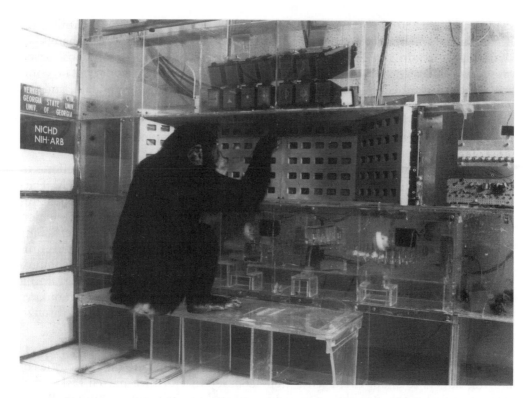

Figure 6.4.   Lana (a chimpanzee) at her computer-monitored keyboard. (Courtesy of F. Kiernan, Yerkes Primate Center, circa 1974.)

units now commercially produced to provide alternative language systems where speech is limited. It is significant that, when the teaching tactics that were generated in the Lana, Sherman and Austin, and Kanzi Projects were extended to special education human populations in need of language assistance, parallel findings were obtained (Romski & Sevcik, 1991; Romski, Sevcik, & Pate, 1988; Romski, Sevcik, & Rumbaugh, 1985). As posited during the inception of the Lana Project, any program that might successfully instate language skills in a species (e.g., *Pan*) otherwise not characterized by language competence should provide insights of benefit to human need (Rumbaugh, 1977). This view has been corroborated by three longitudinal studies—symbolic and language skills have been cultivated in children and young adults who otherwise had failed to learn language. Their achievements ranged from the mastery of a small symbol vocabulary to formulating requests, making comments on surrounding events, engaging in conversations, expressing social graces, and communicating in the workplace and community (Romski & Sevcik, 1991).

COMPUTERS AND PROGRESS IN ANIMAL MODEL RESEARCH
Many of the findings reviewed earlier have been made possible through technological advances in the use of computers. Two of the more important ones have been the development of the computer-monitored keyboard (Rumbaugh, 1977) for language research and the development of the Language Research Center's Computerized Test System (LRC-CTS), which presents any of a wide variety of tasks to an equally broad array of primates and humans in a video-formatted context (Richard-

son, Washburn, Hopkins, Savage-Rumbaugh, & Rumbaugh, 1990; Rumbaugh, Richardson, Washburn, Savage-Rumbaugh, & Hopkins, 1989; Rumbaugh & Williams, 1992). In the LRC-CTS, stimuli are generated, selected, and positioned on-screen randomly and may either move about or remain stationary. The computer and software control all aspects of each task, the collection of data, and the delivery of pellets and associated auditory feedback to reinforce correct responses. Consideration now is given to specific advances enabled by computers and by the LRC-CTS and to the ways in which these advances have served to broaden our understanding of the roots of human competence.

The development of the LRC-CTS is best understood in light of past efforts to automate the manually operated Wisconsin General Test Apparatus (WGTA) (Harlow, 1949). Numerous attempts had been made to automate the WGTA for the investigation of learning and memory in primates (for a review, see Meyer, Treichler, & Meyer, 1965). Such attempts basically failed, however, because the efficient learning and performance by the subjects in WGTA-conducted research was uniformly lost. In contrast, the LRC-CTS constitutes a system that does not compromise the subjects' performances, even on Harlow's classic learning-set training (Washburn & Rumbaugh, 1992b). Performance levels reported for rhesus monkeys tested in the LRC-CTS have been comparable or superior to those obtained through use of the WGTA (Washburn, Hopkins, & Rumbaugh, 1989).

Rhesus Super-Learning
Even the rhesus monkey has demonstrated its ability to calculate the trajectories of moving targets to shoot them with high accuracy in video-formatted task situations, a predictor-operator ability thought previously to be uniquely human (Washburn & Rumbaugh, 1992a). Such skill entails attention to multiple dimensions of a complex test—the loci of the target, target speed, elevation of the target relative to the subject's turret, and the calculation of a vector that, given the observed "bullet speed," will interdict the target with precision.

In addition, Washburn and Rumbaugh (1991) reported that rhesus monkeys readily learn the ordinal ranks of the Arabic numerals 0–9 in a fashion that suggests a matrix of relative values. In tests, the monkeys were able to choose the larger of two numerals on several *novel* pairings of those numerals. This complex relational learning occurred without penalty of choice during training in that, *regardless* of which numeral was selected, the monkeys got a corresponding quantity of pellets of food. They were not required to choose the larger numeral to be rewarded (see Figure 6.5).

Complex abilities of these kinds may be viewed as emergent, qualitatively unique properties provided by the quantitative enhancements of the brain, discussed earlier. Although prevalent in humans and great apes, such abilities are not uniquely theirs. Rhesus monkeys and, to a lesser degree, capuchin monkeys surely have some claim to them. However, to date, no one has reported other than the most constrained expressions of these kinds of competence in the smaller New and Old World monkeys or in the prosimians, in which the brain and cortex are relatively smaller and simpler. Indeed, even the probability that such subjects can learn to use the joystick to execute other than the simpler video-formatted tasks is low (Andrews & Rosenblum, 1994).

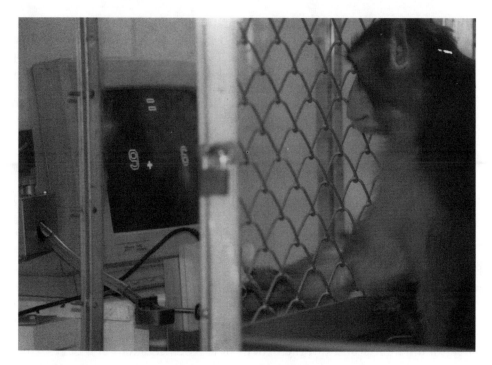

Figure 6.5.   A rhesus monkey at work on the LRC-CTS on the number task. (Courtesy of D.A. Washburn and J. Gulledge.)

Overview of the LRC-CTS

Research with the LRC-CTS has revealed a number of other interesting findings:

- Rhesus monkeys readily learn a battery of 30 or more tasks that range among learning, memory, eye–hand coordination, prediction, planning, and vigilance; and they can switch rapidly between these tasks in routine testing.
- Rhesus monkeys work best in social contexts, in the presence of other monkeys with whom they are familiar.
- Rhesus monkeys prefer to work for incentives through use of the LRC-CTS rather than receive incentives for free.
- Rhesus monkeys' performance on the TI and the number of trials that they work each day are the best psychometric and performance predictors, respectively, of training performance on a comprehensive battery of tasks.
- Rhesus monkeys who respond quickly and have short choice reaction times are generally better in making two-choice decisions than are those who are slower.
- Numerals are treated by the rhesus monkeys as symbols, indicated, for instance, by symbolic distance effects revealed in performance on relative numerousness tasks.
- Rhesus monkeys manifest characteristics of selective attention similar to those of humans (e.g., Strooplike interference, stimulus movement effects, and pop-out versus set-size effects in visual search).

- Rhesus monkeys have the capacity to maintain visual forms or sequences in working memory and show disruption by variables such as distractor activity.
- Unlike chimpanzees and humans, rhesus monkeys appear to process visuospatial stimuli equally well with either the left or the right cerebral hemisphere (Hopkins & Morris, 1989; Hopkins, Washburn, & Rumbaugh, 1990).
- Handedness for joystick manipulation is strongly established in rhesus monkeys, and right-handed monkeys tend to be more facile learners than left-handed monkeys (Hopkins, Washburn, Berke, & Williams, 1992).
- Rhesus monkeys, like humans and dolphins, show evidence of monitoring their uncertainty and similar metacognitive abilities (Schull, Smith, Washburn, & Shields, 1994).
- Rhesus monkeys remember sequences of stimuli at levels comparable to 5- to 7-year-old children.
- Rhesus monkeys learn icons that represent various tasks, and work more quickly and accurately when they can choose tasks on which to work.

The LRC-CTS software maintains an animal's attention and permits subjects to pace their own work. Generally, the screen is without movement and sound *until* the monkey uses the joystick. Subjects work and rest ad libitum during each test day; thus, data are obtained when each subject is motivated. It is common for subjects to produce 1,000–2,000 responses a day, which enables them to participate in a number of different studies to the benefit of their enrichment and of research as well.

These and other findings discussed previously indicate that manifest intelligence of animals is in no small measure contingent upon the technology and testing procedures employed in training and assessment. In turn, it is suggested that the rhesus monkey's proficiency in the kinds of tasks discussed earlier, coupled with brain imaging technology and the cost-effectiveness of the LRC-CTS for intensive behavioral assessments, offers great opportunity for future research that will help identify the individual and coordinated roles of various brain structures as they function in support of the prefrontal cortex and manifest behavioral flexibility (Armstrong, 1990a, 1990b; Mirsky, 1996; Pribram, 1991; Rakic, 1988).

CONCLUSIONS

The order Primates provides a broad and somewhat orderly array of about 200 species that differ widely in morphology, body weight, brain size and cortical complexity, and degrees of encephalization (Martin, 1990). Their study is vital to our understanding of human competence.

The evolution and development of the primate brain and perhaps the prefrontal cortex in particular provides for enhancement of 1) motor repertoires, relational learning, controlled attention, memory, and transfer of learning to an adaptive advantage; 2) learning by observation rather than action; and 3) learning of comprehensive, overarching relationships rather than specific associative responses.

With advanced brain complexity, the structure of early environmental patterns of stimuli and styles of rearing can have differential and pervasive effects on the development of specific cognitive skills, interests, and social preferences that might not be manifest until later stages of development. Similarly, the emergence of speech comprehension and advanced levels of symbolic operations that provide the foundations of language are clearly dependent upon early language-structured rearing experiences—even in apes.

REFERENCES

Andrews, M., & Rosenblum, L.A. (1994). Automated recording of individual performance and hand preference during joystick-task acquisition in group-living bonnet macaques (*Macaca radiata*). *Journal of Comparative Psychology, 108,* 358–362.

Andrews, P., & Martin, L. (1987). Cladistic relationships of extant and fossil hominoids. *Journal of Human Evolution, 16,* 101–108.

Armstrong, E. (1990a). Evolution of the brain. In G. Paxinus (Ed.), *The human nervous system* (pp. 1–16). New York: Academic Press.

Armstrong, E. (1990b). The limbic system and culture: An allometric analysis of the neocortex and limbic nuclei. *Human Nature, 2,* 117–136.

Barkley, R.A. (1996). Linkages between attention and executive functions. In G.R. Lyon & N.A. Krasnegor (Eds.), *Attention, memory, and executive function* (pp. 307–325). Baltimore: Paul H. Brookes Publishing Co.

Bates, E. (1993). Comprehension and production in early language environment: A commentary on Savage-Rumbaugh, Murphy, Sevcik, Brakke, Williams, & Rumbaugh, "Language comprehension in ape and child." *Monographs of the Society for Research in Child Development, 58*(2–3), 222–242.

Bates, E., Thal, D., & Marchman, V. (1991). Symbols and syntax: A Darwinian approach to language development. In N.A. Krasnegor, D.M. Rumbaugh, R.L. Schiefelbusch, & M. Studdert-Kennedy (Eds.), *Biological and behavioral determinants of language development* (pp. 29–65). Hillsdale, NJ: Lawrence Erlbaum Associates.

Bruner, J. (1972). Nature and uses of immaturity. *American Psychologist, 27,* 687–708.

Bryan, G.K., & Riesen, A.H. (1989). Deprived somatosensory-motor experience in stumptailed monkey neocortex: Dendritic spine density and dendritic ring of layer IIIb pyramidal cells. *Journal of Comparative Neurology, 286,* 208–217.

Byrne, R.W. (1996). Relating brain size to intelligence in primates. In P.A. Mellars & K.R. Gibson (Eds.), *The early human mind* (pp. 49–56). Cambridge, CA: McDonald Institute for Archaeological Research.

Cooper, H.M. (1980). Ecological correlates of visual learning in nocturnal prosimians. In P. Charles-Dominique, H.M. Cooper, A. Hladik, C.M. Hladik, E. Pages, G.F. Pariente, A. Petter-Rousseaux, J.J. Peter, & A. Schilling (Eds.), *Nocturnal Malagasy primates* (pp. 191–203). New York: Academic Press.

Darwin, C. (1871). *The descent of man—and selection in relation to sex.* London: Murray.

Davenport, R.K. (1979). Some behavioral disturbances of great apes in captivity. In D. Hamburg & E.R. McCown (Eds.), *The great apes* (pp. 341–356). Menlo Park, CA: Benjamin/Cummings.

Davenport, R.K., & Rogers, C.W. (1970). Intermodal equivalence of stimuli in apes. *Science, 168,* 279–280.

Davenport, R.K., Rogers, C.W., & Rumbaugh, D.M. (1973). Long-term cognitive deficits in chimpanzees associated with early impoverished rearing. *Developmental Psychology, 9,* 343–347.

Deacon, T.W. (1997). *The symbolic species.* New York: Norton.

de Lillo, C., & Visalberghi, E. (1994). Transfer index and mediational learning in tufted capuchins (cebus-apella). *International Journal of Primatology, 15,* 275–288.

Descartes, R. (1956). *Discourse on method* (L.J. Lafleur, trans.). New York: Liberal Arts Press. (Original work published 1637)

Finlay, B.L., & Darlington, R.B. (1995). Linked regularities in the development and evolution of mammalian brains. *Science, 265,* 1578–1584.

Fouts, R.S., & Fouts, D.H. (1989). Loulis in conversation with the cross-fostered chimpanzees. In R.A. Gardner, B.T. Gardner, & T.E. Van Cantfort (Eds.), *Teaching sign language to chimpanzees* (pp. 293–307). New York: State University of New York Press.

Gardner, R.A., & Gardner, B.T. (1969). Teaching sign language to a chimpanzee. *Science, 165,* 664–672.

Gardner, R.A., Gardner, B.T., & Van Cantfort, T.E. (Eds.). (1989). *Teaching sign language to chimpanzees.* New York: State University of New York Press.

Gibson, K. (1986). Cognition, brain size, and the extraction of embedded food resources. In J. Else & P.C. Lee (Eds.), *Primate ontogeny, cognition, and social behavior.* Cambridge, England: Cambridge University Press.

Golinkoff, R.M., Hirsh-Pasek, K., Cauley, K.M., & Gordon, L. (1987). The eyes have it: Lexical and syntactic comprehension in a new paradigm. *Journal of Child Language, 14,* 23–45.

Greenfield, P., & Savage-Rumbaugh, E.S. (1991). Imitation, grammatical development, and the invention of protogrammar by an ape. In N.A. Krasnegor, D.M. Rumbaugh, R.L. Schiefelbusch, & M. Studdert-Kennedy (Eds.), *Biological and behavioral determinants of language development* (pp. 235–258). Hillsdale, NJ: Lawrence Erlbaum Associates.

Greenfield, P., & Savage-Rumbaugh, E.S. (1993). Comparing communicative competence in child and chimp: The pragmatics of repetition. *Journal of Child Language, 20,* 1–26.

Greenough, W.T., Black, J.E., & Wallace, C.S. (1987). Experience and brain development. *Child Development, 58,* 539–559.

Greenough, W.T., Withers, G.S., & Wallace, C.S. (1990). Morphological changes in the nervous system arising from behavioral experience: What is the evidence that they are involved in learning and memory? In L.R. Squire & E. Lindenlaub (Eds.), *The biology of memory* (Symposia Medica Hoechst, Vol. 23, pp. 59–84). Stuttgart, Germany: F.K. Schattauder Verlag.

Harlow, H.F. (1949). The formation of learning sets. *Psychological Review, 56,* 51–65.

Herman, L.M., Pack, A.A., & Morrel-Samuels, P. (1993). Representational and conceptual skills of dolphins. In H. Roitblat, L.M. Herman, & P.E. Nachtigall (Eds.), *Language and communication: Comparative perspectives* (pp. 403–442). Hillsdale, NJ: Lawrence Erlbaum Associates.

Hopkins, W.D., & Morris, R.D. (1989). Laterality for visual-spatial processing in two language trained chimpanzees (*Pan troglodytes*). *Behavioral Neuroscience, 103,* 227–234.

Hopkins, W.D., Morris, R.D., Savage-Rumbaugh, E.S., & Rumbaugh, D.M. (1992). Hemispheric priming by meaningful and nonmeaningful symbols in language-trained chimpanzees (*Pan troglodytes*): Further evidence of a left hemisphere advantage. *Behavioral Neuroscience, 106,* 575–582.

Hopkins, W.D., Washburn, D.A., Berke, L., & Williams, M. (1992). Behavioral asymmetries of psychomotor performance in rhesus monkeys: A dissociation between hand-preference and skill. *Journal of Comparative Psychology, 106,* 392–397.

Hopkins, W.D., Washburn, D.A., & Rumbaugh, D.M. (1990). Processing of form stimuli presented unilaterally to humans, chimpanzees (*Pan troglodytes*), and monkeys (*Macaca mulatta*). *Behavioral Neuroscience, 104,* 577–584.

Jerison, H.J. (1985). On the evolution of mind. In D.A. Oakley (Ed.), *Brain and mind* (pp. 1–31). London: Methuen.

Kennedy, J.S. (1992). *The new anthropomorphism.* Cambridge, England: Cambridge University Press.

Kintz, B.L., Foster, M.S., Hart, J.O., O'Malley, J.J., Palmer, E.L., & Sullivan, S.L. (1969). A comparison of learning sets in humans, primates, and subprimates. *Journal of General Psychology, 80,* 189–204.

Koehler, W. (1925). *The mentality of apes.* New York: Harcourt, Brace.

Krasnegor, N.A., Rumbaugh, D.M., Schiefelbusch, R.L., & Studdert-Kennedy, A.M. (Eds.). (1991). *Biological and behavioral determinants of language development.* Hillsdale, NJ: Lawrence Erlbaum Associates.

Krech, D., Rosenzweig, M.R., & Bennett, E.L. (1962). Relations between brain chemistry and problem solving among rats raised in enriched and impoverished environments. *Journal of Comparative and Physiological Psychology, 55,* 801.

Le Gros Clark. (1959). *The antecedents of man.* Edinburgh: Edinburgh University Press.

Lock, A. (Ed.). (1978). *Action, gesture to symbol: The emergence of language.* New York: Academic Press.

Lock, A. (1980). *The guided reinvention of language.* New York: Academic Press.

Martin, R.D. (1990). *Primate origins and evolution: A phylogenetic reconstruction.* London: Chapman and Hall.

Matsuzawa, T. (1990). *The perceptual world of a chimpanzee.* Project no. 63510057, Kyoto University, Kyoto, Japan. Inuyama, Aichi, 484 Japan.

Meador, D.M., Rumbaugh, D.M., Pate, J.L., & Bard, K.A. (1987). Learning, problem solving, cognition, and intelligence. In G. Mitchell (Ed.), *Comparative primate biology: Vol. 2. Behavior and ecology* (pp. 17–83). New York: Alan R. Liss.

Menzel, E.W., Jr., Davenport, R.K., & Rogers, C.M. (1970). The development of tool using in wild-born and restriction-reared chimpanzees. *Folia Primatologica, 12,* 273–283.

Meyer, D.R., Treichler, F.R., & Meyer, P.M. (1965). Discrete trial training techniques and stimulus variables. In A.M. Schrier, H.F. Harlow, & F. Stollnitz (Eds.), *Behavior of nonhuman primates* (Vol. 1, pp. 1–49). New York: Academic Press.

Miles, L. (1990). The cognitive foundations for reference in a signing orangutan. In S.T. Parker & K.R. Gibson (Eds.), *"Language" and intelligence in monkeys and apes: Comparative developmental perspectives* (pp. 511–539). New York: Cambridge University Press.

Mirsky, A.F. (1996). Disorders of attention: A neuropsychological perspective. In G.R. Lyon & N.A. Krasnegor (Eds.), *Attention, memory, and executive function* (pp. 71–95). Baltimore: Paul H. Brookes Publishing Co.

Napier, J.R., & Napier, P.H. (1994). *The natural history of primates.* Cambridge, MA: MIT Press.

Nelson, K. (1985). *Making sense: The acquisition of shared meaning.* New York: Academic Press.

Nelson, K. (1986). *Event knowledge: Structure and function in development* (pp. 293–296). Hillsdale, NJ: Lawrence Erlbaum Associates.

Oden, D.L., Thompson, R.K.R., & Premack, D. (1990). Infant chimpanzees spontaneously perceive both concrete and abstract same/different relations. *Child Development, 61,* 621–631.

Parker, S.T., & Gibson, K.R. (Eds.). (1990). *"Language" and intelligence in monkeys and apes: Comparative developmental perspectives.* New York: Cambridge University Press.

Patterson, F.L., & Linden, E. (1981). *The education of Koko.* New York: Holt, Rinehart & Winston.

Pepperberg, I.M. (1993). Cognition and communication in an African grey parrot (*Psittacus erithacus*): Studies on a nonhuman, nonprimate, nonmammalian subject. In H. Roitblat, L.M. Herman, & P.E. Nachtigall (Eds.), *Language and communication: Comparative perspectives* (pp. 221–248). Hillsdale, NJ: Lawrence Erlbaum Associates.

Premack, D., & Premack, A.J. (1983). *The mind of an ape.* New York: Norton.

Pribram, K. (1991). *Brain and perception: Holonomy and structure in figural processing* (p. 388). Hillsdale, NJ: Lawrence Erlbaum Associates.

Rakic, P. (1988). Specification of cerebral cortical areas. *Science, 241,* 170–176.

Richardson, W.K., Washburn, D.A., Hopkins, W.D., Savage-Rumbaugh, E.S., & Rumbaugh, D.M. (1990). The NASA/LRC computerized test system. *Behavior Research Methods, Instruments, & Computers, 22,* 127–131.

Roitblat, H.L., Herman, L.M., & Nachtigall, P.E. (Eds.). (1993). *Language and communication: Comparative perspectives.* Hillsdale, NJ: Lawrence Erlbaum Associates.

Romski, M.A., & Sevcik, R.A. (1991). Patterns of language learning by instruction: Evidence from nonspeaking persons with mental retardation. In N.A. Krasnegor, D.M. Rumbaugh, R.L. Schiefelbusch, & M. Studdert-Kennedy (Eds.), *Biological and behavioral determinants of language development* (pp. 429–495). Hillsdale, NJ: Lawrence Erlbaum Associates.

Romski, M.A., Sevcik, R.A., & Pate, J.L. (1988). The establishment of symbolic communication in persons with severe retardation. *Journal of Speech and Hearing Disorders, 53,* 94–107.

Romski, M.A., Sevcik, R.A., & Rumbaugh, D.M. (1985). Retention of symbolic communication skills in five severely retarded persons. *American Journal of Mental Deficiency, 89,* 313–316.

Rumbaugh, D.M. (1970). Learning skills of anthropoids. In L. Rosenblum (Ed.), *Primate behavior: Developments in field and laboratory research* (pp. 231–245). New York: Academic Press.

Rumbaugh, D.M. (1971). Evidence of qualitative differences in learning among primates. *Journal of Comparative and Physiological Psychology, 76,* 250–255.

Rumbaugh, D.M. (1977). *Language learning by a chimpanzee: The LANA project.* New York: Academic Press.

Rumbaugh, D.M., Hopkins, W.D., Washburn, D.A., & Savage-Rumbaugh, E.S. (1991). Comparative perspectives of brain, cognition, and language. In N.A. Krasnegor, D.M. Rumbaugh, R.L. Schiefelbusch, & M. Studdert-Kennedy (Eds.), *Biological and behavioral determinants of language development* (pp. 145–164). Hillsdale, NJ: Lawrence Erlbaum Associates.

Rumbaugh, D.M., & Pate, J.L. (1984). The evolution of cognition in primates: A comparative perspective. In H.L. Roitblat, T.G. Bever, & H.S. Terrace (Eds.), *Animal cognition* (pp. 569–585). Hillsdale, NJ: Lawrence Erlbaum Associates.

Rumbaugh, D.M., Richardson, W.K., Washburn, D.A., Savage-Rumbaugh, E.S., & Hopkins, W.D. (1989). Rhesus monkeys *(Macaca mulatta)*, video tasks, and implications for stimulus-response spatial contiguity. *Journal of Comparative Psychology, 103,* 32–38.

Rumbaugh, D.M., Savage-Rumbaugh, E.S., & Washburn, D.A. (1994). Learning, prediction, and control with an eye to the future. In M.M. Haith, J.B. Benson, R.J. Roberts, Jr., & B.F. Pennington (Eds.), *The development of future–oriented processes* (pp. 119–138). Chicago: University of Chicago Press.

Rumbaugh, D.M., & Williams, S. (1992). Human factors, psychological factors, and affirmation of continuity. *International Journal of Comparative Psychology, 5,* 205–209.

Sarich, V.M. (1983). Retrospective on hominoid macromolecular systematics. In R.L. Ciochon & R.S. Corruccini (Eds.), *New interpretations of ape and human ancestry* (pp. 137–150). New York: Plenum.

Savage-Rumbaugh, E.S. (1986). *Ape language: From conditioned response to symbol.* New York: Columbia University Press.

Savage-Rumbaugh, E.S. (1991). Language learning in the bonobo: How and why they learn. In N.A. Krasnegor, D.M. Rumbaugh, R.L. Schiefelbusch, and M. Studdert-Kennedy (Eds.), *Biological and behavioral determinants of language development* (pp. 209–233). Hillsdale, NJ: Lawrence Erlbaum Associates.

Savage-Rumbaugh, E.S., Brakke, K.E., & Hutchins, S.S. (1992). Linguistic development: Contrasts between co-reared *Pan troglodytes* and *Pan paniscus.* In T. Nishida, W.C. McGrew, P. Marler, M. Pickford, & F.B.M. de Waal (Eds.), *Topics in primatology* (pp. 51–66). Tokyo: University of Tokyo Press.

Savage-Rumbaugh, E.S., & Lewin, R. (1994). *Kanzi: At the brink of the human mind.* New York: John Wiley & Sons.

Savage-Rumbaugh, E.S., Murphy, J., Sevcik, R.A., Brakke, K.E., Williams, S., & Rumbaugh, D.M. (1993). Language comprehension in ape and child. *Monographs of the Society for Research in Child Development, 58*(3–4, Serial No. 233).

Savage-Rumbaugh, E.S., Pate, J.L., Lawson, J., Smith, S.T., & Rosenbaum, S. (1983). Can a chimpanzee make a statement? *Journal of Experimental Psychology: General, 112,* 457–492.

Savage-Rumbaugh, E.S., Sevcik, R.A., & Hopkins, W. (1988). Symbolic cross-modal transfer in two species of chimpanzees *(Pan paniscus* and *P. troglodytes). Child Development, 59,* 617–625.

Schull, J., Smith, J.D., Washburn, D.A., & Shields, W.E. (1994). Uncertainty monitoring in rhesus monkeys. In J.R. Anderson, J.J. Roeder, B. Thierry, & N. Herrenschmidt (Eds.), *Current primatology: Behavioral neuroscience, physiology, and reproduction* (Vol. III, pp. 101–109). Strasbourg, France: Université Louis Pasteur.

Schusterman, R.L., Gisiner, R., Grimm, B.K., & Hanggi, E.B. (1993). Behavior control by exclusion and attempts at establishing semanticity in marine mammals using match-to-sample. In H. Roitblat, L.M. Herman, & P.E. Nachtigall (Eds.), *Language and communication: Comparative perspectives* (pp. 249–274). Hillsdale, NJ: Lawrence Erlbaum Associates.

Semendeferi, K. (1994). *Evolution of the hominoid prefrontal cortex: A quantitative and image analysis of areas 13 and 10.* Doctoral dissertation, University of Iowa, Ames.

Semendeferi, K., Damasio, H., & Van Hoesen, G.W. (1994). Evolution of the frontal lobes. An MRI study on apes and humans. *Society for Neurosciences Abstracts, 20,* 578.7.

Sibley, C.G., & Ahlquist, J.E. (1987). DNA hybridization evidence of hominoid phylogeny: Results from an expanded data set. *Journal of Molecular Evolution, 26,* 99–121.

Terrace, H.S. (1979). *Nim.* New York: Alfred A. Knopf.

Thorndike, E.L. (1970). *Animal intelligence.* Darien, CT: Hafner. (Original work published 1911).

Tomasello, M., Savage-Rumbaugh, E.S., & Kruger, A.C. (1993). Imitative learning of action on objects by children, chimpanzees, and educated chimpanzees. *Child Development, 64,* 1688–1705.

Toth, N., Shick, K.D., Savage-Rumbaugh, E.S., Sevcik, R.A., & Rumbaugh, D.M. (1993). *Pan the tool-maker: Investigations into the stone tool-making and tool-using capabilities of a bonobo (Pan paniscus). Journal of Archaeological Science, 20,* 81–91.

Tuttle, R.H. (1986). *Apes of the world: Their social behavior, communication, and ecology.* Park Ridge, NJ: Noyes Publications.

Velichkovsky, B., & Rumbaugh, D.M. (Eds.). (1996). *Communicating meaning.* Hillsdale, NJ: Lawrence Erlbaum Associates.

Washburn, D.A., Hopkins, W.D., & Rumbaugh, D.M. (1989). Automation of learning-set testing: The video-task paradigm. *Behavior Research Methods, Instruments, & Computers, 21,* 281–284.

Washburn, D.A., & Rumbaugh, D.M. (1991). Ordinal judgments of numerical symbols by macaques *(Macaca mulatta). Psychological Science, 2,* 190–193.

Washburn, D.A., & Rumbaugh, D.M. (1992a). Comparative assessment of psychomotor performance: Target prediction by humans and macaques *(Macaca mulatta). Journal of Experimental Psychology: General, 121,* 305–312.

Washburn, D.A., & Rumbaugh, D.M. (1992b). The learning skills of rhesus revisited. *International Journal of Primatology, 12,* 377–388.

Zimmerman, R.R., & Torrey, C.C. (1965). Ontogeny of learning. In A.M. Schrier, H.F. Harlow, & F. Stollnitz (Eds.), *Behavior of nonhuman primates* (pp. 405–447). New York: Academic Press.

Development of the Prefrontal Cortex: Evolution, Neurobiology, and Behavior
edited by Norman A. Krasnegor, Ph.D., G. Reid Lyon, Ph.D.,
and Patricia S. Goldman-Rakic, Ph.D.
copyright © 1997   Paul H. Brookes Publishing Co., Inc.
Baltimore • London • Toronto • Sydney

7

Language and the Prefrontal Cortex

Christiana M. Leonard

Communication with symbols is a hallmark of humanity. Chimpanzees can be taught to use symbols (see Chapter 6), but human children soon outstrip them in the size of their repertoire as well as the varieties of their symbol combinations and the purposes to which they are put (Bickerton, 1990). Oral communication is a specialized biological function and as such is dependent on a specialized biological substrate—the cerebral cortex in the banks of the sylvian (i.e., lateral) fissure of the left hemisphere. These brain areas surround the auditory cortex on the superior temporal gyrus and the premotor cortex for the mouth in the precentral gyrus (Figure 7.1). These regions are referred to as Wernicke's and Broca's areas, in honor of the neurologists who first identified their crucial roles in language function. Broca's area is part of the prefrontal cortex, the human brain region that has evolved the furthest from its homologue in nonhuman primates (Zilles, 1990).

Evolution is driven by structural and functional variation (Dawkins, 1977). It is the thesis of this chapter that differences in the anatomical organization of Wernicke's and Broca's areas contribute to differences in linguistic skill as well as differences in the speed of language development in individual children. It is now possible to investigate this kind of brain–behavior correlation as a result of modern improvements in imaging techniques. Evidence is presented here that Wernicke's and Broca's areas are smaller in children with specific language impairment and that the size of these regions is related to a number of individual characteristics, such as handedness, phonemic awareness, and fluency.

This chapter was supported by the March of Dimes Social and Behavioral Research Services Grant 93-551, NIDCD R01-2922, the National Science Foundation, and a grant from the Medical Research Service of the Veterans Administration to John M. Kuldau.

It is a pleasure to thank the colleagues, parents, and children who participated in these studies—in particular John M. Kuldau, Linda J. Lombardino, Laurie Mercado-Gauger, Anne L. Foundas, Janice C. Honeyman, Douglas Jones, Mary Ellen Bentham, Chrissy Meyer, Mark Eckert, Lisa Rowe, Erin Gautier, Sam Browd, Melissa Mahoney, Tim Lucas, Ralph Rios, and Laura Phillips.

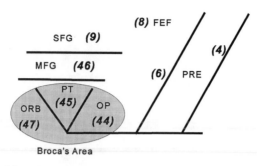

(a)

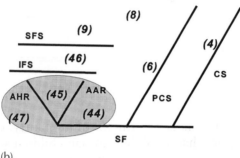

(b)

Figure 7.1.   Schematic illustration of the relationship between frontal lobe areas visible on the lateral surface. Shaded area denotes the core of Broca's area (inferior frontal gyrus on the left). (a) Common area names with Brodmann's numbers in parentheses. (b) Sulci of the frontal lobe. Abbreviations: AAR, anterior ascending ramus; AHR, anterior horizontal ramus; CS, central sulcus; FEF, frontal eye fields; IFS, inferior frontal sulcus; MFG, middle frontal gyrus; OP, pars opercularis; ORB, pars orbitalis; PCS, precentral sulcus; PRE, precentral gyrus; PT, pars triangularis; SF, sylvian (lateral) fissure; SFG, superior frontal gyrus; SFS, superior frontal sulcus.

NEURAL SUBSTRATE OF LANGUAGE

In 95% of right-handed individuals, language functions are controlled by the left hemisphere (left hemisphere dominance) (Rasmussen & Milner, 1975). It is rare for adults to suffer aphasia (a language disorder) after a right-sided lesion. What is the evidence that this functional lateralization is due to anatomical specializations within Broca's and Wernicke's areas? This proposition rests on three forms of evidence: comparative anatomy, language function after brain disease, and brain activation during functional imaging.

If the brains of chimpanzees and humans are compared, two major anatomical specializations unique to humans are noted in the temporal and frontal opercula (lids of the insula). There is a large bulge (the transverse gyrus of Heschl) in the superior surface of the human temporal lobe that is not present in nonhuman primates. This is the primary auditory cortex, that is, the first cortical target for ascending fibers carrying information about sounds. The fact that this bulge is unique to humans suggests that the cortical maps for hearing are much larger and more detailed than in other primates. The obvious implication is that the human auditory cortex has undergone differentiation for the detection of subtle differences in sounds that are essential for the rapid perception and decoding of speech (Liberman, 1982; Molfese & Buhrla, 1985; Tallal, Miller, & Fitch, 1993). Although it seems reasonable to suppose that acoustic perceptual deficits contribute to some forms of aphasia, the systematic study of the anatomical basis of complex auditory perception is still in its infancy.

The inferior frontal gyrus (Broca's area) and the planum temporale in the posterior superior temporal gyrus (Wernicke's area) are connected by a prominent bundle of fibers called the arcuate fasciculus. The Wernicke-Geschwind model of language proposes that thoughts are translated into word images in the posterior language cortex of Wernicke's area of the left hemisphere and carried forward to the inferior frontal gyrus by the arcuate fasciculus to Broca's area, where speech utterances are generated.

One powerful reason for believing that language functions are located in the perisylvian region is that these regions are larger in the left hemisphere (Geschwind & Levitsky, 1968; Musiek & Reeves, 1990; Penhune, Zatorre, MacDonald, & Evans, 1996; Von Economo & Horn, 1930; Witelson & Paillie, 1973). We have found that anatomical asymmetry of the planum temporale is related to the side of language dominance (Foundas, Leonard, Gilmore, Fennell, & Heilman, 1994, 1996). Anatomical asymmetries in the anterior perisylvian region were reported to be less robust (Witelson & Kigar, 1988), although several studies found a population bias toward left asymmetry there as well (Foundas, Leonard, & Heilman, 1995; Foundas et al., 1996). We believe that individual differences in these asymmetries are functionally important and related to individual differences in fluency and phonemic awareness. Data from our laboratory supporting this contention are presented after a brief review of the relevant background literature.

FLUENCY

The major factor differentiating the adult acquired aphasia that results from anterior lesions from that resulting from posterior lesions is fluency (Kimura, 1993). Patients with lesions in Wernicke's area speak fluently, but the communication value of their utterances is greatly degraded. They create words (i.e., neologisms) and make meaningless substitutions. This is thought to be because access to the lexicon relating phonemic structure and word meaning has been destroyed (Caplan, 1992). This view is consistent with animal data suggesting that the auditory association cortex of Wernicke's area is composed of a series of maps, each one of which enhances the perception of a particular type of auditory feature (Seldon, 1985).

"Broca's aphasics," in contrast to Wernicke's, have great difficulty generating words and connected discourse. They have particular trouble with the small words (e.g., functors or closed class words) that are necessary for syntactic organization. Broca's area is frequently referred to as the *motor speech area*. This suggests the erroneous view that the region contains motor directions for laryngeal and tongue movements. However, damage to Broca's area does not produce nonfluent, effortful, telegraphic speech because it has destroyed motor programs. Rather, speech is telegraphic because the ability to generate meaningful sentences has been compromised (Blumstein, Burton, Baum, Waldstein, & Katz, 1994; Lukatella, Shankweiler, & Crain, 1995).

Broca's aphasics have sometimes been called *agrammatical,* as if the lesion had destroyed the files containing syntactic rules. Experiments comparing linguistic impairments in Broca's and Wernicke's aphasics (Bates & Thal, 1991; Blumstein, 1995) modified this view. It is now thought that anterior and posterior lesions do not destroy different types of language *knowledge* (e.g., syntax, semantics); rather, they affect language *processing* or access to linguistic stores in different ways. These experiments suggest that neural mechanisms in Broca's area may be aided in the selection of responses by activation of generalization gradients for phonologically, syntactically, and semantically related words. When Broca's area is destroyed, access to or interpretation of these gradients is disrupted, the selection process becomes effortful, and language becomes nonfluent. In support of this thesis, imaging studies (Cohen & Bookheimer, 1994; Frith, Friston, Liddle, & Frackowiak, 1991; Mazoyer et al., 1993) demonstrated that blood flow increases in the left-middle and inferior frontal gyri during word generation and rhyming tasks.

DEVELOPMENT OF THE NEURAL SUBSTRATE FOR LANGUAGE

The exclusive dependence of language on left hemisphere mechanisms develops gradually during childhood, but the two hemispheres have different potentials to support language, even at birth (Best, Hoffman, & Glanville, 1982; Molfese, Freeman, & Palermo, 1975; Previc, 1991). Children are less likely to become aphasic after brain damage than are adults (Aram, 1988; Lenneberg, 1967). They do, however, show subtle language deficits, particularly in the area of grammar, after early left hemisphere damage (Dennis & Whitaker, 1976; Eisele & Aram, 1994). This capacity for reorganization apparently declines gradually during childhood and adolescence. Some fraction of anomalous (right or mixed) dominance may result from such early cerebral reorganization (Geschwind & Galaburda, 1987; Kinsbourne, 1988; Satz, Strauss, & Whitaker, 1990).

A large multicenter study (Bates, Dale, & Thal, 1995) reported that there is one brain region where even early damage has severe effects on language development. Early left posterior (i.e., Wernicke's) lesions produce effects similar to Broca's area lesions in adults. In contrast, no asymmetry in deficits was found following early anterior lesions. This finding supports the view that the left posterior cortex has unique processing mechanisms that are essential for efficient processing of linguistic stimuli. The left and right anterior cortices appear to be more equipotential than the posterior perisylvian areas. It is possible that the reason why Broca's area appears specialized for language processing in adults is that it has privileged access to language input from the ipsilateral posterior language cortex, not that it contains specialized language modules itself. This view of the function of Broca's area is consistent with a current theoretical formulation of the general functions of the frontal lobes.

FUNCTION OF THE FRONTAL LOBES

Historically, the prefrontal cortex has been considered to be silent "association" cortex, quite different in function from more caudal "motor" frontal lobe regions. However, Passingham (1993) brought together a wide range of clinical and neuroscience data to suggest that all regions rostral to the central sulcus operate in a similar mode. In his view, the premotor, motor, and prefrontal cortices all guide the selection and generation of responses. What differentiates each frontal lobe subregion is the type of response selected and the internal or external eliciting stimuli. The motor cortex (Brodmann's area 4) generates fractionated musculoskeletal responses on the basis of kinesthetic information, as in the cortical reflexes guiding precision grasp. The premotor cortex (area 6) generates coordinated responses that are contingent on exteroreceptive cues—a right turn signaled by a green arrow, whereas a red arrow signals left, for example. The frontal eye fields (area 8) generate orienting responses on the basis of *internally* generated information, as in visual search. The dorsolateral prefrontal cortex (areas 46 and 9) generates behavioral sequences on the basis of "willed action" (Frith et al., 1991) or "inner representations" (Goldman-Rakic, 1988)—a decision to lift a particular cup after a delay because of a memory concerning a peanut. The orbitofrontal cortex (areas 11–14), in contrast, is connected to limbic system structures concerned with emotion, reward, and punishment and selects behavioral patterns on the basis of their reinforcement history—avoidance of areas associated with punishment, for example. In a brief last chapter, Passingham (1993) speculated that Broca's area functions similarly to the rest of the frontal lobe in that it generates speech movements on the basis of internal and external cues.

This synthesis is based, by and large, on the results of anatomical, physiological, and neuropsychological experiments in monkeys. Passingham (1993) found it harder to conceptualize the role of the frontal cortex in language because there are no nonhuman homologues. What knowledge we have amassed about language and the brain is due, in large part, to the clinical analysis of human patients with neurological and mental disease. One line of research that has shed light on the role of the frontal lobes in selecting language responses comes from study of the symptoms of schizophrenia. Many of these symptoms can be characterized as examples of inappropriate response selection. A series of imaging studies in schizophrenia has documented decreased word fluency and decreased blood flow in the frontal lobes during response selection tasks that involve generating verbal responses (Frith et al., 1991; Liddle et al., 1992). There are no reports, however, of gross morphological abnormalities in the frontal lobes of schizophrenics (Breier et al., 1992). Our laboratory has been collecting data on frontal lobe structure and function in patients with schizophrenia to test the hypothesis that subtle individual differences in these structures are related to different symptoms and cognitive deficits in schizophrenia. After a review of prefrontal anatomy and some of the biobehavioral variables that must be considered in these studies, I present evidence that anatomical differences in Broca's area contribute to individual differences in skill at generating verbal responses.

ANATOMY OF BROCA'S AREA

Like the temporal operculum, the human frontal operculum is markedly different from that of the chimpanzee. The area between the dorsolateral prefrontal cortex and the orbitofrontal cortex has undergone dramatic expansion. This area, called the inferior frontal gyrus, lies anterior to the premotor and motor cortices on the upper bank of the sylvian (lateral) fissure and is composed of three subdivisions: the pars opercularis (area 44), the pars triangularis (area 45), and the pars orbitalis (area 47) (Figure 7.1). Two prominent sulci that are unique to humans demarcate these regions. The pars triangularis is formed by the anterior ascending ramus (AAR) and the anterior horizontal ramus (AHR) of the sylvian fissure. Anterior to the AHR lies the pars orbitalis. Posterior to the AAR lies the pars opercularis. Figures 7.2–7.4 give examples of Broca's area in normal right-handed children and adults.

It is interesting that Broca's area is situated at the confluence of the premotor, dorsolateral prefrontal, and orbitofrontal cortices (see Figure 7.1). Each of the three subregions (pars opercularis, triangularis, and orbitalis) lies next to one of Passingham's major frontal lobe functional zones. The pars opercularis lies next to the premotor cortex, the pars triangularis next to the dorsolateral prefrontal cortex, and the pars orbitalis next to the orbitofrontal cortex. Perhaps a key to understanding the role of Broca's area in language generation will lie in an analysis of the differences among these three regions. Verbal responses may be generated by the pars opercularis on the basis of conditional cues in the environment; by the pars triangularis on the basis of internal representations or "willed actions" (Goldman-Rakic, 1988); and by the pars orbitalis on the basis of goals, feelings, and stored experiences. At present, there is little evidence to support these hypotheses, but they suggest possible functional imaging experiments.

ANATOMICAL ASYMMETRY IN THE PREFRONTAL CORTEX

After an extensive review of postmortem data, Witelson and Kigar (1988) concluded that there was no overall anatomical evidence for leftward asymmetry of Broca's area, although isolated studies had reported lateralized effects. In a magnetic resonance imaging (MRI) structural study, however, Foundas et al. (1996) found that the surface area of the pars triangularis was larger on the left in 9 of 10 epilepsy patients with language lateralized to the left hemisphere by a Wada test. The one patient in whom language was controlled by the right hemisphere had a larger pars triangularis on the right. Therefore, only 1 of 11 patients had asymmetry of the pars triangularis that was inconsistent with his or her language dominance. Foundas and colleagues (1995) also found that leftward asymmetry is stronger in right- than

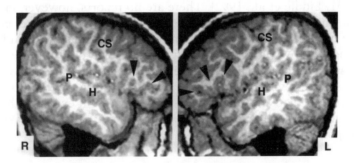

Figure 7.2.　Right (R) and left (L) parasagittal images of the brain of a 6-year-old girl. Pars triangularis (indicated by arrowheads) is larger on the left than on the right (refer to Figure 7.1 for orientation). In this and subsequent such figures, the images are of 1-mm-thick sagittal sections that have been rotated into the anterior commissive–posterior commissive plane and reformatted to correct for head tip in the coronal and axial planes. Right hemisphere sections are 45 Talairach mm lateral to the midline, and left hemisphere sections are 46 Talairach mm lateral. The central sulcus (CS), Heschl's gyrus (H), and the planum (P) are labeled for reference. The central sulcus is relatively easy to identify in sagittal sections because it generally divides two parallel gyri (containing the motor and somatosensory representations of the body). The images were acquired in a Siemens 1T Magnetom with an MPRage "Turboflash" gradient echo, volumetric sequence with the following parameters: repetition time, 10 milliseconds; echo time, 4 milliseconds; flip angle, 10°; matrix, 130 × 256; field of view, 25 cm; one acquisition, 1.25- or 1.4-mm-thick sections. The scan time for this sequence is 6 minutes, and sedation is not required to keep normal children still.

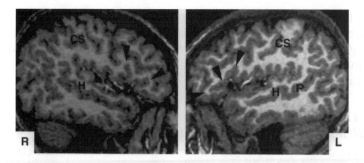

Figure 7.3.   Right (R) and left (L) parasagittal images of a 12-year-old boy with a larger pars triangularis on the left than on the right. (See legend for Figure 7.2 for further description and scan parameters.) The central sulcus (CS), Heschl's gyrus (H), and planum (P) are labeled for reference.

left-handed individuals. There have been no MRI investigations of possible asymmetries in the pars opercularis or pars orbitalis.

Leftward asymmetry in the gross size of perisylvian structures is presumably due to greater cell number, greater cell size, or both. Hayes and Lewis (1995) measured the size of cells in the pars triangularis in a postmortem study and found that the largest pyramidal cells on the left were larger than the largest such cells on the right, although the mean cell size did not differ. In a small sample, Scheibel (1984) reported that the dendritic branching of pyramidal cells is bushier on the left.

One reason for thinking that asymmetry of perisylvian structures is related to language function is that asymmetry is reported to be less in two groups of subjects who are less functionally lateralized—left-handed individuals and women (Foundas et al., 1995; Kulynych, Vladar, Jones, & Weinberger, 1994; Penhune et al., 1996; Steinmetz, Volkmann, Jancke, & Freund, 1991). There have been recurring suggestions that language is represented bilaterally in the posterior cortex of women (McGlone, 1980). Kimura (1993) reported, however, that women are *more* dependent than men on left *anterior* cortex. In an imaging report, Shaywitz et al. (1995) found that a rhyming task activated the prefrontal cortex in the left hemisphere of men but produced bilateral activation in women, a finding inconsistent with that of Kimura (1993). The Foundas studies cited above used both men and women, and, although no significant sex difference was found, the women did tend to be less asymmetrical in both anterior and posterior regions. It is important to remember that there is great individual variation in the size,

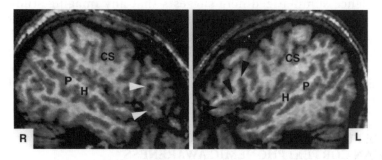

Figure 7.4.   Right (R) and left (L) images of the brain of a 46-year-old man. The pars triangularis (indicated by arrowheads) is larger on the left than on the right. (See legend for Figure 7.2 for further description and scan parameters.)

shape, and, probably, function of these regions that transcends variation resulting from gender, handedness, or both. Brain–behavior correlations must be investigated in large numbers of subjects with well-documented behavioral profiles. The next section reviews some behavioral features that should be assessed in structure–function investigations.

BRAIN ASYMMETRY, HAND
PREFERENCE, AND LANGUAGE DEVELOPMENT

In all cultures, 90% of the people are right-handed (dextral) (Annett, 1985; Corballis, 1991). Individuals who do not use their right hand consistently (adextral) have more minor physical anomalies (Yeo, Gangestad, & Daniel, 1993) and are overrepresented in all groups with developmental disabilities as well as in gifted populations (Coren & Halpern, 1991; Obler & Fein, 1988). Most theories on the origin of adextrality (Annett, 1985; Corballis, 1991; Kinsbourne, 1988; Satz, Strauss, & Whitaker, 1990) propose that some individuals are adextral because of brain damage, whereas other cases are "natural" or "familial." Many individuals in both groups probably have left or bilateral language localization (Rasmussen & Milner, 1975; Strauss, Gaddes, & Wada, 1987). The cortical programs for skilled movement (praxis) do not appear to be tied to a particular hemisphere and are located opposite the preferred hand (Kimura, 1993).

Geschwind and Galaburda (1987) developed an elaborate theory linking anatomical and behavioral asymmetries, fetal testosterone, handedness, learning disabilities, and the immune system. They hypothesized that fetal androgens delay growth of the left planum, permitting the earlier-developing right hemisphere to develop greater within-hemisphere expansion and interconnectivity. This hypothesis was proposed to explain the delayed language development of boys and their increased susceptibility to pathology and left-handedness. There is no evidence for or against a lateralized cortical response to androgens, although Nordeen and Yahr (1982) found an asymmetrical response in the rodent hypothalamus.

Kimura (1992) documented a population bias toward rightward asymmetry in the testes and leftward asymmetry in the breasts. Subjects with larger right-sided body structures, regardless of gender, performed relatively better on "right hemisphere" spatial tests, whereas subjects with larger left-sided structures performed better on "left hemisphere" language tests. Sex hormones were proposed to influence neural and somatic development on the same side, in spite of the well-known crossed connections between brain and body.

The evidence summarized here suggests that any imaging study of brain–behavior correlations should match subjects at least on the basis of handedness and gender. Because studying all possible combinations would enormously increase sample size, most investigators have settled on studying right-handed men. Such studies give an incomplete picture of the complex relations between functional and structural asymmetry. In our studies, we attempt to study left- as well as right-handed people and women as well as men.

LANGUAGE FUNCTION OF THE POSTERIOR
PERISYLVIAN CORTEX: PHONEMIC AWARENESS

A major difference between animal and human modes of communication is the size and combinatorial power of the fundamental auditory units—phonemes, syllables, and words (Liberman, 1982). The formation of phoneme categories is a process fundamental to the acquisition of language. Phoneme boundaries are perceived as categorical, even though there are no physical features of the sound stimulus that define the boundary (Liberman, 1982). When the phenomenon of categorical perception was originally discovered, it was thought to be the cornerstone of a uniquely human language acquisition device. However, this hope was soon dashed by demonstrations (Kuhl & Miller, 1975; Morse, Molfese, Laughlin, Linnville, & Wetzel, 1987) that categorical perception was a general property of the mammalian auditory system. It appears, however, that individual differences in the ability to conceptualize and manipulate phonemes are related to the rate of development of linguistic and reading skill. Children with deficits in the ability to rhyme or conceptualize phonemes are at risk for reading disability and school failure (Wagner & Torgesen, 1987). We have evidence (Leonard et al., 1996) that delays in the development of phonemic awareness in normal children are associated with symmetry of the planum temporale in Wernicke's area.

Deficits in the ability to conceptualize phonemes and an associated symmetry of the planum temporale may also be a risk factor for the development of more serious mental disturbances, such as schizophrenia. Studies of clinic records (Manzano, Zabala, & Borella, 1992) have identified a higher-than-expected rate of language and learning disabilities in children later diagnosed as having schizophrenia. We have found a significant deficit in phoneme awareness in adults with schizophrenia (Gautier, Kuldau, Weis, Leonard, & Mancuso, 1995). There have also been several reports of anomalous asymmetry in the posterior perisylvian cortex in this group (reviewed in Petty et al., 1995). The fact that schizophrenia and learning disability share some linguistic deficits and anomalous anatomy raises the interesting possibility that the probability of schizophrenia may be elevated in families with a history of learning disabilities. This possibility could be investigated in epidemiological studies.

It is unclear to what extent a more fundamental auditory processing deficit may be related to deficient phonemic awareness. Tallal (Tallal, Miller, & Fitch, 1993) has been a vigorous proponent of the view that a left hemisphere–based ability to discriminate short sounds is fundamental to the acquisition of phonemic awareness and that deficits in this auditory perceptual ability characterize children with both dyslexia and specific language impairment (SLI). Molfese, however, showed that both the left and the right hemispheres contribute to the discrimination of linguistically important acoustic information (Molfese & Buhrla, 1985). Evidence collected by Wright (Wright et al., 1996a, 1996b), a psychoacoustician collaborating with our laboratory, also suggests that the relation between acoustic perception and linguistic skill may be complex. In her experiments, auditory perceptual deficits were not necessarily correlated with deficits in phonemic awareness. Children with SLI had deficits in discriminating brief stimuli that were worse than would be expected for their level of phonemic awareness, whereas some dyslexics with very poor phonemic abilities had normal auditory perceptual function (Wright & Lombardino, unpublished data). This finding is particularly interesting because Galaburda, Sherman, Rosen, Aboitiz, and Geschwind (1985) reported postmortem evidence that dyslexics had symmetry of the planum temporale, a finding that several groups replicated in SLI (Gauger, Lombardino, & Leonard, in press; Jernigan, Hesselink, Sowell, & Tallal, 1990; Plante, Swisher, Vance, & Rapcsak, 1991). It is possible that the postmortem tissue that Galaburda and associates examined may have come from patients with linguistic impairments in addition to dyslexia. Language impairments may cover a continuum from those associated with primary acoustic processing deficits and symmetry of the total planum to reading problems whose anatomical correlates may be more heterogeneous or subtle. Reading problems encountered by children with SLI may have a different neurobiological substrate from those in "pure" dyslexia.

LANGUAGE FUNCTION OF THE FRONTAL LOBES

The idea that the function of Broca's area depends on its input from the posterior perisylvian cortex is consistent with Passingham's (1993) view that the frontal cortex acts as a response selection mechanism as well as with human research started by Baddeley (1986) and animal research by Goldman-Rakic and Friedman (1991). Baddeley (1990) developed the concept of "working memory" to describe the process of "temporarily holding and manipulating information as part of a wide range of essential cognitive tasks such as learning, reasoning and comprehending" (p. 67). Baddeley explored one aspect of working memory in great detail, the phonological loop, which is

> a phonological store that is capable of holding speech-based information and an articulatory control process based on inner speech. Memory traces within the phonological store are assumed to fade and become unretrievable after about one-and-a-half to two seconds. The memory trace can however be refreshed by a process of reading off the trace into the articulatory control process which then feeds it back into the store, the process underlying subvocal rehearsal. The articulatory control process is also capable of taking written material, converting it into a phonological code and registering it in the phonological store. (p. 72)

The crucial aspect of this working memory that distinguishes it from long-term memory is its limited capacity. It is possible to fill up or overload the articulatory loop, either by giving it too much information at one time or by asking it to perform two concurrent tasks. If the distracting task is visuospatial in nature, then the articulatory loop functions normally. However, if phonological decoding or encoding is required, then performance deteriorates. Baddeley theorized that the phonological loop evolved for speech production and comprehension. He has performed a series of interesting experiments with Gathercole showing that children whose language development is compromised have deficits in this aspect of working memory (Gathercole & Baddeley, 1989).

Baddeley was not particularly concerned with the anatomical locations of these components of the phonological loop. Many neurobiologically oriented investigators, however, have found his ideas useful for the interpretation of the results of their functional imaging studies. There is substantial evidence that the left prefrontal region is indeed involved in subvocal speech and rehearsal (Caplan, 1995; Demonet et al., 1992; Demonet, Price, Wise, & Frackowiak, 1994; Grasby et al., 1994; Paulesu, Frith, & Frackowiak, 1993). In fact, the inferior or middle frontal gyrus is activated by almost every language task that has been attempted (Howard et al., 1992; Petersen, Fox, Posner, Mintun, & Raichle, 1988; Price et al., 1994), including reading studies in which no vocal response was required. The conclusion from one functional imaging study of reading was that "subjects were automatically adopting a phonological strategy to perform a lexical decision task, a finding that could not be readily predicted from psychological studies" (Price et al., 1994, p. 1255).

Both Broca's area and the dorsolateral prefrontal cortex are activated during reading; subvocal rehearsal; and phonological, lexical, and syntactic decisions. Are there separate modules in these areas that are devoted to each of these tasks? Table 7.1 gives the Talairach coordinates (Talairach & Tournoux, 1988) that have been published in six functional activation studies (Demonet et al., 1992, 1994; Grasby et al., 1994; Paulesu et al., 1993; Petersen, Fox, Snyder, & Raichle, 1990; Price et al., 1994). Two things stand out: 1) the large expanse of frontal cortex that is activated during language tasks and 2) the great variety of tasks that have activated these regions. There is certainly nothing in Table 7.1 that supports the idea of separate specialized modules. However, there is probably no critical evidence against it. Demonet and co-workers (1992, 1994) considered that the same region had been activated in their two studies, even though the peak activations were separated by 1.5 cm. Considering the warping, filtering, and averaging that is necessary to analyze positron emission tomography data, it is probably premature to make conclusions about functional localization. As the functional MRI studies using these paradigms become more prevalent, it should be possible to map the functional activation onto individual sulci and make intraindividual comparisons of the loci and the intensity of activation for different tasks (Sereno et al., 1995). Ultimately, one would hope to correlate individual differences in structure with individual differences in language processing capacity, in both normal and impaired populations.

LANGUAGE DEVELOPMENT IN CHILDREN

The subsystems of language—phonology, semantics, syntax, and pragmatics—develop gradually. Early in development, language is used solely as a social-interactive tool that serves to transmit thoughts. Later, however, language becomes the focus of thought as an object in and of itself (e.g., the use of language as metaphor) in addition to a tool for social communication. These later language skills have been described as metalinguistic abilities and are judged to be crucial to early academic success. Van Kleeck (1994) defined metalinguistic ability as a skill in language awareness whereby the child is able to "reflect consciously on the nature and properties of language" (p. 53). Phonemic awareness—the ability to reflect on and manipulate the sound segments of the language—is a metalinguistic skill. Rhyming is an early metalinguistic skill, blending and segmenting sounds in words are later developing metalinguistic skills, and transposing letters in words to create new words (e.g., *pot → top*) is an even later metalinguistic accomplishment. Constructing arbitrary sentences on demand also depends on metalinguistic ability. Most functional imaging studies tap metalinguistic knowledge. Metalinguistic tasks may be particularly dependent on functional and anatomical asymmetries. We have evidence (Leonard et al., 1996) that the metalinguistic skill of phonemic awareness may develop more rapidly in children with leftward asymmetry of the planum temporale in Wernicke's area.

Early language skills do not develop synchronously in most children (Bates & Thal, 1991). Receptive ability usually precedes expressive fluency. Most normal 2- to 4-year-old children demonstrate a large advantage in receptive over expressive vocabulary. Our pilot data suggest that metalinguistic and linguistic skills also develop asynchronously in our school-age population. The working hypothesis in our laboratory is that the serious language disorders seen in autism, various genetic syndromes, specific language impairment, and schizophrenia represent the ex-

Table 7.1. Talairach coordinates of voxels with significant activation reported in the left frontal lobe in six functional imaging studies

Coordinates[a]	Region[b]	Task	Subtracted task	Reference
−46,2,16	Precentral sulcus (area 6)	Working memory task	No distracting task	Paulesu et al. (1993)
−54,8,16	Pars opercularis (area 44)	Silent viewing	False fonts	Price et al. (1994)
−40,4,28	Pars opercularis (area 44)	Phoneme monitoring	Detect rising pitch	Demonet et al. (1994)
−44,6,28	Pars opercularis (area 44)	Lexical decision	False fonts	Price et al. (1994)
−48,4,36	Middle frontal gyrus (area 46)	Lexical decision	Reading aloud	Price et al. (1994)
−32,14,28	Inferior frontal sulcus (area 46)	Reading aloud	False fonts	Price et al. (1994)
−32,16,28	Inferior frontal sulcus (area 46)	Lexical decision	False fonts	Price et al. (1994)
−30,22,28	Inferior frontal sulcus (area 46)	Lexical decision	Reading aloud	Price et al. (1994)
−52,18,20	Pars triangularis (area 45)	Phoneme monitoring	Detect rising pitch	Demonet et al. (1992)
−52,20,16	Pars triangularis (area 45)	Lexical decision	False fonts	Price et al. (1994)
−52,20,16	Pars triangularis (area 45)	Lexical decision	Reading aloud	Price et al. (1994)
−24,48,−8	Middle frontal gyrus (area 46)	Repeating heard words, activation increases with list length	Repeating heard words	Grasby et al. (1994)
−29,43,0	Middle frontal gyrus (area 46)	Decoding seen word	Fixating word	Petersen et al. (1990)
−40,26,−12	Pars orbitalis (area 47)	Remembering lists of heard words; activation decreases	Repeating heard words	Grasby et al. (1994)
−38,28,−16	Pars orbitalis (area 47)	Silent viewing	False fonts	Price et al. (1994)
−46,22,−4	Pars orbitalis (area 47)	Silent viewing	False fonts	Price et al. (1994)

[a]The coordinates are given in the order x (− is left), y (− is posterior to the anterior commissure), and z (− is inferior to the intercommissural plane).

[b]In most cases, the corresponding region in the right hemisphere showed decreased or with no activation. The region listed is where the activated pixel would fall in a typical brain.

tremes of asynchronous language development resulting from uncoupling of different language modules. We propose that this uncoupling is caused by errors in neural development that cause miswiring and anomalous size and asymmetry.

SPECIFIC LANGUAGE IMPAIRMENT AND THE BRAIN

Specific language impairment is a serious developmental disability. Locke (1994) proposed that children with SLI may suffer from a general maturational lag in brain development. Locke's theory postulates that, because of this maturational lag, children with SLI 1) are not able to store a critical mass of utterances sufficient to activate analytical mechanisms needed for the development of grammar and 2) miss the possibility of establishing grammar during the "critical period." Acquisition of the rules of grammar is essential for normal language development (Bates & Thal, 1991). Three studies (Gauger et al., in press; Jernigan et al., 1990; Plante et al., 1991) have reported symmetry or reversed, rightward asymmetry in the posterior language regions in children with SLI. This anatomical symmetry/reversed asymmetry could be a sign of anomalous or slowed brain development that interferes with left hemisphere specialization. Individual differences in the rate of cerebral differentiation may also account for the variability seen in individual response to brain damage (Aram, 1988; Thal et al., 1991) and the exceptional language abilities that are sometimes found in children with other developmental delays (Bellugi, Wang, & Wang, 1993; Obler & Fein, 1988).

Experimental Studies from Our Laboratory

The examination of differences in brain structure between developmentally delayed and control populations is difficult. There are many biological factors that contribute to variation in brain and behavior in the developing population. The complex relationship among gender, handedness, brain structure, and age complicates every developmental investigation. When we initiated an MRI study of children with SLI 2 years ago, we proposed to compare each impaired child with a matched control. We quickly discovered that the range of variation in control anatomy was so large that the behavioral correlates of this variability would be an interesting subject of study in its own right.

Our research group has been interested in correlating different rates of language development to developmental changes in the planum and pars triangularis. Because the prefrontal cortex continues to myelinate into the fourth decade of life (Brody, Kinney, Kloman, & Gilles, 1987; Hassink, Hiltbrunner, Muller, & Lutschg, 1992; Yakovlev & LeCours, 1967), it is a likely candidate to show developmental changes during childhood. Table 7.2 gives the demographic characteristics and language scores of the 5- to 13-year-old children studied in this project. They were recruited by a letter to a demographically diverse public school and by word of mouth. An attempt was made to recruit participants who exhibited a wide range of language and nonverbal IQ scores. Twenty percent of the sample were African Americans. When initial examination of the data suggested that there was an unexpectedly high number of young left-handed girls, left-handed boys were recruited to balance the adextral group for gender.

Language and Brain Structure in Normal Children   The children received a neurolinguistic battery of standardized tests. The Lindamood Auditory Conceptualization test (LAC; Lindamood & Lindamood, 1979) was also given. The LAC assesses

Table 7.2.   Demographic variables and language scores of subject group

Subjects (n)[a]	Age	HQ[c]	TONI	LAC	WA	PC	FS	OD
				Average score[b] (standard deviation)				
DM (16)	9.2	96%	107	72	102	101	8.2	9.8
	(2.0)	(7%)	(11)	(23)	(12)	(12)	(3.0)	(2.3)
DF (11)	9.5	96%	113	74	98	106	10.4	9.5
	(1.3)	(6%)	(15)	(19)	(10)	(12)	(4.0)	(2.3)
AM (7)	8.6	−17%	99	65	112	109	8.1	9.9
	(2.5)	(51%)	(12)	(32)	(17)	(15)	(1.9)	(3.2)
AF (6)	7.6	−18%	106	71	113	110	8.8	10.5
	(1.8)	(56%)	(9.9)	(20)	(15)	(5)	(1.7)	(2.4)

[a]D, dextral; A, adextral; M, male; F, female.

[b]HQ, handedness quotient (> 75%; Kimura, 1993); TONI, test of nonverbal intelligence; LAC, Lindamood Auditory Conceptualization test; WA, word attack; PC, passage comprehension; FS, CELF–R test of formulated sentences; OD, CELF–R test of oral directions. The mean standard score is 100 for the TONI, WA, and PC and 10 for the OD and FS. The LAC scores are raw scores; grade norms but not age norms are published.

[c]Two adextral groups have significantly lower quantitative handedness scores ($p < .0001$). No other test scores were significantly different, although there was a trend ($p = .06$) for the left-handed participants to have significantly higher word attack scores.

the ability to conceptualize the phonemic structure of language by the manipulation of colored blocks that symbolize phonemes. Hand preference was assessed with a modified Edinburgh battery (Briggs & Nebes, 1974). Several anatomical structures were traced and measured on computer images of each brain: 1) the area and length of the midsagittal section (Schaefer et al., 1990) and the width of each hemisphere; 2) the area of the corpus callosum (Witelson, 1989); and 3) the surface area of the banks of the horizontal and vertical plana in Wernicke's area (Leonard, Voeller, et al., 1993) and the surface area of the pars triangularis in the frontal lobe.

The pars triangularis was measured by tracing the sulci indicated by the two arrowheads in Figures 7.2–7.4 on every sagittal section between the lateral Talairach coordinates (x) of 39 and 52, summing the individual surface areas, and multiplying by the image thickness (1–1.4 mm) to obtain the total surface area in each hemisphere. Several modifications in the measurement technique were necessary to ensure reliability:

1. The brains were reformatted to correct for tip in the sagittal, axial, and coronal planes.
2. The sections were paged through to identify the pars triangularis on every section before beginning measurement.
3. Sections 2 mm apart were displayed during the measuring procedure to demonstrate how the structure was changing from medial to lateral.
4. Lines at Talairach coordinates 20 anterior and 10 superior were displayed on every image to facilitate differentiation of the diagonal sulcus and the AAR (Foundas et al., 1995).
5. The location of the measured wedge was shifted medially or laterally by one to three sections to ensure measurement of the pars triangularis at its maximal extent.

Still, in about one quarter of the cases, no clear-cut triangular-shaped region could be identified. In these cases, the sulci anterior and closest to the crosshairs were measured.

Age, Handedness, and Gender Effects in Controls   Adextrals were slightly but not significantly younger than the dextrals and showed a trend toward better scores on some language tests. The dextral girls had somewhat but not significantly higher nonverbal IQ scores, higher formulated sentence scores, and lower word attack scores than the other groups. As can be seen from the standard deviations in Table 7.2, there was a wide range of performance on every test. Although their mean non-verbal IQ score was higher than 100, the children demonstrated language abilities that cover a wide range. The size of some structures on the right side decreased slightly with age (the pars triangularis is graphed against age in Figure 7.5). The exciting question of whether the age-related increase in asymmetry is related to pruning on the right is currently being investigated in a longitudinal study.

Handedness and gender were significantly related to some aspects of brain anatomy (Table 7.3). Girls had smaller brain widths and midsagittal areas; and adextrals had wider right hemisphere widths, smaller corpus callosa, and longer vertical plana on the right. Surprisingly, in view of the literature on adults (Foundas et al., 1995; Jancke, Schlaug, Huang, & Steinmetz, 1994; Steinmetz et al., 1991; Witelson & Kigar, 1992), the adextral children in our sample did not have symmetrical horizontal plana. Because this particular group of adextrals showed a trend toward superior language skills, it is possible that by chance our sample includes atypically asymmetrical and linguistically skilled adextrals. A previous study also found that skilled early readers tend to be ambidextrous (Mamen, 1987). It will be

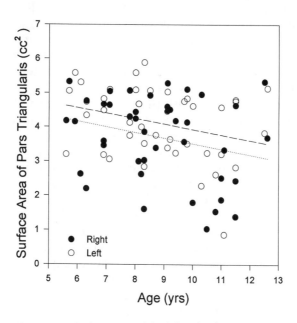

Figure 7.5.   Surface areas of the left and right pars triangularis plotted against age in 40 control children. There is a gradual (nonsignificant) decrease in size with age. Individual differences at any one age are far greater than the possible developmental change, however.

Table 7.3.   Selected brain structure measurements in subject group

Subjects (n)[a]	Average size[b] (standard deviation)					Asymmetry coefficient[c]			
	Mid[d] (cm²)	CC[e] (cm²)	CC/Mid (cm²)	LH[d] (cm)	RH[d,e] (cm)	H	V[e]	H&V	PT[e]
DM (16)	156	6.33	0.041	6.5	6.5	29%	−28%	10%	23%
	(9)	(0.7)	(0.005)	(0.3)	(0.2)	(41%)	(68%)	(32%)	(38%)
DF (11)	148	6.12	0.041	6.2	6.3	32%	−35%	10%	18%
	(6)	(0.7)	(0.005)	(0.1)	(0.2)	(28%)	(57%)	(18%)	(42%)
AM (7)	153	5.86	0.038	6.5	6.7	38%	−61%	0%	−16%
	(11)	(1.0)	(0.007)	(0.3)	(0.2)	(31%)	(56%)	(12%)	(39%)
AF (6)	149	5.2	0.034	6.3	6.4	51%	−124%	−13%	16%
	(6)	(0.9)	(0.005)	(0.3)	(0.3)	(39%)	(67%)	(15%)	(69%)

[a]D, dextral; A, adextral; M, male; F, female.

[b]Mid, area of midsagittal section; CC, area of corpus callosum; LH, width of left hemisphere; RH, width of right hemisphere.

[c]Asymmetry coefficient calculated using the formula $(L − R)/[(L + R)/2]$. H, horizontal bank of planum temporale; V, vertical bank of planum temporale; PT, pars triangularis.

[d]Gender effect significant, $p < .05$.

[e]Handedness effect significant, $p < .05$.

interesting to follow these children over time to see whether either their dextrality or their structural asymmetry weakens.

The only structure to show the predicted symmetry in adextrals was the pars triangularis: The mean coefficient of asymmetry $\{(L−R)/[(L+R)/2]\}$ for the adextrals was .01. The mean asymmetry for the dextrals was .26, which was significantly different from 0 (paired $t = 2.68$, $p < .01$; see Figure 7.6). Whether children with larger brain structures on the right are more likely to become adextral or use of the left hand leads to increased size of right brain structures is an interesting question that will also be examined in our longitudinal study.

We found no consistent relationships between the size and asymmetry of the pars triangularis and any of the language variables. There were a few scattered correlations, but not more than would have been expected by chance given the number of tests that were performed. We have preliminary evidence that the lack of brain–behavior correlation may be due to inappropriate test selection (see following).

Prefrontal Structure in Specific Language Impairment   A study (Gauger et al., in press) from the University of Florida Health Sciences Center laboratory compared language structures in 11 children diagnosed as having SLI and 19 control children matched on age, gender, handedness, and socioeconomic status (a subset of the control children discussed previously). The children with SLI all scored more than 1 standard deviation below the mean on two tests of expressive or receptive language and were in special classrooms for students with language impairment. Their nonverbal IQ scores were within 1 standard deviation of normal.

There were two major findings in the SLI group: 1) the left pars triangularis was significantly smaller, and 2) the total planum (i.e., horizontal and vertical banks) was symmetrical. The right pars triangularis and all other brain structures were equivalent in the two groups. Figures 7.7 (see p. xxxiv), 7.8, and 7.9 show examples of the prefrontal regions in these children. The prefrontal regions on both sides

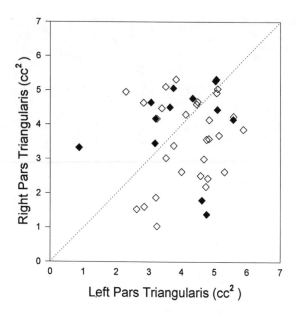

Figure 7.6.   The size of the right pars triangularis as a function of the left in 40 dextral (◇) and adextral (◆) control children. The line defines equality between the two sides. Dextrals but not adextrals have a significant leftward asymmetry.

appear poorly developed, and there is very little myelin apparent. This pattern was not characteristic of all children with SLI but was frequent enough to cause a significant difference in group means.

There were no mean differences in the rate of myelination, mainly because of the wide degree of variation in both groups. Myelin development is also being examined in our longitudinal study. The children with SLI had no gross anomalies such as lissencephaly or microgyria (Barkovich, Koch, & Carrol, 1991), although there were subtle anomalies in sulcal patterns of the sylvian fissure. Clark and Plante (1995) reported that the prefrontal regions of adults in families with SLI are characterized by anomalous sulci. After seeing their report, we have started to examine our cases, and, in fact, the brains shown in Figures 7.7 (see page xxxiv), 7.8, and 7.9 do show evidence of extra sulci. We have not yet analyzed this difference quantitatively in all subjects.

Fluency and the Pars Triangularis   We had not included an explicit test of word fluency in our neurolinguistic battery when we started the study, thinking that this feature of language would be tapped by the standardized tests. We do, however, administer Thurstone's test of word fluency, the Controlled Oral Word Association test (COWA) (Benton & Hamsher, 1989), to our sample of schizophrenics and adult controls. In the interests of having comparable data from as wide a sample as possible, we have started to administer this test to our children as well. In this test, subjects are asked to generate as many words as they can beginning with designated letters. They are given 1 minute for each letter. We currently have data from 51 subjects (19 schizophrenics, 6 children with SLI, 15 adult controls, and 11 child controls).

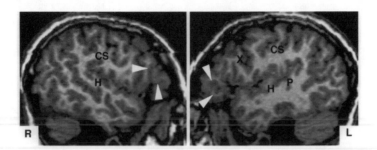

Figure 7.8.   Two parasagittal images of the brain of an 11-year-old boy with SLI. The pars triangularis is poorly developed on both sides but especially on the left. Note presence of extra sulci (indicated by X). These sulci are not the AAR because they disappear in more medial sections, as reported by Clark and Plante (1995). (See legend for Figure 7.2 for further description and scan parameters.)

Initially we analyzed the data for the adults and the children separately. In both samples, regression analysis showed that the size of the left and right pars triangularis contributed significantly and independently to the prediction of fluency. The left side was related positively and the right side negatively, just as predicted. In adults, verbal IQ and handedness quotient also contributed independent, significant positive effects. With the addition of a negative contribution from age, 59% of the variance in fluency score was predicted by these five factors. No other brain measures contributed significantly.

In children, nonverbal IQ score (we did not have a measure of verbal IQ score on a sufficient number of subjects) did not contribute significantly. Age had a highly significant effect, and handedness had a negative effect. With the addition of the positive contribution of the left pars triangularis and the negative contribution of the right pars triangularis, 87% of the variance in word fluency was explained by these four factors.

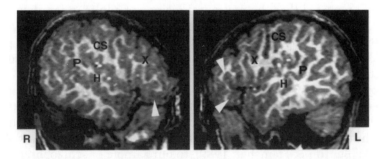

Figure 7.9.   Two parasagittal images of the brain of a 6-year-old girl with SLI. This brain was small, with the language areas being particularly reduced in size. Note the extremely small size of the pars triangularis as well as the pars orbitalis. This was the only one of the 11 children with SLI examined who had any obvious radiological abnormalities. Children with SLI frequently have difficulty keeping still in the scanner. Note that, in spite of the obvious motion artifact visible above X on the right, the fine details of cortical morphology can still be discerned. (See legend for Figure 7.2 for further description and scan parameters.)

The success of the regression analysis in predicting the aspect of fluency may, in part, be due to an interaction with intelligence. When the population is divided at the mean (IQ score = 105 in this sample), only individuals with high intelligence show the predicted relationship between pars triangularis asymmetry and fluency (Figure 7.10). This interaction occurred in both patients and controls. When the relationship among intelligence, fluency, and pars triangularis asymmetry was probed further in the adults, it was revealed that, in the group with lower-than-average intelligence, there were positive correlations of fluency from *both* the left and the right pars triangularis, whereas, in adults with higher intelligence, there was the expected negative correlation between the size of the right pars triangularis and fluency—that is, the smaller the right pars triangularis, the higher the fluency score. This interaction between intelligence and the relation between fluency and pars triangularis asymmetry may underlie the independent contributions of IQ score and pars triangularis in the regression analysis.

The relation among intelligence, learning disability, and mental illness is complex and is not discussed further here. On the basis of these limited data, cause, effect, and correlation cannot be distinguished. Perhaps individuals of lower intelligence are using both pars triangulares to promote fluency and thus fail to capitalize on the functional advantages of structural asymmetry. The risk of learning disability, schizophrenia, or both may increase with decreased intelligence because less

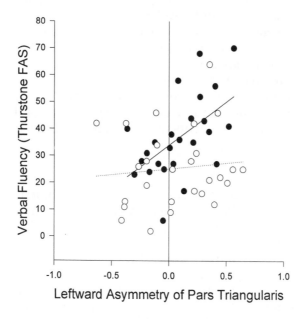

Figure 7.10.   Fluency and asymmetry of the pars triangularis. In subjects with above-average intelligence, for the group there is a significant correlation between verbal fluency and leftward asymmetry (solid circles) (IQ > 105, $r = .54$, $p < .005$). No such relation is found in subjects with below-average intelligence (open circles) (IQ < 105, $r = .01$, $p = $ NS). The subject group includes patients with schizophrenia and SLI and age-matched controls. The interaction between pars triangularis asymmetry and intelligence holds for both diagnosed and control populations.

advantage is taken of the lateralized properties of various anatomical specializations. Clearly, the influence of IQ score must be assessed in all brain–behavior studies. The current practice of using volunteer control groups with IQ scores more than 1 standard deviation superior to those in the group with disabilities (Giedd et al., 1996; Schultz et al., 1994) should be reassessed.

POSSIBILITIES FOR FUTURE RESEARCH

What is the role of the prefrontal cortex in language development? The data presented previously suggest that size and asymmetry differences are related to function, but they do not address the actual role that these areas play in the acquisition of language function. The work of Passingham, Baddeley, Goldman-Rakic, and the researchers using functional imaging points to a vital prefrontal role in the formulation of thoughts and utterances. How can we become more specific in our questions? One interpretation of the functional imaging studies is that the traditional categories of language (i.e., semantics, phonology, syntax, morphology, pragmatics) that emerge from philosophical and behavioral studies of language may not be appropriate for neurobehavioral studies. Goldman-Rakic and her colleagues (see Chapter 2) showed the power of mapping techniques borrowed from visual neuroscience (Allman, 1987) for elucidating the function of the sulcus principalis (area 46) in the prefrontal cortex. A map of intended locations was found that predicted the target of a monkey's later saccade (i.e., its internal representation or "thought"). Jackendoff (1987) made a powerful case for the spatial origins of syntax; he pointed out that almost all prepositions (the crucial functors eliminated in Broca's aphasia) describe spatial relations. Engel et al. (1994) devised a powerful paradigm for rapidly mapping complete visual areas in human imaging experiments. This technique could, in principle, be adapted for any sensory system. Could it be used to investigate a phoneme map in the planum or a word sequence map in the pars triangularis? A major challenge for cognitive neurobiologists through the turn of the 21st century will be to design experiments that assess the mapping functions of the human frontal association cortex.

BRAIN–BEHAVIOR RELATIONS

The children with SLI in our studies show a variability in brain structure equivalent to that of the controls. We do not yet have a large enough sample to determine whether different types of language impairment are characterized by different patterns of brain morphology. One of the problems that plagues the field of MRI morphometry is the relatively minor nature of the volume and structural differences that are found on MRI in patients with devastating cognitive or behavioral problems (Flaum et al., 1995; Jernigan et al., 1990; Leonard, Martinez, Weintraub, & Hauser, 1995; Leonard, Voeller, et al., 1993; Leonard, Willliams, et al., 1993). Furthermore, there is rarely more than a modest correlation between the size or location of a particular anomaly and the nature of the cognitive deficit. We and others have rationalized our findings as indicating biological risk factors for anomalous cognitive development. There is accumulating evidence in schizophrenia that prenatal insults alter brain development so that vulnerability to developmental experiences is increased (Cannon & Marco, 1994; Lipska, Jaskiw, & Weinberger, 1993; see also Chapter 10). The altered brain structures do not cause the behavior deficits; rather, they are evidence that early brain damage has occurred that altered the developmental trajectory. The behavioral response depends on the nature of the genetic background and other prenatal and postnatal factors. These findings have doused with disappointing complexity the naive hope that MRI would reveal "holes in the brain." These hopes were initially raised when the first neuropathological study on dyslexia found the same anomaly in eight consecutive cases (Galaburda, 1989). It was thought that MRI was a potential diagnostic tool—that there might be structural landmarks for each developmental disability and that the painstaking steps necessary for differential behavioral diagnoses could go the way of frontal lobotomy, insulin shock, and other outdated techniques. There is now overwhelming evidence that children with learning disabilities do not have "holes in the brain." No subsequent studies have found a one-to-one correlation between behavioral symptoms and MRI or postmortem pathology in learning disabilities. We must reconcile ourselves to the realization that the relationship between brain structure as currently visualizable on MRI and behavioral symptoms will probably not be direct.

CONCLUSIONS

Our studies of brain structure in populations with various forms of language impairment have produced these major findings:

- Leftward asymmetry of the pars triangularis and the planum temporale predicts the side of functional language localization (Foundas et al., 1994, 1996).
- Leftward asymmetry of the pars triangularis and the planum temporale is greater in right-handed than left-handed individuals (Foundas et al., 1995).
- Extra and missing gyri are more frequent in populations with genetic anomalies, dyslexia, SLI, and schizophrenia (C. Leonard, unpublished data; Leonard et al., 1995; Leonard, Voeller, et al., 1993; Leonard, Williams, et al., 1993; Mercado, 1995).
- Phonemic awareness is greater in young children with leftward asymmetry of the planum temporale (Leonard et al., 1996). Children with SLI have significantly less asymmetrical total plana as a result of reduced size on the left.
- Verbal fluency correlates with leftward asymmetry of the pars triangularis in individuals with above-average intelligence.
- Asymmetry of the pars triangularis is reduced in children with SLI as a result of reduced size on the left (Gauger et al., in press).

In each case the brain–behavior correlations are complex and involve the interaction of biobehavioral variables such as gender, handedness, age, and intelligence. The task now must be to devise the imaginative experimental designs and data analysis that will be necessary to unravel the epigenetic trajectory of biopsychosocial development.

REFERENCES

Allman, J. (1987). Maps in context: Some analogies between visual cortical and genetic maps. In L. Vaina (Ed.), *Matters of intelligence* (pp. 369–393). Dordrecht, The Netherlands: D. Reidel.

Annett, M. (1985). *Left and right brain: The right shift theory.* London: Lawrence Erlbaum Associates.

Aram, D. (1988). Language sequelae of unilateral brain lesions in children. In F. Plum (Ed.), *Language, communication and the brain* (pp. 171–198). New York: Raven Press.

Baddeley, A. (1986). *Working memory.* New York: Oxford University Press.

Baddeley, A. (1990). *Human memory.* Needham, MA: Allyn & Bacon.

Barkovich, A., Koch, T., & Carrol, C. (1991). The spectrum of lissencephaly: Report of ten patients analyzed by magnetic resonance imaging. *Annals of Neurology, 30,* 139–146.

Bates, E., Dale, P., & Thal, D. (1995). Individual differences and their implications for theories of language development. In P. Fletcher & B. MacWhinney (Eds.), *Handbook of child language* (pp. 96–163). Oxford, England: Basil Blackwell.

Bates, E., & Thal, D. (1991). Associations and dissociations in child language development. In J. Miller (Ed.), *Research on child language disorders* (pp. 147–168). Austin, TX: PRO-ED.

Bellugi, U., Wang, P., & Wang, T. (1993). Williams syndrome: An unusual neuropsychological profile. In S. Broman & J. Grafman (Eds.), *Atypical cognitive deficits in developmental disorders: Implications for brain function* (pp. 23–56). Hillsdale, NJ: Lawrence Erlbaum Associates.

Benton, A.L., & Hamsher, K. de S. (1989). *Multilingual aphasia examination: III. Controlled word association* (2nd ed.). Iowa City, IA: AJA Associates, Inc.

Best, C., Hoffman, H., & Glanville, B. (1982). Development of ear asymmetries for speech and music. *Perception and Psychophysics, 31,* 75–85.

Bickerton, D. (1990). *Language and species.* Chicago: University of Chicago Press.

Blumstein, S. (1995). The neurobiology of the sound structure of language. In M. Gazzaniga (Ed.), *The cognitive neurosciences* (pp. 915–930). Cambridge, MA: MIT Press.

Blumstein, S., Burton, M., Baum, S., Waldstein, R., & Katz, D. (1994). The role of lexical status on the phonetic categorization of speech in aphasia. *Brain and Language, 46,* 181–197.

Breier, A., Buchanon, R., Elkashef, A., Munson, R., Kirkpatrick, B., & Gellad, F. (1992). Brain morphology and schizophrenia: A magnetic resonance imaging study of limbic, prefrontal cortex, and caudate structures. *Archives of General Psychiatry, 49,* 921–926.

Briggs, G., & Nebes, R. (1974). Patterns of hand preference in a student population. *Cortex, 11,* 230–238.

Brody, B., Kinney, H., Kloman, A., & Gilles, F. (1987). Sequence of central nervous system myelination in human infancy. I. An autopsy study of myelination. *Journal of Neuropathology and Experimental Neurology, 46,* 283–301.

Cannon, T., & Marco, E. (1994). Structural brain abnormalities as indicators of vulnerability to schizophrenia. *Schizophrenia Bulletin, 20,* 89–99.

Caplan, D. (1992). *Language: Structure, processing and disorders.* Cambridge, MA: MIT Press.

Caplan, D. (1995). The cognitive neuroscience of syntactic processing. In M. Gazzaniga (Ed.), *The cognitive neurosciences* (pp. 871–879). Cambridge, MA: MIT Press.

Clark, M., & Plante, E. (1995). Morphology of the inferior frontal lobe in language impaired adults. *Cognitive Neuroscience Society Annual Meeting, 2,* 9.

Cohen, M.S., & Bookheimer, S.Y. (1994). Localizing of brain function using magnetic resonance imaging. *Trends in Neurosciences, 17,* 268–277.

Corballis, M. (1991). *The lopsided ape.* New York: Oxford University Press.

Coren, S., & Halpern, D. (1991). Left-handedness: A marker for decreased survival fitness. *Psychological Review, 109,* 90–106.

Dawkins, R. (1977). *The selfish gene.* Oxford, England: Oxford University Press.

Demonet, J., Chollet, F., Ramsay, S., Cardebat, D.N., Nesopoulous, J.L., Wise, R., Rascol, A., & Frackowiak, R. (1992). The anatomy of phonological and semantic processing in normal subjects. *Brain, 115,* 1753–1768.

Demonet, J., Price, C., Wise, R., & Frackowiak, R. (1994). A PET study of cognitive strategies in normal subjects during language tasks: Influence of phonetic ambiguity and sequence processing on phoneme monitoring. *Brain, 117,* 671–682.

Dennis, M., & Whitaker, H. (1976). Language acquisition following hemidecortication: Linguistic superiority of the left over the right hemisphere. *Brain and Language, 3,* 404–433.

Eisele, J., & Aram, D. (1994). Comprehension and imitation of syntax following early hemisphere damage. *Brain and Language, 48,* 320–325.

Engel, S., Rumelhart, D., Wandell, B., Lee, A., Glover, G., Chichilnisky, E., & Shadlen, M. (1994). FMRI of human visual cortex. *Nature, 369,* 525.

Flaum, M.S., Swayze, V.W., O'Leary, D., Yuh, W., Ehrhardt, J., Arndt, S., & Andreasen, N. (1995). Effects of diagnosis, laterality, and gender on brain morphology in schizophrenia. *American Journal of Psychiatry, 152,* 704–714.

Foundas, A., Leonard, C., Gilmore, R., Fennell, E., & Heilman, K. (1994). Planum temporale asymmetry and language dominance. *Neuropsychologia, 32,* 1225–1231.

Foundas, A., Leonard, C., Gilmore, R., Fennel, E., & Heilman, K. (1996). The pars triangularis and speech and language lateralization. *Proceedings of the National Academy of Sciences of the United States of America, 93,* 719–722.

Foundas, A., Leonard, C., & Heilman, K. (1995). Morphological cerebral asymmetries and handedness: The pars triangularis and planum temporale. *Archives of Neurology, 52,* 501–508.

Frith, C., Friston, K., Liddle, P., & Frackowiak, R. (1991). Willed action and the prefrontal cortex in man: A study with PET. *Proceedings of the Royal Society of London, Series B: Biological Sciences, 244,* 241–246.

Galaburda, A.M. (1989). Ordinary and extraordinary brain development: Anatomical variation in developmental dyslexia. *Annals of Dyslexia, 39,* 67–79.

Galaburda, A., Sherman, G., Rosen, G., Aboitiz, F., & Geschwind, N. (1985). Developmental dyslexia: Four consecutive cases with cortical anomalies. *Annals of Neurology, 18,* 222–223.

Gathercole, S., & Baddeley, S. (1989). Development of vocabulary in children and short-term phonological memory. *Journal of Memory and Language, 28,* 200–213.

Gauger, L.M., Lombardino, L.J., & Leonard, C.M. (in press). Brain morphology in children with specific language impairment. *Journal of Speech and Hearing Research.*

Gautier, E., Kuldau, J., Weis, A., Leonard, C., & Mancuso, A. (1995). Schizophrenia and the temporal lobe: A replication. *New Research of the American Psychiatric Association,* 115.

Geschwind, N., & Galaburda, A. (1987). *Cerebral lateralization: Biological mechanisms, association and pathology.* Cambridge, MA: MIT Press.

Geschwind, N., & Levitsky, W. (1968). Human brain: Left–right asymmetries in temporal speech region. *Science, 161,* 186–187.

Giedd, J., Castellanos, F., Kozuch, P., Casey, B., Kaysen, D., & Rapoport, J. (1996). Quantitative magnetic resonance imaging of human brain development: Ages 5–18. *Cerebral Cortex, 6,* 551–560.

Goldman-Rakic, P. (1988). Topography of cognition: Parallel distributed networks in primate association cortex. *Annual Review of Neuroscience, 11,* 137–156.

Goldman-Rakic, P., & Friedman, H. (1991). The circuitry of working memory revealed by anatomy and metabolic imaging. In H. Levin, H. Eisenberg, & A. Benton (Eds.), *Frontal lobe function and dysfunction* (pp. 72–91). New York: Oxford University Press.

Grasby, P., Frith, C., Friston, K., Simpson, J., Flectcher, P., Frackowiak, R., & Dolan, R. (1994). A graded task approach to the functional mapping of brain areas implicated in auditory-verbal memory. *Brain, 117,* 1271–1282.

Hassink, R., Hiltbrunner, B., Muller, S., & Lutschg, J. (1992). Assessment of brain maturation by T2-weighted MRI. *Neuropediatrics, 23,* 72–74.

Hayes, T.L., & Lewis, D.A. (1995). Anatomical specializations of the anterior motor speech area. *Brain and Language, 49,* 289–308.

Howard, D., Patterson, K., Wise, R., Brown, W., Friston, K., Weiller, C., & Frackowiak, R. (1992). The cortical localization of the lexicons: Positron emission tomography evidence. *Brain, 115,* 1769–1782.

Jackendoff, R. (1987). *Consciousness and the computational mind.* Cambridge, MA: MIT Press.

Jancke, L., Schlaug, G., Huang, Y., & Steinmetz, H. (1994). Asymmetry of the planum parietale. *NeuroReport, 5,* 1161–1163.

Jernigan, T., Hesselink, J., Sowell, E., & Tallal, P. (1990). Cerebral morphology on MRI in language and learning-impaired children. *Archives of Neurology, 48,* 539–545.

Kimura, D. (1992, August). Body asymmetry and cognitive function. *The University of Western Ontario Department of Psychology Research Bulletin.*

Kimura, D. (1993). *Neuromotor mechanisms of human communication.* New York: Oxford University Press.

Kinsbourne, M. (1988). Sinistrality, brain organization, and cognitive deficits. In D. Molfese & S. Segalowitz (Eds.), *Brain lateralization in children: Developmental implications* (pp. 259–280). New York: Guilford Press.

Kuhl, P., & Miller, J. (1975). Speech perception by the chinchilla: Voiced-voiceless distinction in alveolar plosive consonants. *Science, 190,* 69–72.

Kulynych, J., Vladar, K., Jones, D., & Weinberger, D. (1994). Gender differences in the normal lateralization of the supratemporal cortex-MRI surface-rendering morphometry of Heschl's gyrus and the planum temporale. *Cerebral Cortex, 4,* 107–118.

Lenneberg, E. (1967). *Biological foundations of language.* New York: John Wiley & Sons.

Leonard, C., Lombardino, L., Mercado, L., Browd, S., Breier, J., & Agee, O. (1996). Cortical asymmetry and cognitive development: A magnetic neuroimaging study. *Psychological Science, 7,* 79–85.

Leonard, C., Martinez, P., Weintraub, B., & Hauser, P. (1995). Magnetic resonance imaging of cerebral anomalies in subjects with resistance to thyroid hormone. *American Journal of Medical Genetics, 60,* 238–243.

Leonard, C., Voeller, K.K., Lombardino, L., Morris, M.K., Alexander, A., Andersen, H., Garofalakis, M., Hynd, G., Honeyman, J., Mao, J., Agee, O., & Staab, E. (1993). Anomalous cerebral structure in dyslexia revealed with magnetic resonance imaging. *Archives of Neurology, 50,* 461–469.

Leonard, C., Williams, C., Nicholls, R., Agee, O., Voeller, K., Honeyman, J., & Staab, E. (1993). Angelman and Prader-Willi syndrome. A magnetic resonance imaging study of differences in cerebral structure. *American Journal of Medical Genetics, 46,* 26–33.

Liberman, A. (1982). On finding that speech is special. *American Psychologist, 37,* 148–167.

Liddle, P., Friston, K., Frith, C., Hirsch, S., Jones, T., & Frackowiak, R. (1992). Patterns of cerebral blood flow in schizophrenia. *British Journal of Psychiatry, 160,* 179–186.

Lindamood, C., & Lindamood, P. (1979). *Lindamood Auditory Conceptualization Test.* Hingham, MA: Teaching Resources.

Lipska, B., Jaskiw, G., & Weinberger, D. (1993). Postpubertal emergence of hyperresponsiveness to stress and to amphetamine after neonatal excitotoxic hippocampal damage; A potential animal model of schizophrenia. *Neuropsychopharmacology, 9,* 67–75.

Locke, J. (1994). Gradual emergence of developmental language disorders. *Journal of Speech and Hearing Research, 37,* 608–616.

Lukatella, K., Shankweiler, D., & Crain, S. (1995). Syntactic processing in agrammatic aphasia by speakers of a Slavic language. *Brain and Language, 49,* 50–76.

Mamen, M. (1987). Laterality patterns in young fluent readers. *Brain and Language, 30,* 81–92.

Manzano, J., Zabala, I., & Borella, E. (1992). Continuité et discontinuité de la psychopathologie: Une étude sur des patients examines comme enfants et comme adultes: L'enfance deteoubles schizophrenes adultes. *Archives Suisses de Neurologie et Psychiatrie, 143,* 5–25.

Mazoyer, B., Tzourio, N., Frak, V., Syrota, A., Murayama, N., Cohen, L., Levrier, O., Salamon, G., Syrota, A., & Mehler, J. (1993). The cortical representation of speech. *Journal of Cognitive Neuroscience, 5,* 467–479.

McGlone, J. (1980). Sex differences in human brain asymmetry: A critical survey. *Behavioral and Brain Sciences, 3,* 215–263.

Mercado, L. (1995). *Brain structure and specific language impairment: An MRI study.* Unpublished doctoral dissertation, University of Florida, Gainesville.

Molfese, D., & Buhrla, R.W. (1985). The right hemisphere and temporal processing of consonant transition duration: Electrophysiological correlates. *Brain and Language, 26,* 49–62.

Molfese, D.L., Freeman, R., Jr., & Palermo, D. (1975). The ontogeny of brain lateralization for speech and nonspeech sounds. *Brain and Language, 2,* 356–368.

Morse, P., Molfese, D., Laughlin, N., Linnville, S., & Wetzel, F. (1987). Categorical perception for voicing contrasts in normal and lead treated rhesus monkeys: Electrophysiological indices. *Brain and Language, 30,* 63–80.

Musiek, F., & Reeves, A. (1990). Asymmetries of the auditory areas of the cerebrum. *Journal of the American Academy of Audiology, 1,* 240–245.

Nordeen, E., & Yahr, P. (1982). Hemispheric asymmetries in the behavioral and hormonal effects of sexually differentiating mammalian brain. *Science, 218,* 391–394.

Obler, L., & Fein, D. (1988). *The exceptional brain: Neuropsychology of talent and special abilities.* New York: Guilford Press.

Passingham, R. (1993). *The frontal lobes and voluntary behavior.* Oxford, England: Oxford University Press.

Paulesu, E., Frith, D., & Frackowiak, R. (1993). The neural correlates of the verbal component of working memory. *Nature, 362,* 342–345.

Penhune, V., Zatorre, R.J., MacDonald, J.D., & Evans, A.C. (1996). Interhemispheric differences in human primary auditory cortex: Probabilistic mapping and volume measurement from MR scans. *Cerebral Cortex, 6,* 661–672.

Petersen, S., Fox, P., Posner, M., Mintun, M., & Raichle, M. (1988). Positron emission tomographic studies of the cortical anatomy of single-word processing. *Nature, 331,* 585–589.

Petersen, S.E., Fox, P.T., Snyder, A.Z., & Raichle, M.E. (1990). Activation of extrastriate and frontal cortical areas by visual words and word-like stimuli. *Science, 249,* 1041–1044.

Petty, R., Barta, P., Pearlson, G., McGilchrist, I., Lewis, R., Tien, A., Pulver, A., Vaughn, D., Casanova, M., & Powers, R. (1995). Reversal of asymmetry of the planum temporale in schizophrenia. *American Journal of Psychiatry, 152,* 715–721.

Plante, E., Swisher, L., Vance, R., & Rapcsak, S. (1991). MRI findings in boys with specific language impairment. *Brain and Language, 41,* 52–66.

Previc, F. (1991). A general theory concerning the prenatal origins of cerebral lateralization in humans. *Psychological Review, 98,* 299–334.

Price, C., Wise, R., Watson, J., Patterson, K., Howard, D., & Frackowiak, R. (1994). Brain activity during reading: The effects of exposure duration and task. *Brain, 117,* 1255–1269.

Rasmussen, T., & Milner, B. (1975). Clinical and surgical studies of the cerebral speech areas in man. In O.C.K.J. Zulch & G.C. Galbraith (Eds.), *Otfrid Foerster Symposium on Cerebral Localization* (pp. 238–257). New York: Springer-Verlag.

Satz, P.S., Strauss, E., & Whitaker, H. (1990). The ontogeny of hemispheric specialization: Some old hypotheses revisited. *Brain and Language, 38,* 596–614.

Schaefer, G., Thompson, J., Bodensteiner, J., Hamza, M., Tucker, R., Marks, W., Gay, C., & Wilson, D. (1990). Quantitative morphometric analysis of brain growth using magnetic resonance imaging. *Journal of Child Neurology, 5,* 127–130.

Scheibel, A.B. (1984). A dendritic correlate of human speech. In N. Geschwind & A.M. Galaburda (Eds.), *Cerebral dominance: The biological foundations* (pp. 43–52). Cambridge, MA: Harvard University Press.

Schultz, R., Cho, N., Staib, L., Kier, L., Fletcher, J., Shaywitz, S., Shankweiler, D., Katz, L., Gore, J., Duncan, J., & Shaywitz, B. (1994). Brain morphology in normal and dyslexic children: The influence of sex and age. *Annals of Neurology, 35,* 732–742.

Seldon, H. (1985). The anatomy of speech perception: Human auditory cortex. In A. Peters & E. Jones (Eds.), *Cerebral cortex* (pp. 273–327). New York: Plenum.

Sereno, M., Dale, A., Tootell, R., Reppas, J., Kwong, K., Belliveau, J., Brady, T., & Rosen, B. (1995). Human visual areas identified by visual field sign on the cortical surface using phase-encoded retinotopic stimulation. *Science, 268,* 889–893.

Shaywitz, B., Shaywitz, S., Pugh, K., Constable, R., Skudlarski, P., Fulbright, R., Bronen, R., Fletcher, J., Shankweiler, D., Katz, L., & Gore, J. (1995). Sex differences in the functional organization of the brain for language. *Nature, 373,* 607–609.

Steinmetz, H., Volkmann, J., Jancke, L., & Freund, H. (1991). Anatomical left–right asymmetry of language related temporal cortex is different in left- and right-handers. *Annals of Neurology, 29,* 315–319.

Strauss, E., Gaddes, W., & Wada, J. (1987). Performance on a free-recall verbal dichotic listening task and cerebral dominance determined by the carotid amytal test. *Neuropsychologia, 25,* 747–753.

Talairach, J., & Tournoux, P. (1988). *Coplanar stereotaxic atlas of the human brain: Three-dimensional proportional system: An approach to cerebral imaging.* New York: Thieme.

Tallal, P., Miller, S., & Fitch, R.H. (1993). Temporal processing in the nervous system: Implications for the development of phonological systems. *Annals of the New York Academy of Sciences, 682,* 27–47.

Thal, D., Marchman, V., Stiles, J., Aram, D., Trauner, D., Nass, R., & Bates, E. (1991). Early lexical development in children with focal brain injury. *Brain and Language, 40,* 491–527.

van Kleeck, A. (1994). Metalinguistic development. In G. Wallach & K. Boller (Eds.), *Language learning in school-age children and adolescents* (pp. 53–98). New York: Maxwell Macmillan.

Von Economo, C., & Horn, L. (1930). Gyral relief, size and cortical architectonics of the suprotemporal surface: Their individual and lateral differences. *Zeitschrift für Gesamte Neurologie und Psychiatry, 130,* 687–757.

Wagner, R., & Torgesen, J. (1987). The nature of phonological processing and its causal role in acquisition of reading skills. *Psychological Review, 101,* 192–212.

Witelson, S. (1989). Hand and sex differences in the isthmus and genu of the human corpus callosum. *Brain, 112,* 799–835.

Witelson, S., & Kigar, D. (1988). Asymmetry in brain function follows asymmetry in anatomical form: Gross, microscopic, postmortem and imaging studies. In F. Boller, J. Grafman, G. Rizzolatti, & H. Goodglass (Eds.), *Handbook of neuropsychology* (pp. 111–142). Amsterdam: Elsevier.

Witelson, S., & Kigar, D. (1992). Sylvian fissure morphology and asymmetry in men and women: Bilateral differences in relation to handedness in men. *Journal of Comparative Neurology, 323,* 326–340.

Witelson, S., & Paillie, W. (1973). Left hemisphere specialization for language in the newborn: Neuroanatomical evidence of asymmetry. *Brain, 96,* 641–646.

Wright, B.A., Lombardino, L.J., King, W.M., Puranik, C.S., Leonard, C.M., & Merzenich, M.M. (1996a). Auditory temporal and spectral resolution in children with language impairment. *Society for Neuroscience Abstracts, 22,* 1852.

Wright, B.A., Lombardino, L.J., King, W.M., Puranik, C.S., Leonard, C.M., & Merzenich, M.M. (1996b). *Deficits in auditory temporal and spectral processing in language-impaired children.* Manuscript submitted for publication.

Yakovlev, P., & LeCours, A. (1967). The myelogenetic cycles of regional maturation of the brain. In A. Minkowski (Ed.), *Regional development of the brain in early life* (pp. 3–70). Oxford, England: Blackwell.

Yeo, R.A., Gangestad, S.W., & Daniel, W.F. (1993). Hand preference and developmental instability. *Psychobiology 21,* 161–168.

Zilles, K. (1990). Cortex. In G. Paxinos (Ed.), *The human nervous system* (pp. 757–802). New York: Academic Press.

Development of the Prefrontal Cortex: Evolution, Neurobiology, and Behavior
edited by Norman A. Krasnegor, Ph.D., G. Reid Lyon, Ph.D.,
and Patricia S. Goldman-Rakic, Ph.D.
copyright © 1997   Paul H. Brookes Publishing Co., Inc.
Baltimore • London • Toronto • Sydney

8

Development of Neuronal Activity in Cortical Regions Underlying Visual Recognition in Monkeys

Hillary R. Rodman and Kristy L. Nace

How do we know what it is that we see? How do we go from birth, having little knowledge of the visual world but a rudimentary capacity for interacting with it, to being sophisticated observers and actors with exquisite ability to identify and utilize the objects and scenes that are crucial to our survival, well-being, and contentment, despite changes in their exact appearance and location relative to other objects and scenes? Primates in particular are gifted at visual pattern recognition. Visual pattern recognition capacity is a complex set of abilities involving perception of identifying characteristics of stimuli, abstraction of features that reliably identify objects under varied or degraded conditions, and generation of signals indicating that a given stimulus has been seen before. In both humans and monkeys, visual pattern recognition is subserved by a ventrally coursing occipito-temporo-frontal system of interconnected cortical areas. In adult primates, these areas contain cells with visual responses that are selective for aspects of stimulus form, responses that are believed to be crucial for recognition behavior. To what extent does the final manifestation of these properties depend on physiological and structural maturation, experience of the visual world, or specific interactions between these factors? In order to understand the relationship between development of neuronal activity in this system and the ontogeny of pattern recognition behavior, we have conducted neurophysiological and anatomical studies in infant monkeys, concentrating on the inferior temporal (IT) cortex, a crucial area for formation and storage of visual object representations. We have been interested, in particular, in the relationship between the prefrontal cortex and IT.

Physiological and connectional studies of inferior temporal cortex in infant monkeys described in this chapter were performed in collaboration with S.P. Ó Scalaidhe, C.G. Gross, T.-M. Woods, A.M. Galioto, N.S. Rebmann, and M. Consuelos and were supported by National Institutes of Health Grants MH-14202 and MH-19420 and by the Sloan Foundation.

The authors thank A. Repp and M. Rosengarten for assistance with the manuscript. Animals for the majority of these studies were obtained with the assistance of the New England Primate Research Center.

CORTICAL SUBSTRATES OF VISUAL RECOGNITION CAPACITY

A major portion of the neocortex of primates is devoted to the processing of visual information. Visual cortical areas of primates can be divided roughly into two streams: an occipitoparietal "dorsal stream" concerned with the analysis of the locations of objects and their movements in space and an occipitotemporal "ventral stream" responsible for the processing and storage of information about their identity—their shape, color, and other salient physical features. Although the two cortical streams are not completely segregated anatomically or functionally, this formulation, first put forth in 1982 by Ungerleider and Mishkin and subsequently elaborated by those authors and other workers, remains a valuable principle in our understanding of visual cortex.

Evidence has appeared for continued segregation of the two major processing streams in the frontal cortex (Barbas, 1988; Webster, Bachevalier, & Ungerleider, 1994; Wilson, Ó Scalaidhe, & Goldman-Rakic, 1993). Therefore, frontal cortex contributes to pattern recognition as well as to spatial cognition and executive function (see also Chapter 2).

Ventral cortical pathways for visual pattern recognition in macaques are diagrammed in Figure 8.1. Analysis of objects and scenes begins in visual area (V)1, where information about edges and about the color and brightness of stimuli is extracted from visual inputs from the thalamus. This information is then sent on to certain subdivisions of area V2. From V2, the object recognition pathway takes a largely ventral, occipitotemporal course (reviewed in Desimone & Ungerleider, 1989; Felleman & Van Essen, 1991; Gross, Rodman, Gochin, & Colombo, 1993). Visual information about objects is sent from V2 to area V4 on the lateral and ventromedial surfaces of the hemisphere and to visual areas TEO and TF just anterior to V4. From these regions, information proceeds forward to area TE, also known as IT cortex, and then to the most ventral and anterior reaches of temporal lobe neocortex, particularly Brodmann's area 36. These areas and adjacent parahippocampal and entorhinal cortices are interconnected with medial temporal lobe structures, most notably the hippocampus, that are crucial for memory of visual objects (Mishkin & Murray, 1994; Zola-Morgan & Squire, 1993). At all stages of the pathway, connections tend to be reciprocal; that is, an area receiving *forward* projections from another earlier in the ventral hierarchy also tends to provide return projections to the "earlier" area. Long-range nonreciprocal connections also exist, such as that from TE back to V1 (Rockland & Van Hoesen, 1994). In addition, the ventral object recognition pathway involves interconnections of temporal areas, such as TEO and TE, with ventral portions of frontal lobe neocortex (Bates, Wilson, Ó Scalaidhe, & Goldman-Rakic, 1994; Seltzer & Pandya, 1989; Webster et al., 1994) and with portions of the superior temporal polysensory area (STP), which appears to contribute to both object and motion analyses on the basis of converging projections from both dorsal and ventral streams (Baizer, Ungerleider, & Desimone, 1991). Furthermore, all areas in the ventral stream are interconnected with subcortical visual structures, most notably the pulvinar and portions of the amygdala, claustrum, and basal ganglia (e.g., Kaas & Huerta, 1988; Webster, Bachevalier, & Ungerleider, 1993). Finally, all areas in the ventral stream are connected with their counterparts and other ventral stream areas of the opposite hemisphere through the corpus callosum or, in the anterior and ventral regions, through the anterior commissure (see Rodman & Consuelos, 1994, and references therein). Presumably, all

A

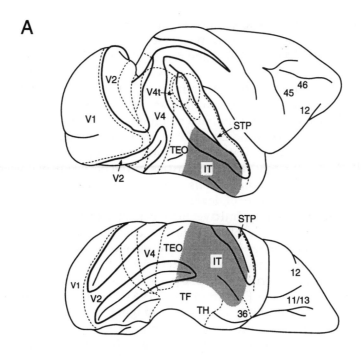

B

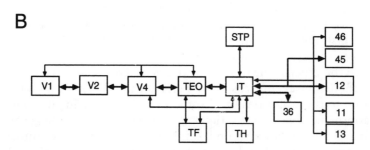

Figure 8.1. Ventral cortical pathways for visual pattern and object recognition in macaques. (A) Location of occipitotemporal visual areas and frontal cytoarchitectonic regions discussed in this chapter, shown on lateral (top) and ventral (bottom) views of a macaque brain in which posterior sulci have been "opened up." Inferior temporal cortex is shaded. (B) Flow diagram illustrating crucial features of the sequence of information processing described in this chapter. Other abbreviations: TEO—visual area TEO; STP—superior temporal polysensory area; V1, V2, V3, V4, V4t—visual areas 1, 2, 3, 4, and transitional 4, respectively; 11, 12, 13, 36, 45, 46, TF, and TH—architectonically defined areas of the temporal and frontal lobes.

of these patterns of connectivity must achieve their mature status prior to full adult functioning of visual pattern recognition capacity.

DEVELOPMENT OF VISUAL RECOGNITION CAPACITY IN PRIMATES

Ontogeny of Pattern Recognition in Humans and Monkeys

Many visual recognition abilities appear to be present early in humans and then take a very long time to mature completely (see Carey, 1992; Johnson, 1994). For example, human infants show a preference for certain types of visual stimuli shortly after birth (Goren, Sarty, & Wu, 1975; Johnson, Dziurawiec, Ellis, & Morton, 1991; Meltzoff & Moore, 1977) and can easily learn long lists of object-pair discriminations at 1 year of age (Overman, Bachevalier, Turner, & Peuster, 1992). However, children require extensive training to learn a more complex visual recognition task, namely, delayed nonmatch to sample (DNMS) (Overman et al., 1992). Moreover, although both adult humans and monkeys can identify visual forms under altered or degraded conditions, children are much poorer at this task (Carey & Diamond, 1977; Diamond & Carey, 1990; Foreman & Hemmings, 1987).

Overall, there are remarkable similarities in the ontogeny of object recognition and other cognitive abilities in humans and macaque monkeys (see Chapter 15). As in humans, the general picture of development of visual pattern and object recognition in macaques is one of primitive early capacity followed by a long period of gradual emergence of adult levels of performance. Like human infants, infant monkeys show a visual preference for novel patterns or objects within the first weeks of life (Bachevalier, 1990; Gunderson & Sackett, 1984; Sackett, 1966). Infant monkeys can solve simple form discriminations (e.g., horizontal versus vertical stripes, circle versus triangle) by 3 weeks (Zimmermann, 1961). Harlow, Harlow, Reuping, and Mason (1960) studied the ability of monkeys ranging in age from 2 months to 1 year to discriminate among small, multidimensional objects and found that all age groups could solve the problem, with progressively older infants requiring correspondingly fewer trials to achieve criterion performance. Bachevalier and colleagues (Bachevalier, 1990) further found that 3- to 4-month-old infant monkeys could learn lists of object-pair discriminations nearly as quickly as adult monkeys. However, they also found that infant monkeys do not even begin to be able to learn the DNMS task until they are approximately 4 months and do not reach adult levels of ability until 2 years of age.

Despite the crucial role of inferior temporal cortex in form recognition in adult primates, there are several reasons to believe that IT cortex does not make its full contribution to these abilities until sometime after early infancy. First, as described above, pattern and object recognition capacity, per se, takes a long time to mature in both humans and monkeys. Second, some *sparing* of form discrimination and recognition capacity follows when lesions of IT cortex occur in monkeys 1 year of age or younger (Bachevalier, 1990; Bachevalier, Brickson, Hagger, & Mishkin, 1990; Raisler & Harlow, 1965). In this respect, IT cortex appears to be comparable with the prefrontal cortex, where early lesions likewise fail to produce impairments in characteristic functions (Goldman, 1971). Moreover, unlike the case for early lesions of dorsolateral frontal cortex, in which deficits appear only as the monkey grows older, neonatal IT cortex damage leads to apparently preserved performance for several years thereafter, at least on the tests of visual object discrimination and recognition examined thus far (Bachevalier & Mishkin, 1988). The sparing induced by early IT lesions, therefore, appears to be lasting, which suggests that other structures are capable of compensating for at least some of the effects of early damage to this region.

Development of Face Recognition

One aspect of pattern recognition that has received a great deal of attention, from both the perspective of cognitive development and that of neural substrates of vision, is the perception and recognition of face stimuli. Adult humans and monkeys alike are highly adept at recognizing and differentiating new and old conspecific faces. Moreover, both human infants and infant monkeys show preferential atten-tiveness to face stimuli in the early postnatal period and can even distinguish indi-viduals and expressions (for a review, see Johnson, 1994; Rodman, 1994; Slater, 1993). Debate continues as to whether these early abilities reflect innate "tem-plates" for faces (Johnson, 1994) or merely attentional biases toward more general types of salient information present in faces (Kleiner, 1993; Slater, 1993). As is the case for other aspects of pattern and object recognition, primitive early capacity is followed by a long period of maturation to adult levels, and encoding strategies for faces used by young children differ from those used by older humans (Carey, 1992; Carey & Diamond, 1977; Ellis, 1992).

Implications for Development of Neuronal Activity

In adult monkeys, cells in the anterior portions of the ventral cortical stream, such as area IT, show patterns of neural response consistent with a high-level role in pat-tern and object recognition (Desimone, Albright, Gross, & Bruce, 1984; Gross et al., 1993; Tanaka, Saito, Fukada, & Moriya, 1991). For example, many neurons in IT cortex and neighboring areas are selective for particular complex objects or feature conjunctions. In particular, although they make up only a small percentage of the overall population of visually responsive IT cells, neurons responding preferentially to face stimuli have received a great deal of attention. Moreover, IT cells that show selectivity often maintain their stimulus preferences over relatively wide regions of visual space. Finally, for many IT neurons in adult monkeys, receptive fields are bi-lateral, straddling the vertical midline; again, stimulus selectivity tends to be simi-lar across the two half-fields as well as within them. How do such properties of IT cells arise ontogenetically? If one assumes that the stimulus selectivity of adult IT cells plays a role in visual pattern and object recognition, one logical possible rea-son for the long time needed for pattern recognition functions to arise may be that cells in infant IT cortex are not very selective until they have a fair amount of spe-cific visual experience, even if they are otherwise physiologically mature. Another possible reason is that cells in infant IT cortex are simply inactive early in life be-cause of an immaturity of cellular mechanisms (e.g., oxidative metabolism) needed to generate action potentials concordant with activation of input pathways. In-activity of IT cells early in life would be consistent with the proposed dominance of subcortical mechanisms of vision in neonatal primates (Dubowitz, Mushin, DeVries, & Arden, 1986; Johnson, 1990). An additional possibility is that the pat-terns of anatomical connectivity of IT cortex, particularly with regard to its inputs from visual structures, show an extended period of maturation. To begin to answer these questions, we have conducted a series of experiments on the physiology and cortical connectivity of temporal cortex (chiefly area IT) in infant monkeys within approximately the first 7 months of life.

PHYSIOLOGICAL STUDIES OF DEVELOPMENT OF TEMPORAL CORTEX

Methods

Neuronal activity was studied in temporal cortex of 17 infant macaques and 3 adult control macaques. Cells were studied both in immobilized animals anesthetized with nitrous oxide (for precise plotting of receptive fields) and in awake monkeys taught to perform a visual fixation task during recording and presentation of stim-uli. The methods used for electrophysiological recording, behavioral training, and general procedures for maintenance of the health and welfare of the infant and adult monkeys have been described previously (Rodman, 1991; Rodman, Ó Scalaidhe, & Gross, 1993). A total of 503 single, isolated neurons were studied in IT cortex. An additional 80 single units were studied in the superior temporal polysensory area (STP). For both the anesthetized and the alert recording experiments, three classes of visual stimuli were used. The first class consisted of three-dimensional complex objects, including a standard set of 16, consisting of head models, monkey dolls, large brushes of various colors, and plastic food objects. The second class consisted of images projected from slides under computer control, including faces, scrambled faces, lines, control objects, and so-called Fourier descriptors (FD stimuli), which varied systematically in boundary curvature (Schwartz, Desimone, Albright, & Gross, 1983). These images subtended 3°–6° of visual angle and were presented at the fovea or, in a few cases, at 4° on the horizontal meridian in the contralateral field. The third class of stimuli consisted of two-dimensional images presented by hand, including bars of light generated with a projector fitted with an adjustable aperture that could be varied in width, length, orientation, and color, as well as pictures of the three-dimensional objects, faces, and other images included in the first two classes of stimuli.

Signal Characteristics of Neurons in Infant Inferior Temporal Cortex
Overall, in alert infant monkeys, more than three fourths of neurons sampled in IT cortex responded to visual stimulation, a proportion comparable with that found in this region in alert adult animals (Figure 8.2). No developmental trend toward greater incidence of responsiveness was observed within the developmental window studied. In contrast, in anesthetized infants, only a very few cells (10%) responded at ages younger than 4 months; significantly fewer neurons responded in monkeys between 4 and 7 months than in adults under comparable conditions. There was a fairly sharp transition at approximately the 4-month point in animals studied longitudinally in repeated sessions under anesthesia (Rodman, Ó Scalaidhe, & Gross, 1993). A similar time course of appearance of responsiveness under anesthesia and an abundance of responses at the earliest ages in the alert state were found for area STP of infant monkeys. For alert infants, despite the similar incidence of responsive neurons, responses of temporal cortex neurons were weaker overall (Figure 8.3A), and latencies to visual response were longer and more variable (Figure 8.3B). Finally, baseline rates of action potential generation in the absence of visual stimulation (i.e., spontaneous activity) were also lower in infant IT cortex than in adult cortex under both anesthetized and alert conditions (Rodman, 1994; Rodman, Ó Scalaidhe, & Gross, 1993).

Encoding of Stimulus Form
General Form Selectivity   Although visually responsive IT neurons were found less frequently in infants (under anesthetized recording conditions) or showed reduced magnitudes of response (under alert recording conditions), the types and incidences of form selectivity observed were similar to those seen under comparable conditions in adult monkeys. At the earliest ages, when we were able to study visually responsive neurons (i.e., approximately 6 weeks in the alert infants), individual IT cells showed responses that were selective for shape, geometrical patterns, color, or specific three-dimensional objects. For example, the selectivity of several infant IT neurons for shape, as defined by boundary curvature, is illustrated in Figure 8.4. These cells were tested with FD stimuli, images that differ systematically in "fre-

Alert

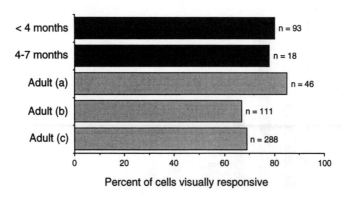

Anesthetized

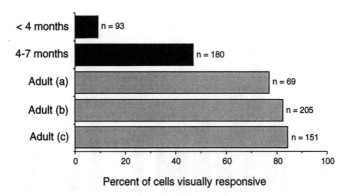

Figure 8.2.   Incidence of visually responsive single neurons in IT cortex in infant and adult macaques. (Top) Awake animals performing a fixation task. Adult data: a, from Rodman, Ó Scalaidhe, and Gross (1993); b, from Gross, Bender, and Gerstein (1979); c, from Richmond, Wurtz, and Sato (1983). (Bottom) Animals under nitrous oxide anesthesia and immobilization. Adult data: a, from Rodman, Ó Scalaidhe, and Gross (1993); b, from Gross, Rocha-Miranda, and Bender (1972); c, from Desimone et al. (1984).

quency," or the number of lobes around the perimeter of the shape; a similar proportion of neurons show tuning of response as a function of FD frequency in alert infant and adult macaques (Rodman, Ó Scalaidhe, & Gross, 1993).

Other neurons responded to a greater variety of images and objects. Figure 8.5 presents distributions of the proportions of tested stimuli that elicited significant responses from individual neurons in the alert infant and adult samples. The distributions do not differ significantly, thereby confirming that IT cells in infant monkeys are about as selective overall as are those in adult monkeys. Note that, although very few IT neurons respond indiscriminately to most of the stimuli tested, only a small percentage respond to only one or two of the images. The greatest proportion responds to a larger subset of the total stimulus set, suggesting that, in both

A

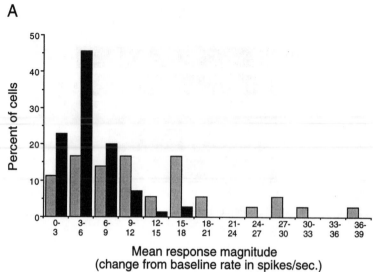

Mean response magnitude
(change from baseline rate in spikes/sec.)

B

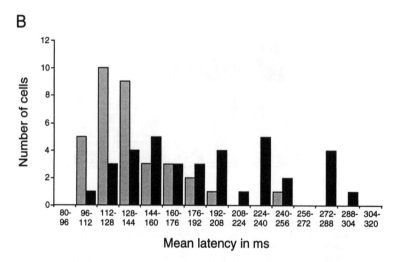

Mean latency in ms

Figure 8.3.   Signaling properties of IT cortex in infant monkeys. (A) Overall mean response magnitude distributions for samples of IT cells in awake infant and adult macaques. (▨ Adult IT [*n* = 36], ■ Infant IT [*n* = 70].) (B) Distributions of mean latencies of visual response of IT cells in awake infant and adult macaques. (▨ Adult IT [*n* = 34], ■ Infant IT [*n* = 36].) (Adapted from Rodman, Ó Scalaidhe, & Gross [1993].)

infant and adult IT cortex, many cells participate in encoding multiple objects in an ensemble fashion (Gochin, Colombo, Dorfman, Gerstein, & Gross, 1994; Gross et al., 1993).

Face Selectivity   One of the most striking characteristics of IT cortex and of the immediately adjacent area STP of adult monkeys is the presence of a small population of neurons that have responses that are selective for aspects of face stimuli. Although these neurons vary in the extent of their preference for faces, they often have little or no response to other tested stimuli, and their selectivity is typically maintained over transformations such as changes in the size, lighting, or spatial frequency content of the face stimulus (reviewed in Gross et al., 1993; Perrett,

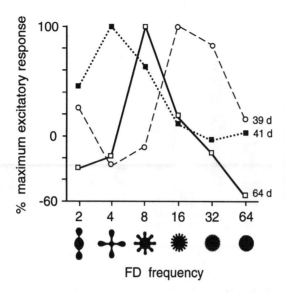

Figure 8.4.   Responses of neurons in IT cortex. Examples of responses of three cells tuned to boundary curvature in IT cortex of awake infant macaques. Age in days (d) at the time of recording is given for each tuning curve. Stimuli were black and white images projected onto a screen and subtended 3°–6° at the fovea. (Adapted from Rodman, Skelly, & Gross [1991].)

Hietanen, Oram, & Benson, 1992; Rolls, 1992). Subsets of face-selective neurons have responses specific for particular facial expressions, types of face view (e.g., profiles), and possibly even particular individuals (Desimone et al., 1984; Hasselmo, Rolls, & Baylis, 1989). Although few investigators now believe that such neurons *individually* provide reliable signals about face identity or even the presence of a significant face stimulus, it remains tenable that face-selective populations are likely to provide "relatively dedicated circuitry" for face processing (for discussion, see Gross et al., 1993) through the use of small neuronal ensembles that are involved more or less exclusively in encoding facial stimuli (e.g., Gross & Sergent, 1992; Young & Yamane, 1992).

Are there neural correlates of the early appearance of rudimentary face recognition capacity in primates? In our studies of temporal cortex, we found neurons selective for aspects of face stimuli in both anesthetized and alert infant monkeys (Rodman, Ó Scalaidhe, & Gross, 1993; Rodman, Skelly, & Gross, 1991). We were not able to systematically evaluate the components of faces that were responsible for the selectivity, but for some such neurons it appeared that components of the faces did contribute to the response as much as the prototypical overall organization. This finding suggested that the response for such neurons was not based on some overall gestalt of the facial configuration but was influenced by other factors differentiating the two faces, such as the ages or expressions of the monkeys depicted or specific structural features of the faces. Other cells did not respond well or at all to a scrambled version of the optimal face; rather, they responded only to particular normal faces.

The cell for which responses are graphed in Figure 8.6, recorded in an alert 3-month-old monkey, illustrates a type of face selectivity we have seen repeatedly in

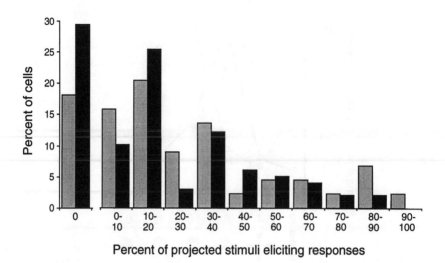

Figure 8.5.   Distributions of percentages of projected stimuli in the standard set eliciting statistically significant responses for IT cells in awake infant and adult macaques. (▒ Adult IT [$n = 44$], ■ Infant IT [$n = 98$].)

both infant and adult IT cortex. This cell was selective specifically for profiles and, in fact, responded only to profiles showing the teeth. Informal testing suggested that, when the teeth from the profile view were seen alone, this was adequate to elicit some response. Because other views with open mouths (e.g., threats, yawns [see Stimuli 8 and 9 and 11 and 12]) and the scrambles did not elicit responses, some combination of a normal profile view and the feature of teeth seemed to be necessary to activate the cell. Moreover, although the cell was sensitive to viewing angle (front view versus side view versus profile), in additional tests, it showed very similar responsiveness to the profile regardless of which way the profile was facing. The cell's response, therefore, was probably not dependent on the precise position of critical elements within the visual world. In other words, although the response did not show invariance over viewing angle, it appeared to show invariance over orientation of the stimulus.

Receptive Fields and Stimulus Invariance
The large, bilateral receptive fields of IT neurons historically found in anesthetized animals have been proposed as a basis for the perceptual equivalence of stimuli regardless of which half-field they fall into. In other words, they have been proposed to "knit together" visual space at the midline. Moreover, the role of IT in perceptual equivalence of objects across retinal translation has been supported and inferred from the tendency of many (although not all) IT cells to show similar stimulus selectivity when stimuli are presented in different locations within the cell's receptive field or at different sizes (Gross & Mishkin, 1977; Lueschow, Miller, & Desimone, 1994; Rolls & Baylis, 1986; Schwartz et al., 1983). To see whether similar receptive field properties are present early in life, we plotted receptive fields of IT neurons in anesthetized infant monkeys with the smallest stimulus that would reliably drive the cell. As in adult monkeys, the majority of IT receptive fields were large and bilateral in infant monkeys (e.g., Figure 8.7; Rodman, 1994; Rodman, Ó Scalaidhe, & Gross, 1993). Median receptive field size and proportions of bilateral

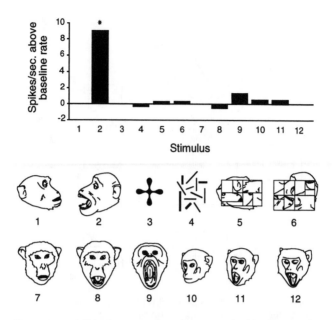

Figure 8.6.   Cell in IT cortex of an alert 3-month-old infant monkey selective for a particular profile view. Stimuli were black and white (3 and 4) or color (1, 2, and 5–12) images projected onto a screen and subtended 3°–6° at the fovea.

fields in infants were not significantly different from those seen in adults (Rodman, Ó Scalaidhe, & Gross, 1993). In our studies of awake infant animals, limited assessments of receptive field sizes suggested that IT fields in infant monkeys were more restricted than were those in adults. It is not yet known whether cells in infant IT cortex show a degree of invariance of selectivity across changes in retinal size or location of the stimulus comparable with that observed in adult IT cortex; however, informal assessments on a few cells indicated that preference for a stimulus was maintained throughout the central 10° for at least some infant IT neurons (see also the previous discussion of face-selective neurons).

CONNECTIONAL STUDIES OF THE DEVELOPMENT OF TEMPORAL CORTEX AND OF TEMPORAL-FRONTAL INTERACTIONS

Methods

To gain additional insight into mechanisms of development of IT cortex, we compared the pattern of cortical inputs present to IT cortex from both hemispheres in the first few months of life with cortical inputs present in adulthood. Retrograde tracers (either wheat germ agglutinin–horseradish peroxidase [WGA–HRP] or cholera toxin B-subunit [CTB]) were injected into the anterior portion of IT cortex of the left hemisphere in 12 macaques ranging from 2 weeks of age to adulthood. For the WGA–HRP cases, sections were processed using tetramethylbenzene (TMB) histochemistry; for CTB cases, sections were processed using standard immunohistochemistry and the avidin-biotin-complex (ABC) method with diaminobenzidine as the chromogen. Additional series of sections were stained with cresyl violet, cytochrome oxidase histochemistry, and the Gallyas myelin stain. Locations and den-

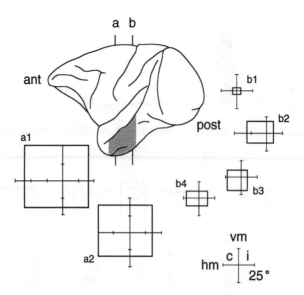

Figure 8.7.   Bilateral receptive fields of IT cortex cells plotted in anesthetized infant monkeys, taken from coronal levels a and b, indicated on the lateral view of the brain. (c, contralateral visual field; i, ipsilateral visual field; hm, horizontal meridian; vm, vertical meridian.) (Adapted from Rodman et al. [1991].)

sities of label were charted onto tracings of neighboring cresyl-stained sections and plotted onto lateral reconstructions of each hemisphere and onto flattened maps of portions of the cortex that had been constructed by using the method of Barbas (1988). Criteria used to assign labels to cortical regions included cytoarchitectonic and myeloarchitectonic transitions as well as sulcal landmarks (see, e.g., legend to Figure 8.9).

Overall Pattern of Retrograde Labeling

Overall, retrogradely labeled cells were found within visual areas V4, TEO, IT, and STP; within the intraparietal sulcus, parahippocampal, and perirhinal cortex; and within the temporal pole, the lateral and ventral frontal cortex, the insula, and the anterior cingulate cortex. Retrograde labeling in the cortex of a 6-week-old infant monkey given an injection of CTB into IT cortex is shown in Figure 8.8. An analysis of the injected cases suggests that the overall pattern of occipitotemporal inputs (i.e., from cortical areas that are exclusively visual in function) is similar in adult monkeys and infants (Rodman & Consuelos, 1994; Rodman, Nace, Woods, Gross, & Rebmann, 1993). In particular, no "exuberant" connectivity was found with posterior visual areas, such as V2, which do not provide input to IT in the adult animal.

Connections with Frontal Cortex

However, some intriguing differences between the pattern of inputs to IT cortex from frontal cortex in adult monkeys and the pattern in infant monkeys are present. Retrograde labeling in frontal cortex after injections of tracers into anterior IT cortex is illustrated in Figures 8.8–8.10. Projections to IT cortex from frontal cortex in both infant and adult monkeys originate from two major sectors. The first sector includes cortex of cytoarchitectonic area 45, the lateral portion of area 12, and a

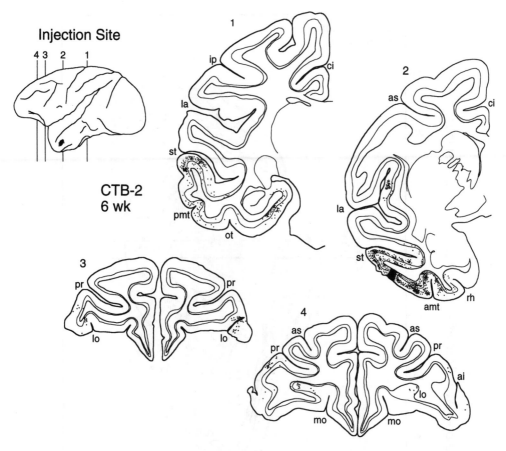

Figure 8.8.   Coronal sections illustrating locations of retrogradely labeled cells in anterior temporal lobe and frontal lobe of a 6-week-old monkey after an injection of CTB into anterior IT cortex. Each dot corresponds to one labeled cell. (ai, inferior arcuate sulcus; amt, anterior medial temporal sulcus; as, superior arcuate sulcus; ci, cingulate sulcus; ip, intraparietal sulcus; la, lateral sulcus; lo, lateral orbital sulcus; mo, medial orbital sulcus; ot, occipitotemporal sulcus; pmt, posterior medial temporal sulcus; pr, principal sulcus; rh, rhinal sulcus; st, superior temporal sulcus.)

portion of lower area 46 on the lateral surface. The second sector consists of a zone of orbital cortex, which comprises parts of cytoarchitectonic areas 11 and 13 and the orbital portion of area 12. Despite the overall similarity, several important differences were seen between the pattern of frontal labeling observed in infant monkeys and that seen in adults (compare Figures 8.9 and 8.10). First, in infant monkeys 7 weeks of age or younger, labeling was found in these sectors within both contralateral and ipsilateral cortices, whereas, in older infants and adults, these projections were strictly ipsilateral. Second, frontal projections to IT cortex originated over a more widespread region of cortex in the youngest infant monkeys, involving substantial portions of areas 8 and 6V, a small zone within area 10, a substantial zone within lower area 46 on the lower bank of the principal sulcus, as well as areas 45, lower 46 on the lateral surface, and 12, 11, and 13. Finally, projections to IT cortex from frontal areas appeared to be quantitatively strongest in the youngest monkeys.

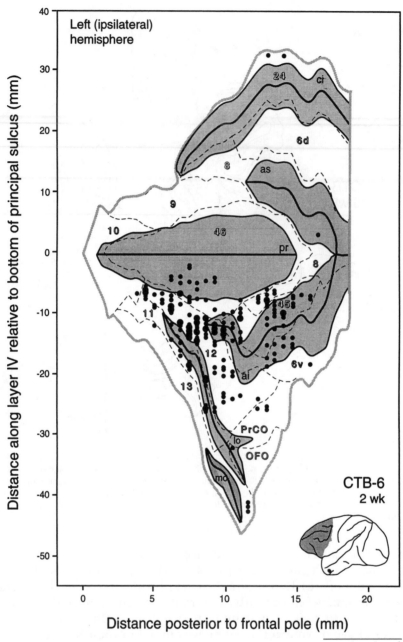

(continued)

Figure 8.9.   Overall pattern of retrograde labeling in frontal cortex after injection of anterior IT cortex in a 3-week-old monkey, shown on flattened reconstructions of each hemisphere. Smaller and larger dots represent less dense and more dense labeling (1–8 cells/300 μm and 9–30 cells/300 μm, respectively; see also Rodman & Consuelos, 1994). The flattened area is indicated on the small lateral view of the brain shown at the bottom of each map. In the flattened maps, sulci are bounded by heavy black lines and shaded gray; cytoarchitectonic divisions are bounded by dotted lines and indicated by hollow letters. Borders of cytoarchitectonic areas in frontal cortex were evaluated with reference to the descriptions of Barbas and Pandya (1989), Carmichael and Price (1994), and Preuss and Goldman-Rakic (1991); nomenclature follows that given by Preuss and Goldman-Rakic (1991). See also legends to Figures 8.1 and 8.8.

Figure 8.9.   (*continued*)

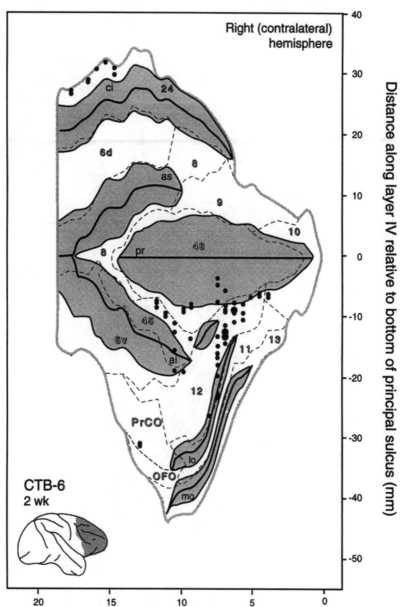

Other Differences in Connectivity Between Infants and Adults

Several additional differences in the cortical connectivity of IT cortex in infant and adult monkeys were apparent in our studies (Rodman & Consuelos, 1994; Rodman, Nace, et al.,1993). For example, we found moderately dense projections to IT cortex from the insular cortex of the ipsilateral hemisphere in the infant monkeys. We also found a sparse to moderately dense bilateral projection from the anterior cingulate cortex, a portion of which is visible in the flat map illustrations of the frontal lobe presented in Figure 8.9, in the animals 2–7 weeks of age. Finally, we found an immature pattern of connectivity between IT cortex and cortex of the rhinal sulcus

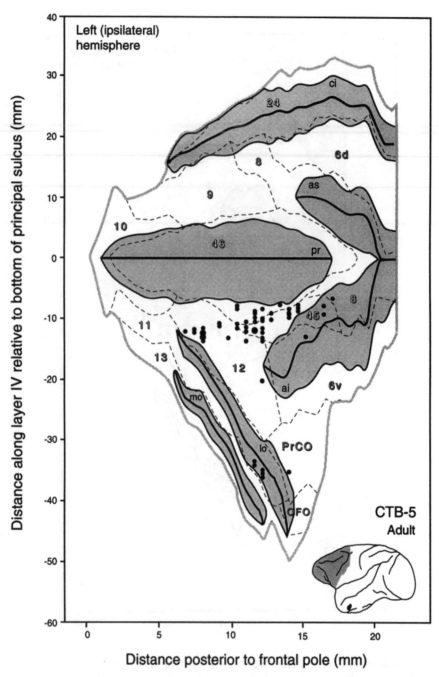

Figure 8.10.   Flattened reconstruction of ipsilateral frontal cortex in an adult monkey illustrating pattern of retrograde labeling after an injection of anterior IT cortex. Because no label was found in the contralateral hemisphere, this hemisphere is not shown. (See also legend to Figure 8.9.)

at 7 weeks, which has also been noted previously by other workers (Webster, Ungerleider, & Bachevalier, 1991). An interesting point about the sources of novel or transient projections to IT cortex in infants is that all of these areas (i.e., frontal, rhinal, insular, and cingulate cortices) themselves are not visual sensory areas but rather areas that have been implicated in memory, attention, and/or affective functions (Rodman & Consuelos, 1994).

SUMMARY AND DISCUSSION

Nature of Signals Deriving from Inferior Temporal Cortex Early in Life

As described in this chapter, in both monkeys and humans, there is a behavioral dissociation between the time at which primitive recognition capacities emerge during infancy and the time at which recognition ability becomes robust. Our data suggest that there is a similar neurophysiological distinction between the time at which certain types of signals become observable within the brain and the time at which they become robust. In other words, although the appropriate signals may be present early on, they may be too weak to support behavior. Our physiological experiments show that the incidence and features of stimulus selectivity shown by alert infant IT neurons are very similar to those of IT cells of both anesthetized and unanesthetized adult monkeys. Within the second month of life (i.e., as early as we could test), individual IT neurons clearly had responses selective for shape (boundary curvature), faces, arbitrary geometrical patterns, or color. Several measures of form selectivity for the alert infant and adult samples indicated that the overall degree of stimulus selectivity did not differ between the two groups. However, the magnitude of responses was reduced overall relative to cells in adult temporal cortex (even for alert infants), and latencies were long and variable. With respect to these phenomena, it should be noted that primate temporal cortex, like other "association" areas, is not fully myelinated until much later than other cortical regions—in fact, not until well after the first year of life in monkeys (Flechsig, 1876; Yakovlev & LeCours, 1967). For example, at 7 months of age, when both striate cortex and extrastriate visual area MT are clearly recognizable in a myelin stain, the dense adult pattern of myelination is just beginning to emerge in IT. This gradual increase in myelination in the postnatal period is likely to be related to the longer latencies seen in infant IT cortex and may also affect the timing of arrival of inputs needed to trigger high rates of action potentials.

Development of Areas Providing Information to
Inferior Temporal Cortex and General Aspects of Cortical Circuitry

The long period of emergence of adultlike levels of pattern recognition capacity (and the emergence of the contribution of IT cortex to these functions) does not appear to be caused in any obvious way by an immaturity of afferent cortical projections providing visual signals. Nonetheless, limited physiological studies provide evidence that, even at the level of striate cortex, there is a protracted postnatal maturation of response properties (Blakemore & Vital-Durand, 1981; Hubel, Wiesel, & LeVay, 1977). Moreover, there is a notable synchrony of overproduction of both synaptic contacts (Rakic, Bourgeois, Eckenhoff, Zecevic, & Goldman-Rakic, 1986) and neurotransmitter receptors (Lidow, Goldman-Rakic, & Rakic, 1991) throughout neocortex within the first 6 months of life in the monkey, and these investigators have suggested that a "critical mass" of functional synapses may be a necessary precondition to mature function of diverse portions of association cortex. The postnatal development of IT, therefore, is likely to reflect developmental mechanisms common to diverse cortical regions (see Bourgeois, Goldman-Rakic, & Rakic, 1994). The low rates of spontaneous activity in infant temporal cortex under both anesthetized and alert conditions also raise the possibility that the relatively weak responses in the infant monkeys may reflect more global characteristics of synaptic or cellular function of cortical cells early in ontogeny. For example, the process of integration of inputs, both stimulus driven and spontaneously active, may be less efficient or faithful than that achieved by adult cortical cells. Alternatively, cortical cells in young monkeys may not be able to utilize energy efficiently enough to allow the rapid depolarization and repolarization of the cell membrane that is required for high rates of action potential generation.

Relationship of the Development of Signals in Inferior Temporal Cortex to the Development of Pattern Recognition

The delayed contribution of IT cortex to visual recognition and the slow development of adult capacity are evidently not due to a nonspecificity of IT responses early in life. Rather, the limited role of IT early in life and the extended maturation of visual recognition learning may reflect the weakness of signals deriving from IT cells in at least the first 6 months of life, as reflected in the cells' weak responses, long latencies, and suppression by anesthesia.

Several other factors may also contribute to both the extended time course of the maturation of visual pattern recognition ability and the specific contribution of temporal cortex to these functions. First, although basic response properties and overall degree of form selectivity in these areas are adultlike early in life, other variables that we have not studied may contribute information about visual objects and may be different in the infant. For example, it has been suggested that selectivity patterns of *groups,* or ensembles, of neurons may convey more information than do those of individual cells (Gochin et al., 1994; Young & Yamane, 1992), and such ensemble activity may be different in the young animal. In addition, attentional and task-related influences known to affect IT responses in adult monkeys (see following) either may not be present or may not be very marked early in ontogeny. There may be, for example, postnatal changes in the efficacy of inputs from chemically specific systems implicated in arousal and attention in adult animals, such as basal forebrain and locus ceruleus; such changes could be due to refinement of input patterns, changes in synaptic numbers, or changes in receptor expression.

Finally, responses of individual adult IT cells appear to play a role not only in representing objects but also in providing specific signals about the novelty, familiarity, or recency of appearance of those objects, information that may help redirect visual attention as well as play a role in memory (reviewed in Desimone, Miller, Chelazzi, & Lueschow, 1994; Gross et al., 1993); such signals may be weak early in ontogeny. Relevant types of signals provided by temporal neurons in adults include 1) passive "habituation" and response suppression to repeated stimulation with a given image; 2) differences in responses to match and nonmatch stimuli in delayed match to sample (DMS) tasks, including enhancement of response when a specific image is anticipated; 3) delay-period activity in DMS tasks, a possible correlate of working memory when an object is not physically present; and 4) changes in stimulus selectivity with either passive experience or explicit learning (Logothetis & Pauls, 1995; Rolls, Baylis, Hasselmo, & Nalwa, 1989; Sakai & Miyashita, 1991). Some of these types of putative memory signals should be amenable to study in infant monkeys. Habituation to repeated stimulus presentation is, in fact, found under passive conditions (i.e., anesthesia) in both adult (Miller, Gochin, & Gross, 1991) and infant monkeys (Rodman, Ó Scalaidhe, & Gross, 1993). In adult monkeys, suppression of responses to stimuli that have become familiar has been reported by several groups (Baylis & Rolls, 1987; Desimone et al., 1994; Riches, Wilson, & Brown, 1991); however, systematic decline of response magnitude with familiarity has not yet been investigated developmentally. Likewise, enhancement of response as a function of attention, task relevance, or expectation (Desimone et al., 1994; Moran & Desimone, 1985; Spitzer & Richmond, 1991) has not been addressed in infant monkeys. With regard to changes in selectivity with experience, it is possible that selectivity patterns of neurons in "high-order" temporal cortex may actually be *less* efficiently modified by experience in the infant and that rapid reorganization of selectivity, itself, is the feature of IT cortex that appears as pattern recognition develops.

Relationship of Inferior Temporal Cortex to Frontal Cortex

The anatomical data presented herein suggested that interactions between IT and nonvisual cortical areas may be important in the emergence of adult levels of visual pattern recognition capacity. In particular, an immature pattern of connections of IT cortex in infant monkeys was seen specifically with portions of cortex known to play a role in visual learning and memory (i.e., frontal, rhinal, cingulate cortices) and with the insula, a polymodal association area. As mentioned previously, there is considerable evidence that the ventral cortical pathway for pattern and object recognition extends into ventral portions of the frontal lobe neocortex. For example, in adult monkeys, lesions of the portions of frontal cortex connected with IT cortex produce impairments in visual recognition (Bachevalier & Mishkin, 1986), and physiological recordings in these regions have demonstrated visual form selectivity similar to that seen in IT cortex (Wilson et al., 1993). Moreover, Fuster, Bauer, and Jervey (1985) used a cortical cooling strategy to show mutual influences between IT cortex and frontal cortex during the performance of a visual discrimination task. These phenomena and other observations led Desimone et al. (1994) to propose that frontal cortex exerts an influence on IT neurons that "primes" them to respond strongly to a stimulus that the monkey is anticipating. It is of interest that, although we have obtained evidence that projections from frontal cortex back to IT cortex are immature during the first few months of life in macaques, projections from IT cortex *to* the frontal lobe appear to be adultlike as early as 1 week of age (Webster et al., 1994). Therefore, the establishment of the mature pattern of feedback from frontal cortex and other anterior cortices to temporal cortex may be one of the final components of the postnatal configuration of the cortical pathway for visual recognition in primates.

FUTURE DIRECTIONS

As described above, IT cells in adult monkeys provide signals about the familiarity, recency, and significance of visual stimuli in terms of selective increments and decrements of response rate and changes in stimulus selectivity, and it would be desirable to know when such signals can first be observed during ontogeny. At an even more fundamental level, much remains to be established regarding the developmental changes that take place in the ability of IT neurons—and neurons in other related regions such as inferior frontal cortices—to represent visual stimuli per se (Rodman, 1994). For example, we still do not know what response properties are truly like in the "beginning" (i.e., close to the moment of birth), and it will be especially important to determine whether features that are clear at 6 weeks, including selectivity for complex objects, are present earlier. A cardinal property of adult IT cells (i.e., the frequent maintenance of selectivity across changes in exact position of the stimulus) has yet to be established in infant monkeys. With regard to the development of face perception, it would be valuable to determine whether the ontogeny of face-selective behavior at the single-unit level mirrors developmental patterns seen behaviorally in the human developmental literature: whether, for example, responses of IT cells are based more on the presence of specific features than on facial configuration early in life. An issue of particular interest is whether there may be sex differences in the development of response properties that mirror sex differences in the emergence of recognition capacity and other cognitive skills (see Chapter 15). Comparing response properties of neurons in IT cortex and related regions in developing males and females may help pinpoint *which* specific ontogenetic changes in response strength, latency, or other variables are critical for development of mature capacity.

Ultimately, what we wish to understand are the mechanisms that translate environmental events (i.e., experience) into changes in the coding and mnemonic abilities of neurons in the developing cortex. We have hypothesized (see also Rodman, Ó Scalaidhe, & Gross, 1993) that rapid, efficient changes in coding ability subsequent to experience may be the property that develops only gradually in "association" cortices and that cells in infants may actually be less malleable; that is, they may shift their properties more slowly. A corollary of this suggestion is that the types of environmental events that produce alterations in neuronal responses are different in infant and adult macaques. For example, early in life, mere association of object components or views by temporal contiguity (as would be the case when scanning different parts of an object with eye movements) may be especially effective in producing neuronal responses that are "conjointly" selective for different components of objects or for particular objects independent of the way the objects are viewed. Experiments measuring the efficacy of changes of selectivity patterns of IT neurons as a function of passive pairing of novel visual stimuli at different times in development would shed light on this question. Future studies of the development of the neural substrates of visual recognition capacity in primates should supplement inquiry at the single-unit level with approaches that can be applied equally to humans and to monkeys, such as noninvasive imaging procedures. Finally, the existing behavioral, electrophysiological, and anatomical data all point to the need for a fuller examination of the specific contributions of the frontal cortex in the development and maintenance of visual recognition functions.

REFERENCES

Bachevalier, J. (1990). Ontogenetic development of habit and memory formation in primates. In A. Diamond (Ed.), *Development and neural bases of higher cognitive functions* (pp. 457–484). New York: Academic Press.

Bachevalier, J., Brickson, M., Hagger, C., & Mishkin, M. (1990). Age and sex differences in the effects of selective temporal lobe lesion on the formation of visual discrimination habits in rhesus monkeys. *Behavioral Neuroscience, 104*, 885–889.

Bachevalier, J., & Mishkin, M. (1986). Visual recognition impairment follows ventromedial but not dorsolateral prefrontal lesions in monkeys. *Behavioral Brain Research, 20*, 249–261.

Bachevalier, J., & Mishkin, M. (1988). Long-term effects of neonatal temporal cortical and limbic lesions on habit and memory formation in rhesus monkeys. *Society for Neuroscience Abstracts, 14*, 1.

Baizer, J.S., Ungerleider, L.G., & Desimone, R. (1991). Organization of visual inputs to the inferior temporal and posterior parietal cortex in macaques. *Journal of Neuroscience, 11*, 168–190.

Barbas, H. (1988). Anatomic organization of basoventral and mediodorsal visual recipient prefrontal regions in the rhesus monkey. *Journal of Comparative Neurology, 276*, 313–342.

Barbas, H., & Pandya, D.N. (1989). Architecture and intrinsic connections of the prefrontal cortex in the rhesus monkey. *Journal of Comparative Neurology, 286*, 353–375.

Bates, J.F., Wilson, F.A.W., O'Scalaidhe, S.O., & Goldman-Rakic, P.S. (1994). Area TE connections with inferior prefrontal regions responsive to complex objects and faces. *Neuroscience Abstracts, 20*, 1054.

Baylis, G.C., & Rolls, E.T. (1987). Responses of neurons in the inferior temporal cortex in short term and serial recognition memory tasks. *Experimental Brain Research, 65*, 614–622.

Blakemore, C., & Vital-Durand, R. (1981). Postnatal development of the monkey's visual system in the fetus and independent life. *CIBA, 86*, 152–171.

Bourgeois, J.-P., Goldman-Rakic, P.S., & Rakic, P. (1994). Synaptogenesis in the prefrontal cortex of rhesus monkeys. *Cerebral Cortex, 4*, 78–96.

Carey, S. (1992). Becoming a face expert. *Philosophical Transactions of the Royal Society of London, B, 335*, 95–103.

Carey, S., & Diamond, R. (1977). From piecemeal to configurational representation of faces. *Science, 195*, 312–314.

Carmichael, S.T., & Price, J.L. (1994). Architectonic subdivision of the orbital and medial prefrontal cortex in the macaque monkey. *Journal of Comparative Neurology, 346*, 366–402.

Desimone, R., Albright, T.D., Gross, C.G., & Bruce, C. (1984). Stimulus selective properties of inferior temporal neurons in the macaque. *Journal of Neuroscience, 4*, 2051–2062.

Desimone, R., Miller, E.K., Chelazzi, L., & Lueschow, A. (1994). Multiple memory systems in the visual cortex. In M.S. Gazzaniga (Ed.), *The cognitive neurosciences* (pp. 475–486). Cambridge, MA: MIT Press.

Desimone, R., & Ungerleider, L.G. (1989). Neural mechanisms of visual perception in monkeys. In R. Boller & J. Grafman (Eds.), *Handbook of neuropsychology* (Vol. II, pp. 267–299). Amsterdam: Elsevier.

Diamond, R., & Carey, S. (1990). On the acquisition of pattern encoding skills. *Cognitive Development, 5*, 345–368.

Dubowitz, L.M., Mushin, J., DeVries, L., & Arden, G.B. (1986). Visual function in the newborn infant: Is it cortically mediated? *Lancet, 1*, 1139–1141.

Ellis, H.D. (1992). The development of face processing skills. *Proceedings of the Royal Society of London, B, 335*, 105–111.

Felleman, D.J., & Van Essen, D.C. (1991). Distributed hierarchical processing in primate cerebral cortex. *Cerebral Cortex, 1*, 1–48.

Flechsig, P. (1876). Die leitungsbahnen im gehirn und ruckenmark des menschen auf grund entwicklungsgeschichtlicher untersuchungen. Liepzig, Germany: Engelmann.

Foreman, N., & Hemmings, R. (1987). The Gollin incomplete figures test: A flexible, computerized version. *Perception, 16*, 543–548.

Fuster, J.M., Bauer, R.H., & Jervey, J.P. (1985). Functional interactions between inferotemporal and prefrontal cortex in a cognitive task. *Brain Research, 330*, 229–307.

Gochin, P.M., Colombo, M., Dorfman, G., Gerstein, G.L., & Gross, C.G. (1994). Neural ensemble coding in inferior temporal cortex. *Journal of Neurophysiology, 71*, 2325–2337.

Goldman, P.S. (1971). Functional development of the prefrontal cortex in early life and the problem of neuronal plasticity. *Experimental Neurology, 32*, 366–387.

Goren, C.C., Sarty, M., & Wu, P.Y.K. (1975). Visual following and pattern discrimination of face-like stimuli by newborn infants. *Pediatrics, 56*, 544–549.

Gross, C.G., Bender, D.B., & Gerstein, G.L. (1979). Activity of inferior temporal neurons in behaving monkeys. *Neuropsychologia, 7*, 215–229.

Gross, C.G., & Mishkin, M. (1977). The neural basis of stimulus equivalence across retinal translation. In S. Harnad, R. Doty, J. Jaynes, L. Goldstein, & G. Krauthamer (Eds.), *Lateralization in the nervous system* (pp. 102–122). New York: Academic Press.

Gross, C.G., Rocha-Miranda, C.E., & Bender, D.B. (1972). Visual properties of neurons in inferotemporal cortex of the macaque. *Journal of Neurophysiology, 35,* 96–111.

Gross, C.G., Rodman, H.R., Gochin, P.M., & Colombo, M.W. (1993). Inferior temporal cortex as a pattern recognition device. In E. Baum (Ed.), *Proceedings of the third annual NEC research symposium* (pp. 47–73). Philadelphia: SIAM Press.

Gross, C.G., & Sergent, J. (1992). Face recognition. *Current Opinion in Neurobiology, 2,* 156–161.

Gunderson, V.M., & Sackett, G.P. (1984). Development of pattern recognition in infant pig-tailed macaques (*Macaca nemestrina*). *Developmental Psychology, 20,* 418–426.

Harlow, H.F., Harlow, M.K., Reuping, R., & Mason, W. (1960). Performance of infant rhesus monkeys on discrimination learning, delayed response, and discrimination learning set. *Journal of Comparative Physiological Psychology, 53,* 113–121.

Hasselmo, M.E., Rolls, E.T., & Baylis, G.C. (1989). The role of expression and identity in the face-selective responses of neurons in the temporal visual cortex of the monkey. *Behavioral Brain Research, 32,* 203–218.

Hubel, D.H., Wiesel, T.N., & LeVay, S. (1977). Plasticity of ocular dominance columns in monkey striate cortex. *Philosophical Transactions of the Royal Society of London, B, 278,* 337–404.

Johnson, M.H. (1990). Cortical maturation and the development of visual attention in early infancy. *Journal of Cognitive Neuroscience, 26,* 81–95.

Johnson, M.H. (1994). Brain and cognitive development in infancy. *Current Opinion in Neurobiology, 4,* 218–225.

Johnson, M.H., Dziurawiec, S., Ellis, H.D., & Morton, J. (1991). Newborns' preferential tracking of face-like stimuli and its subsequent decline. *Cognition, 40,* 1–19.

Kaas, J.H., & Huerta, J.F. (1988). The subcortical visual system of primates. In H. Steklis & J. Erwin (Eds.), *Comparative primate biology* (Vol. 4, pp. 327–391). New York: Alan R. Liss.

Kleiner, K.A. (1993). Specific vs. non-specific face recognition device. In B. de Boysson-Bardies, S. de Schonen, P. Jusczyk, P. MacNeilage, & J. Morton (Eds.), *Developmental neurocognition: Speech and face processing in the first year of life* (pp. 103–108). Dordrecht, The Netherlands: Kluwer Academic Publishers.

Lidow, M.S., Goldman-Rakic, P.S., & Rakic, P. (1991). Synchronized overproduction of neurotransmitter receptors in diverse regions of the primate cerebral cortex. *Proceedings of the National Academy of Sciences, 88,* 10,218–10,221.

Logothetis, N.K., & Pauls, J. (1995). Psychophysical and physiological evidence for viewer-centered object representations in the primate. *Cerebral Cortex, 5,* 270–288.

Lueschow, A., Miller, E.K., & Desimone, R. (1994). Inferior temporal mechanisms for invariant object recognition. *Cerebral Cortex, 4,* 523–531.

Meltzoff, A.N., & Moore, M.K. (1977). Imitation of facial and manual gestures by human neonates. *Science, 98,* 75–78.

Miller, E.K., Gochin, P.M., & Gross, C.G. (1991). Habituation-like decrease in the responses of neurons in inferior temporal cortex of the macaque. *Visual Neuroscience, 7,* 357–362.

Mishkin, M., & Murray, E.A. (1994). Stimulus recognition. *Current Opinion in Neurobiology, 4,* 200–206.

Moran, J., & Desimone, R. (1985). Selective attention gates visual processing in the extrastriate cortex. *Science, 229,* 782–784.

Overman, W., Bachevalier, J., Turner, M., & Peuster, A. (1992). Object recognition versus object discrimination: Comparison between human infants and infant monkeys. *Behavioral Neuroscience, 106,*15–29.

Perrett, D.I., Hietanen, J.K., Oram, M.W., & Benson, P.J. (1992). Organization and function of cells responsive to faces in the temporal cortex. *Philosophical Transaction of the Royal Society of London, B, 335,* 23–30.

Preuss, T.M., & Goldman-Rakic, P.S. (1991). Myelo- and cytoarchitecture of the granular frontal cortex and surrounding regions in the strepsirhine primate Galago and the anthropoid primate Macaca. *Journal of Comparative Neurology, 310,* 429–474.

Raisler, R.L., & Harlow, H.F. (1965). Learned behavior following lesions of posterior association cortex in infant, immature and preadolescent monkeys. *Journal of Comparative Physiological Psychology, 60,* 167–174.

Rakic, P., Bourgeois, J.P., Eckenhoff, M.E.F., Zecevic, N., & Goldman-Rakic, P.S. (1986). Concurrent overproduction of synapses in diverse regions of the primate cerebral cortex. *Science, 232,* 232–235.

Riches, I.P., Wilson, F.A.W., & Brown, M.W. (1991). The effects of visual stimulation and memory on neurons of the hippocampal formation and the neighboring parahippocampal gyrus and inferior temporal cortex of the primate. *Journal of Neuroscience, 11,* 1763–1779.

Richmond, B.J., Wurtz, R.H., & Sato, T. (1983). Visual responses of inferior temporal neurons in awake rhesus monkey. *Journal of Neurophysiology, 50,* 1415–1432.

Rockland, K.S., & Van Hoesen, G.W. (1994). Direct temporal-occipital feedback connections to striate cortex (V1) in the macaque monkey. *Cerebral Cortex, 3,* 300–313.

Rodman, H.R. (1991). Methods for repeated recording in visual cortex of anesthetized and awake behaving infant monkeys. *Journal of Neuroscience Methods, 38,* 209–222.

Rodman, H.R. (1994). Development of temporal cortex in the monkey. *Cerebral Cortex, 4,* 484–498.

Rodman, H.R., & Consuelos, M.C. (1994). Cortical projections to anterior inferior temporal cortex in infant macaque monkeys. *Visual Neuroscience, 11,* 119–133.

Rodman, H.R., Nace, K.L., Woods, T.M., Gross, C.G., & Rebmann, N.S. (1993). Transient inputs to inferior temporal cortex in infant macaques. *Society for Neuroscience Abstracts, 19,* 972.

Rodman, H.R., Ó Scalaidhe, S.P., & Gross, C.G. (1993). Visual response properties of neurons in temporal cortical visual areas of infant monkeys. *Journal of Neurophysiology, 70,* 1115–1136.

Rodman, H.R., Skelly, J.P., & Gross, C.G. (1991). Stimulus selectivity and state dependence of activity in inferior temporal cortex of infant monkeys. *Proceedings of the National Academy of Sciences of the United States of America, 88,* 7572–7575.

Rolls, E.T. (1992). Neurophysiological mechanisms underlying face processing within and beyond the temporal cortical visual areas. *Philosophical Transaction of the Royal Society of London, B, 335,* 11–21.

Rolls, E.T., & Baylis, G.C. (1986). Size and contrast have only small effects on the responses to faces of neurons in the cortex of the superior temporal sulcus of the monkey. *Experimental Brain Research, 65,* 38–48.

Rolls, E.T., Baylis, G.C., Hasselmo, M.E., & Nalwa, V. (1989). The effect of learning on the face selective responses of neurons in the cortex in the superior temporal sulcus of the monkey. *Experimental Brain Research, 76,* 153–164.

Sackett, G.P. (1966). Development of preference for differentially complex patterns by infant monkeys. *Psychonomic Science, 6,* 441–442.

Sakai, K., & Miyashita, Y. (1991). Neural organization for the long-term memory of paired associates. *Nature, 354,* 152–155.

Schwartz, E.L., Desimone, R., Albright, T.D., & Gross, C.G. (1983). Shape recognition and inferior temporal neurons. *Proceedings of the National Academy of Sciences of the United States of America, 80,* 5776–5778.

Seltzer, B., & Pandya, D.N. (1989). Frontal lobe connections of the superior temporal sulcus in the rhesus monkey. *Journal of Comparative Neurology, 281,* 97–113.

Slater, A.M. (1993). Visual perceptual abilities at birth: Implications for face processing. In B. de Boysson-Bardies, S. de Schonen, P. Jusczyk, P. MacNeilage, & J. Morton (Eds.), *Developmental neurocognition: Speech and face processing in the first year of life* (pp. 125–134). Dordrecht, the Netherlands: Kluwer Academic.

Spitzer, H., & Richmond, B.J. (1991). Task difficulty: Ignoring, attending to, and discriminating a visual stimulus yield progressively more activity in inferior temporal neurons. *Experimental Brain Research, 83,* 340–348.

Tanaka, K., Saito, H.A., Fukada, Y., & Moriya, M. (1991). Coding visual images of objects in the inferotemporal cortex of the macaque monkey. *Journal of Neurophysiology, 66,* 170–189.

Ungerleider, L.G., & Mishkin, M. (1982). Two cortical visual systems. In D.J. Ingle, M.A. Goodale, & R.J.W. Mansfeld (Eds.), *Analysis of visual behavior* (pp. 549–586). Cambridge, MA: MIT Press.

Webster, M.J., Bachevalier, J., & Ungerleider, L.G. (1993). Subcortical connections of inferior temporal areas TE and TEO in monkeys. *Journal of Comparative Neurology, 335,* 73–91.

Webster, M.J., Bachevalier, J., & Ungerleider, L.G. (1994). Connections of inferior temporal areas TEO and TE with parietal and frontal cortex in macaque monkeys. *Cerebral Cortex, 4,* 470–483.

Webster, M.J., Ungerleider, L.G., & Bachevalier, J. (1991). Connections of inferior temporal areas TE and TEO with medial temporal-lobe structures in infant and adult monkeys. *Journal of Neuroscience, 11,* 1095–1116.

Wilson, F.A.W., Ó Scalaidhe, S.P., & Goldman-Rakic, P.S. (1993). Dissociation of object and spatial processing domains in primate prefrontal cortex. *Science, 260,* 1955–1958.

Yakovlev, P.I., & LeCours, A.R. (1967). The myelogenetic cycles of regional maturation of the brain. In A. Minkowski (Ed.), *Regional maturation of brain in early life* (pp. 3–70). Philadelphia: Davis.

Young, M.P., & Yamane, S. (1992). Sparse population coding of faces in the inferotemporal cortex. *Science, 256,* 1327–1331.

Zimmermann, R.R. (1961). Analysis of discrimination learning capacities in the infant rhesus monkey. *Journal of Comparative Physiological Psychology, 54,* 1.

Zola-Morgan, S., & Squire, L.R. (1993). Neuroanatomy of memory. *Annual Review of Neuroscience, 16,* 547–563.

Development of the Prefrontal Cortex: Evolution, Neurobiology, and Behavior
edited by Norman A. Krasnegor, Ph.D., G. Reid Lyon, Ph.D.,
and Patricia S. Goldman-Rakic, Ph.D.
copyright © 1997   Paul H. Brookes Publishing Co., Inc.
Baltimore • London • Toronto • Sydney

9

Frontal and Attentional Mechanisms Regulating Distress Experience and Expression During Infancy

Catherine Harman and Nathan A. Fox

CEREBRAL ASYMMETRY, EMOTION, AND EMOTION REGULATION

A variety of data from a number of sources suggest that the two hemispheres of the brain may be differentially involved in the expression of different emotions. These data, reviewed in detail elsewhere (Silberman & Weingartner, 1986), are derived from three sources: 1) cases of individuals with unilateral cerebral damage; 2) cases of individuals who undergo testing with the sodium amytal procedure (the Wada test); and 3) studies of normal and clinical populations that utilize different neuroimaging techniques, including regional cerebral blood flow, positron emission tomography (PET) scanning, and brain electrical activity. The data from these sources are not always consistent. Indeed, there are two prominent interpretations of these data, one that advocates a valence hypothesis and another that claims that the expression of emotion is under unilateral control (Borod, 1992). The valence hypothesis, briefly stated, is that specific regions of the left and right hemispheres are responsible for coordinating the motor, facial, and other expressive aspects of certain emotions (Davidson, 1992; Fox, 1991, 1994). The frontal region is consistently associated with differential involvement in emotional expression, although the precise areas of such involvement within the frontal region are often left unstated. Underlying this asymmetry of expressive control is the notion that the functional significance of this asymmetry lies along the psychological-motivational continuum of approach–withdrawal. Simply stated, it is hypothesized that areas of the left frontal region are involved in the control of expression of emotions associated with approach behavior (i.e., positive emotions), and areas of the right frontal region are involved in the control of expression of emotions associated with withdrawal behavior (i.e., negative emotions). Data from several studies utilizing electroencephalographic (EEG) indices of regional brain activation from infants, children, and adults seem to support these contentions (Davidson, Ekman, Saron, Senulis, &

Friesen, 1990; Dawson, Grofer-Klinger, Panagiotides, Spieker, & Frey 1992; Fox & Davidson, 1984; Jones & Fox, 1992).

A corollary to the valence hypothesis, proposed by Fox (1994), is that the functional significance of frontal asymmetry for emotion involves the regulation of affective expression rather than the control of expression per se. Fox based this hypothesis on a reexamination of the data from unilateral brain damage and Wada test patients. By and large, individuals suffering unilateral stroke or brain damage or undergoing the Wada procedure did not display impairment in the ability to produce individual expressions, but rather lost the ability to control voluntarily the expression of certain emotions. Therefore, Fox (1994) proposed, the left and right frontal regions may be directly involved in the regulation and control of expressions associated with either approach or withdrawal behavior.

DEVELOPMENTAL FACTORS

Much research describes the behavior changes that occur during the first years of life that reflect the development of emotion regulation (Fox, 1994). In addition, a number of researchers have speculated on the cognitive strategies that develop during this time period that may be directly involved in emotion regulation. For example, Rothbart and Posner (1985) proposed that individual differences in attention, distractibility, or both may be related to the infant's ability to self-soothe. Infants who are easily distracted when distressed may be better able to calm themselves. Similarly, Thompson (1994) discussed the role of verbal skills for the toddler and preschool child as useful in assisting the distressed child to regulate his or her affect. In addition, Fox (1991) suggested that skills hypothesized to be subserved by the frontal region (e.g., the ability to switch set and maintain cognitive flexibility, the ability to hold representations in working memory in the face of distraction, certain verbal analytical skills) may be critical for the young child in developing successful regulatory skills. A number of these frontal skills have been associated with areas of the left frontal region. Therefore, Fox (1991) speculated that, in older children, individual differences in left or right frontal activation may in fact reflect an ability to make use of certain verbal skills necessary for emotion regulation.

INFANT AND CHILD TEMPERAMENT

Research by Fox and colleagues extended these notions regarding the differential control of emotional expression by areas of the left or right frontal region to the study of individual differences in infant and child temperament. The literature on adult clinical populations suggests that adults who display signs of depression or who are highly anxious exhibit unique patterns of anterior cerebral activation. For example, Henriques and Davidson (1991) reported that depressed adults were more likely to exhibit greater relative right frontal EEG activation even after remission of depression. Heller (1993) found that highly anxious adults displayed a greater right hemifield preference on the chimeric faces test, a measure of hemispheric activation. These authors argued that a pattern of resting right frontal activation underlies the disposition to express negative emotions in certain individuals.

Based upon these studies with adults, Fox, Bell, and Jones (1992) reasoned that a similar pattern of anterior frontal EEG activation may underlie the behavior of infants who display a particular temperamental pattern of behavior reflecting negative affect and distress. That is, if one could identify a group of infants who exhibit a disposition of negative affect and distress, then one would expect these infants to also exhibit a pattern of frontal activation consonant with that temperament. Behavioral research with temperamentally inhibited children provided an opportunity to test this hypothesis. Previous work by Kagan and colleagues (Kagan, Reznick, & Gibbons, 1989; Kagan, Reznick, Snidman, Gibbons, & Johnson, 1988) identified a group of children during the second year of life who were extremely fearful and vigilant when confronted with novel situations. Kagan et al. identified the behavior patterns of infants who would later exhibit, as toddlers and preschoolers, the characteristics of behaviorally inhibited children. These patterns included a unique response to visual and auditory stimuli as infants (i.e., a high degree of motor arousal and a high-intensity expression of negative affect with a corresponding inability to soothe. Data from Kagan's lab suggested that infants who exhibited these patterns were likely to display inhibited, fearful, and vigilant behavior as toddlers and preschoolers (Kagan, Reznick, & Gibbons, 1989).

In an effort to examine the underlying physiology of these highly distressed infants, Fox and colleagues undertook a study that identified a group of 4-month-old infants who displayed the particular pattern of high motor arousal and high negative affect and distress. More than 300 infants were observed in their homes while they sat in a quiet alert state and were presented with a series of novel auditory and visual stimuli. Their responses were coded for motor activity and affect. Those infants displaying high degrees of motor activity and negative affect in response to the stimuli were subsequently brought into the laboratory when they were 9 months of age and again at 24 months of age. At the 9- and 24-month assessments, EEG was recorded. At 24 months of age, the children were observed in a playroom, during which time their responses to a series of novel events were observed. Analysis of the 9-month EEG data revealed that infants who at 4 months of age displayed a high degree of motor activity and negative affect and who were difficult to soothe exhibited greater relative right frontal EEG activation compared with other infants (Calkins, Fox, & Marshall, 1995). A significant number of these infants, at 24 months of age, exhibited behavioral signs of fearfulness and inhibition. In fact, the best predictor of behavioral inhibition at age 24 months was temperamental pattern at 4 months of age and stable right frontal EEG activation across the 4- to 24-month age period (Calkins et al., 1995).

The data from this research suggest that infants who are prone to distress are likely to display a pattern of right frontal activation. These infants are also likely to exhibit inhibited, fearful, and vigilant behavior as toddlers. What these data do not address are the underlying cognitive and neural systems that may be involved in such temperamental dispositions. Left unanswered is whether infants exhibiting a negative disposition also display differences in those cognitive strategies or processes that are important for regulation of distress (e.g., attentional processes, verbal regulative strategies).

The remainder of this chapter presents a discussion of a model for the underlying cognitive and neural basis for regulation of distress in infants. We begin with a brief review of Posner and Peterson's (1990) model of attention and the three subnetworks of the human attention system. Following this review, we outline issues in the development of attention and emotion regulation, with emphasis on the neural bases of obligatory attention. Finally, we discuss a model system for understanding the infant's developing ability to handle distress. We hope that the information provided in this discussion may be linked to the behavioral and psychophysiological data on individual differences in disposition to distress to enable us to ultimately understand the behavioral and psychophysiological characteristics of behaviorally inhibited infants and children.

NEURAL BASES FOR THE REGULATION OF DISTRESS

Among the first challenging developmental tasks for the human infant is the regulation of distress expression, that is, control over fussing and crying. Although it is difficult to quantify the marked decrease in negative emotional expression over the first years of life, St. James-Roberts and Halil (1991) used maternal diaries to determine the cumulative amount of time per day in which British middle-class infants engaged in fussing and crying. One- to three-month-old infants cried an average of 121 minutes per day, whereas this expression declined to an average of 54 minutes per day by 10–12 months of age. Certainly, the decrease in negative emotional expression involves the interaction between postnatal neural maturation and socialization processes. Among the factors thought to be involved in the decrease in negative emotional expression is the development of the infant's ability to attend to objects in the environment in a flexible manner. Therefore, study of the development of attention, including the neural bases of attention, may shed some light on understanding changes in the regulation of emotional distress. In order to describe changes in the development of attention, it is first necessary to review one particular model that we have used to understand the neural substrates of attentional processes.

Posner and Peterson's Model of Attention

Posner and Peterson (1990) developed a theory of attention in which the neural substrates of attention are emphasized. Three principles concerning the nature of attention have guided Posner and Peterson's analyses of the neuroanatomy and neurophysiology of attention. First, experiments in which multiple sensory modalities are stimulated have demonstrated that the attention network is anatomically separate from data processing systems. When sensory modalities are simultaneously stimulated, processing within any one sensory modality is compromised. Because stimulation of one modality causes interference with and interruption of data processing in any other modality, a common mechanism or central system must subserve multiple modalities. A primary function of this central system is to establish processing priorities among input sources, especially the sensory modalities. Therefore, attention systems interact with data processing systems yet maintain distinct identities. They have specific functions—in the present example, selecting a modality in which sensory data will be given processing priority—that cannot be accounted for by the isolated functioning of any one modality.

The second principle is that the substrates of attention are best conceived of as networks of neuroanatomical areas distributed throughout the brain. They are not discretely localized areas or structures. The spatial distribution or web of attentional substrates allows attention to support and enhance the functioning of the entire central nervous system, including sensory channel monitoring and processing, interoceptive information processing, motor control, propositional thought, language, and imagery. Two common misconceptions about attention are refuted by the principle that the neural substrates of attention are spatially distributed. First, it is tempting to conceptualize attention as a central control mechanism (i.e., a homunculus). Emphasizing the distributed nature of the physiological substrates of attention lessens this temptation. Second, theorists have attempted to explain the phenomenon of attention as an epiphenomenon of brain functioning as a whole. Clearly, a system with a distributed yet distinct neural substrate is not an epiphenomenon of global cortical functioning.

The final principle guiding Posner and Peterson's conceptualization is the premise that attention can be decomposed into functional components and that each functional component can be mapped onto a specific neural substrate. Just like other neural mechanisms, attention is a collection of specific circuits performing specific functions, with these circuits and component functions operating in concert to produce complex operations.

Three Subnetworks of the Human Attention System

Posner and Peterson (1990) delineated three subnetworks of the human attention network using a variety of methodologies, primarily PET. These three subsystems are an anterior attention subnetwork, a posterior attention subnetwork, and a vigilance subnetwork. The anterior and posterior attention subnetworks are named according to their regions of cerebral localization; the vigilance subnetwork is named for its functional role.

Posterior Subnetwork: Neural Bases and Function   The neural substrates of the posterior attention subnetwork include the parietal lobes, the superior colliculus, and the thalamus—more specifically, the pulvinar nucleus of the thalamus. This system functions to enhance the sensory processing of stimuli at particular locations, operating in conjunction with mechanisms that control the orienting of sensory organs. Once a particular location is selected, the sensory organs are oriented to it, and the attributes of stimuli from that location are enhanced. Thus, the posterior attention subnetwork operates exclusively on external or environmental information.

Posner and colleagues specified the particular functions of each of the neural substrates of the posterior attention subnetwork (Posner, Inhoff, Friedrich, & Cohen, 1987). The elaboration of stimuli at a particular location involves three component processes: 1) maintaining engagement at a particular location, 2) disengagement from that location upon selection of another location, and 3) the actual shifting of the index of attention from one location to another. Maintaining engagement at a particular location is primarily subserved by the parietal lobes. Disengagement is primarily subserved by the pulvinar nuclei of the thalamus, and the superior colliculus shifts the index of attentional focus from one location to another.

Anterior Subnetwork: Neural Bases and Function   The neural substrates of the anterior attention subnetwork include regions of the frontal lobes and anterior regions of the paralimbic cortex, most notably the right dorsolateral prefrontal cortex and the anterior cingulate gyrus. The anterior cingulate is a major output of the limbic system, suggesting an important role for this structure in influencing emotional experience and expression. It has long been recognized that the limbic system, particularly the amygdala, is crucial to emotional processes. At least one function of the anterior attention subnetwork is to detect target information, that is, to match the representation of a goal state, or a desired state, to a current state or sensory input. Unlike the posterior attention subnetwork, which primarily enhances the processing of stimuli from the external environment, the anterior attention subnetwork utilizes internal data from memory storage in addition to current input from sensory processing systems.

The evidence for the claim that the anterior attention subnetwork functions as a target detection mechanism was the demonstration, using PET, that the anterior cingulate was active during a semantic target detection task (Peterson, Fox, Posner, Mintun, & Raichle, 1988). Subjects were required to detect target words from streams of visually presented words. PET scans showed that blood flow in the anterior cingulate was a function of the number of targets presented. Although this task required primarily the visual and semantic domains, Posner and Peterson (1990) believed it to be more general, serving target detection from sensory processing systems as well as the semantic network and information stored in memory. Its role in consciousness may be to carry a model of the state of the world and to detect deviations from those expectations.

Vigilance Subnetwork: Neural Bases and Function   Finally, the vigilance subnetwork has been identified as being involved in maintaining the alert state over substantial durations, on the order of seconds and minutes, in contrast to milliseconds. The neural substrates of this subnetwork include the brainstem area known as the locus ceruleus (LC) and the cortex of the right frontal lobe, with the LC supplying norepinephrine to the right frontal cortex. The data supporting this claim include the finding that damage to the right frontal cortex results in a compromised ability to maintain the alert state (Coslett, Bowers, & Heilman, 1987) and that right lateral midfrontal cortical activation increases during tasks requiring auditory vigilance (Cohen et al., 1988). In the emotional domain, LC cells are particularly responsive to threatening or aversive stimuli, suggesting an important role for this system in the fear state (Grant, Aston-Jones, & Redmond, 1988).

Subnetwork Interaction   Although the subnetworks are distinct, certainly they interact. Posner and Peterson (1990) suggested that the anterior and posterior subnetworks are hierarchically organized such that the anterior subnetwork dominates the posterior subnetwork. Typically, the anterior subnetwork selects targets based on schema stored in the semantic network, passing control to the posterior subnetwork when attention to the environment is required. Goldman-Rakic (1988) explicated the neuroanatomical architecture of the connections between the anterior and posterior subnetworks, which consist of alternating bands of cells emerging from the posterior parietal lobe and connecting to the dorsolateral prefrontal cortex. Behavior studies show that the vigilance subnetwork attenuates the functions of both the anterior and the posterior subnetworks. When vigilance subnetwork activity increases, anterior attention subnetwork activity decreases and posterior subnetwork activity increases. The decrease in anterior subnetwork activity likely corresponds to the clearing of conscious awareness in order to speed detection and responding to particular targets. The posterior attention subnetwork activation likely corresponds to enhancing data processing of environmental stimuli in order to speed target detection. Thus, the vigilance subnetwork, like the posterior subnetwork and unlike the anterior subnetwork, primarily influences processing of external stimuli.

DEVELOPMENT OF ATTENTION AND EMOTION REGULATION

Because the tripartite model of the attention network of the human brain is a relatively recent conceptualization, little work has been done to elucidate the developmental trajectories of particular subnetworks. Posner and colleagues, however, have made substantial progress in understanding the development of the posterior attention subnetwork, specifically the development of orienting capacities.

Development of the Orienting Response

The human infant is not maximally capable of efficient orientation at birth. This capacity develops sometime between 3 and 6 months of age (Clohessy, Posner, Rothbart, & Vecera, 1991). One component function of orienting that shows development between 3 and 6 months of age is inhibition of return. Inhibition of return is the bias of the visual system against returning fixation to locations that have recently been inspected. This bias facilitates orientation to novel locations, thereby maximizing the area of visual space monitored. Inhibition of return can be demonstrated by presenting a unilateral target to a subject, followed by the presentation of bilateral targets. The bilateral targets are identical both to one another and to the unilateral stimulus. Subjects typically orient more frequently to the side opposite that of the unilateral target presentation. Infants 6 months of age and older show adult-level inhibition of return in this paradigm; infants 3 months of age do not show normal inhibition of return (Clohessey et al., 1991). When targets are presented at 30° eccentricities, 3-month-old infants show a perseverative pattern, more frequently returning gaze to the location of the unilateral target. However, 3-month-olds do show inhibition of return when targets are presented at 10° eccentricities (Harman, Posner, Rothbart, & Thomas-Thrapp, 1994). These results show that 3-month-old infants do not demonstrate mature visual orienting.

Role of the Orienting Response in Promoting Soothing

The orienting response comprises a set of neurophysiological, physiological, and behavioral responses that function to enhance information processing by setting the human organism to be optimally receptive to information from the environment (Sokolov, 1960). Behavioral activity is quieted as the orienting response is "accompanied by the characteristic freezing or suppression of other activity during the alerting period" (Pavlov, 1928, as summarized in Stechler & Latz, 1966, p. 517). Orienting to external stimuli is associated with heart rate deceleration, which opposes the heart rate acceleration that occurs as a response to and manifestation of distress. Richards and Casey (1991) reported that, in addition to heart rate deceleration, changes in heart rate variability are also associated with intensive attention to external stimuli. In their study, heart rate variability of 14-, 20-, and 26-week-old infants decreased while the infants were attending to visual and auditory stimuli and returned to prestimulus levels approximately 5 seconds following attention termination. Richards and Casey argued that these findings are consistent with a model of parasympathetic vagal activity on the heart in which vagal firing is increased during sustained attention and inhibited during attention termination.

The association between attention and parasympathetic activity invites speculation about other parasympathetic responses associated with intensive attention that may promote soothing in the infant. Co-occurring relations between attention and heart rate variability may increase with age during the first year of life, which may contribute to the increasing soothability of the infant during the first year. The central nervous system controls of attention and cardiac function are similarly lateralized. Posner and Peterson (1990) cited data from several sources suggesting that vigilance tasks depend on activation of right frontal lobe areas. These sources include lesion, split brain, and neuroimaging studies. The neurotransmitter involved in this activity may be norepinephrine because the structures in both the frontal lobes and the posterior part of the brain maximally innervated by norepinephrine are precisely those that have been shown to mediate spatial attention. Norepinephrine innervation arising in the LC has also been found to be lateralized on the right in the frontal lobes. Robinson (1985) found that lesions of the right frontal lobe produce bilateral depletion of norepinephrine, whereas lesions of the left frontal lobe produce unilateral left norepinephrine depletion. Yanowitz, Preston, and Abildskov (1966) (as cited in Lane & Schwartz, 1987) provided evidence that sympathetic cardiac control is right lateralized in dogs. Stimulation of the right stellate ganglion produces increases in heart rate, whereas stimulation of the left stellate ganglion does not affect heart rate.

Obligatory Attention: Vulnerability to Distress

Distress during infancy may arise from the difficulty infants have in averting their gaze from particular objects. Several researchers have observed extraordinarily long gaze fixations in infants 2 months of age or younger. Friedman (1972) reported that 2-month-olds fixated on checkerboards for a mean of 55 seconds during 60-second trials. Stechler and Latz (1966) observed visual fixations of up to 54 minutes in neonates, terming this phenomenon *obligatory attention*. The link between visual and affective behavior is seen in the observation that these extended gaze fixations were often terminated by hard crying. Tennes, Emde, Kisley, and Metcalf (1972) observed extended fixations that terminated in hard crying and general distress in 2-month-old as well as in 4- to 5-week-old infants. They described the sequence of events as follows. First, the infants orient to the stimulus. During this initial orientation, their activity level decreases. The orienting and decreased activity lasts for 10–30 seconds, after which activity level increases and the infant becomes fussy. This terminates in hard crying, and the infant finally turns his or her head away, closes his or her eyes, or both. Curiously, this gaze termination is often followed by a return to the stimulus, as if the infant is stimulus-bound or stimulus-driven.

In a study designed to examine the ability of 2-, 3-, and 4-month-olds to disengage visual attention, Johnson, Posner, and Rothbart (1991) demonstrated that 2- and 3-month-olds have difficulty in averting their gaze from visual stimuli. In contrast, 4-month-olds exhibit proficiency on this task. The infants were presented with a visual stimulus. Once the infants fixated the stimulus, bilateral peripheral stimuli were presented 30° to either side of fixation. The probability of the infants' averting their gaze within 8 seconds of peripheral stimulus onset was calculated. For the trials on which the infants disengaged visual attention, latency to disengage was also calculated. These disengagement measures were related to scores on the Infant Behavior Questionnaire (IBQ) (Rothbart, 1981). A significant positive correlation of .50 was obtained between the probability of disengaging from the central stimulus and the infant's score on the IBQ scale of Soothability. Significant negative correlations were also found between probability of disengaging and scores on the IBQ scales of Fear (−.39) and Frustration (−.47).

Reports of emotion regulation via gaze aversion are common, including both the avoidance of distressing stimulation and the avoidance of stimulation that may be too exciting. For example, Stechler and Latz (1966) described an infant interacting with her mother. When the infant showed signs of extreme excitement, she turned her head away from the mother, demonstrating the proclivity to avoid stimulation that may be too arousing. Infants who cannot yet walk or even crawl are incapable of physically removing themselves from situations in which they find stimuli aversive, noxious, annoying, or arousing. The development of eye movement control appears to facilitate emotional regulation.

As a final note, obligatory attention may have paradoxical effects on infant state regulation. Although infants who are prone to fixate on distressing stimuli for long durations may show elevated distress relative to infants who can quickly switch their gaze, these long orienting durations can also be used to promote soothing. Wolff (1987) demonstrated that, if an infant's gaze could be maintained, soothing would be achieved by extended fixations to nondistressing stimuli. Although it may be difficult to promote orienting, once orienting is achieved, it may aid in soothing.

Neural Bases of Obligatory Attention

Johnson (1990) proposed that obligatory attention in infancy is due to the asynchronous development of subsystems of the visual system. Four of these systems and the functions they mediate are as follows:

1. The *SC Pathway*, a pathway from the retina to the superior colliculus (SC), is thought to be involved in the generation of eye movements toward simple, easily discriminable stimuli, and is fed mainly by the peripheral visual field.
2. An *inhibitory pathway* inhibits collicular input from several cortical areas via the substantia nigra and basal ganglia. Schiller (1985) proposed that this pathway ensures regulation of collicular activity by top-down mechanisms.
3. The *FEF pathway* is a cortical pathway that converges both broadband and color-opponent streams of processing in the frontal eye fields (FEF). It is involved in the detailed and complex analysis of visual stimuli such as the temporal sequencing of eye movements within complex arrays.
4. The *MT pathway* is a cortical pathway that goes to the SC both directly from the primary visual cortex and also via the middle temporal area (MT). This pathway is exclusively driven by the broadband or magnocellular system and may be involved in the smooth tracking of moving objects.

The competency of each of these systems depends on the maturational state of the neural structures subserving them. Johnson (1990) proposed that only the SC pathway is mature at birth. The next pathway to develop, at 1 month of age, is the inhibitory pathway. By this age, lower Layer IV of the primary visual cortex has matured, allowing functional connectivity of the projection to the basal ganglia and substantia nigra.

The behavioral implications of this maturational sequence are that newborn infants are capable of eye movements driven by the SC pathway. One month later, these movements are inhibited because of the maturation of the inhibitory pathway. Yet the pathways that excite the oculomotor system and initiate eye movements, the FEF and MT pathways, remain immature. Therefore, the oculomotor system is weighted in favor of inhibition, giving rise to the extended orienting observed in infants beginning around the age of 1 month.

Role of Distraction in the Regulation of Distress

Some studies have been done on the use of distraction to soothe infants. Wolff (1987), reporting on informal experiments with newborn to 10-week-old infants, demonstrated notable effects on behavioral state using visual distraction. When crying infants were presented with a large target to look at, they oriented to the target and momentarily ceased crying. Diffuse motor activity was also suspended. If the target was removed as soon as the infant stopped crying, the infant immediately resumed crying. However, if the target was moved around slowly such that the infant was induced to track it and maintain fixation, the infant often remained soothed when the target was finally removed. Halsted (1989) studied the calming effects of soap bubbles presented to 3-, 6-, 10-, and 13-month-old infants. Prior to the presentation of the soap bubbles, distress was induced using a black and white checkerboard with small squares (i.e., high spatial frequency and bold contrasts). Of the infants who became distressed while viewing the checkerboard, a substantial percentage were soothed after watching the bubbles: 33% of the 3-month-olds, 67% of the 6-month-olds, 90% of the 10-month-olds, and 75% of the 13-month-olds. Soothing was assessed by both behavioral level of distress and heart rate. Heart rate decreased while viewing the bubbles. An interesting developmental finding was also noted. The 3-month-olds who did soothe in response to bubbles took nearly three times as long to soothe (mean, 15.4 seconds) as did infants at the other three ages (mean, 4.57 seconds).

Several types of auditory distraction have been identified as effective soothers, among them white noise (Brackbill, 1973; Brackbill, Adams, Crowell, & Gray, 1966; Wolff, 1966) and the sound of the human heart (Brackbill et al., 1966). Characteristics of noise that seem to have differential effects include high volumes in excess of 75 dB (Birns, Blank, Bridger, & Escalona, 1965; Palmquist, 1975; Tullock, Brown, Jacobs, Prugh, & Green, 1964). Demonstrations have also been offered showing that low-pitched tones are more effective as soothers than high-pitched tones (Birns et al., 1965; Stubbs, 1934). Finally, continuous sounds are more effective than intermittent tones, which are no better, or even worse, than no intervention (Birns et al., 1965; Brackbill, 1972; Wolff, 1966).

A MODEL SYSTEM FOR STUDYING
THE INTERACTION OF ATTENTION AND DISTRESS

Harman, Rothbart, and Posner (1995) developed a model system to study how attention deployment and regulation influences distress expression and distress experience. Using the model system, the use of distraction to soothe human infants was investigated. The method consists of encouraging an infant who is fussing or crying to orient to an environmental event such as a toy or television display. There were three primary goals for this series of studies. First, several findings relating attention control to the expression and experience of negative emotions motivated the development of a model system for studying such relations. Second, amounts of distress expression (i.e., fussing, crying) significantly decline during early infancy. The coincidence of this reduction in distress expression with the maturation of the human attention network suggests that attention network functioning may significantly influence distress expression, a hypothesis warranting investigation. Third, the results of these studies can be appreciated for their practical value in developing optimal techniques to soothe human infants.

Infants were chosen as the population for the model system because of their characteristics of both distress and attention. Distress in infants is relatively easy to induce because infants are so much more vulnerable to distress than older children and adults. Once induced, distress expression in the infant is overt and therefore quantifiable by direct observation. An older child or adult may be distressed but show no or few overt signs of distress, in contrast to the facial expressions, vocalizations, and motor patterns of infants, who have relatively little regulation over their emotional expression. The attention systems of the infant are functionally immature, and there is a period at approximately 4 months of age during which the posterior attention subnetwork, associated with involuntary orienting, is functioning in a fairly mature fashion while the anterior attention subnetwork, associated with voluntary orienting, is not. The precise age range of the period during which the anterior attention subnetwork remains relatively immature has not yet been determined. The significance of the asynchronous development between involuntary and voluntary orienting systems is that, from 3 to 6 months of age, orienting behavior is more strongly influenced by the environment than it is by voluntary control (i.e., will). Therefore, 3- to 6-month-old infants are easily influenced by other people, such as parents, or by environmental events to orient to specific stimuli. The combination of vulnerability to distress and malleability of orienting of the human infant during the first year of life provides a unique opportunity for studying the interaction of distress and negative emotionality in the human.

In Harman et al.'s (1995) paradigm, distress is induced in 3- to 6-month-old infants using high levels of visual and auditory stimulation presented on three computer screens. The computer screen display—consisting of simple, multicolored shapes accompanied by a continuous, randomly paced series of computer-generated bleeps—induces distress in about half of the infants exposed to it. Following distress induction, the infants are presented with stimuli known or thought to be soothing to the human infant. In this manner, the effects of orientation on distress expression can be observed.

Empirical Results Obtained Using the Model System

In a first study using this model system, Harman and co-workers (1995) induced distress in infants using the procedure described previously, then presented a series of distractors to them (i.e., a baby rattle, a brass bell, soap bubbles, a small animal toy). The distractors were each presented for 10 seconds, with 10-second pauses between distractors. It was found that orientation to the soothing stimuli greatly diminished distress behavior. The babies decreased or ceased negative vocalizations, negative facial expressions, and diffuse motor movements. Their faces became calm or neutral, they quieted, and their motor movements became coordinated or ceased altogether. However, immediately following withdrawal of the distractors, the infants resumed distress expression at levels identical to those observed prior to distraction (see Figure 9.1). Based on this finding, Harman and colleagues postulated the existence of a *distress keeper*, a mechanism or system that maintains a "distressed status." During distraction, orienting behavior dominates the behavior of the infant; upon termination of distraction, however, the distress-keeping mechanism reinstates distress expression. At least three possibilities exist concerning the relationship between the maintenance of distress and attentional distraction. First, there is the possibility that the activation of the mechanism that maintains distress decays as it normally would, but the distress is not apparent during distraction. A second possibility is that attentional distraction, in addition to blocking overt manifestations of distress, accelerates decay of the activation of the mechanism that maintains distress. Finally, it may be that distraction contributes to the maintenance of distress, as if some finite quantity of distress must be discharged before the distressed state is allowed to decay.

Consistent with the third possibility is a finding by Wolff (1987), who, while observing infants in their homes, noted that a small number of babies cried after be-

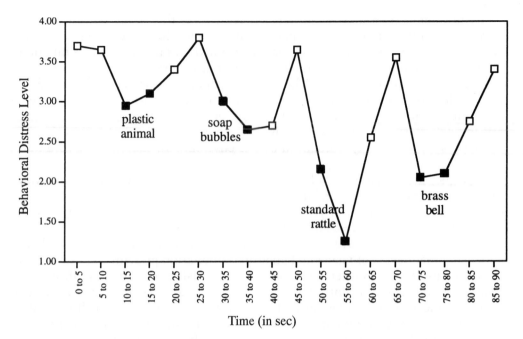

Figure 9.1.   Behavioral distress level plotted as a function of time. (Darkened boxes indicate the presence of distraction.)

ing fed and put to bed, just before falling asleep. Their mothers believed that "they just needed to cry it out" and did not attempt to soothe their infants when the infants cried at this time. The crying lasted 1–3 minutes, followed by sleep. Skeptical that the crying was "okay for them," Wolff conducted some casual experiments in which he attempted to soothe the infants in this situation. His soothing interventions, picking up the babies and holding them or visually distracting them, were successful in eliciting quiet, oriented attentiveness. However, when he terminated the soothing intervention, the infant resumed crying. The overall effect was one of prolonging the infants' awake state (up to 30 minutes), rather than promoting sleep through soothing.

In a second experiment, the duration for which the distress keeper would remain activated was explored. Distraction intervals of 10, 30, and 60 seconds were compared. No effect of the duration of the distraction was found; infants expressed just as much distress following 10 seconds of distraction as they did following 1 full minute of distraction (see Figure 9.2). The distress levels of infants following all three distraction intervals were similar to the distress levels of infants in whom distress was induced but to whom no soothing intervention, distraction or otherwise, was provided followed distress induction. From this, it is concluded that the distress keeper is at least robust enough to reinstate distress following 1 minute of inhibition of distress expression.

A third study examined the contributions of the anterior and posterior attentional subnetworks to the soothing-during-distraction phenomenon. Within the cortex, there is evidence of separation between the structures and systems subserving identity and location processing (Ungerleider & Mishkin, 1982). Location signals are processed by dorsal structures, including the posterior parietal cortex and the SC, and are therefore closely allied with the posterior attention subnetwork.

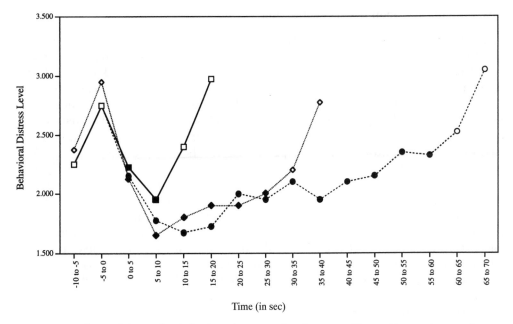

Figure 9.2.   Behavioral distress levels for three distraction durations. (———□———, 10 seconds; ⋯⋯◇⋯⋯, 30 seconds; - - - -○- - - -, 60 seconds.) (Darkened symbols indicate the presence of distraction.)

Identity information is processed by temporal and anterior substrates, most markedly the inferior temporal cortex. Thus, identity processing is closely allied with the anterior attention subnetwork. To address the question of which subnetworks, anterior, posterior, or both, are involved in the phenomenon of soothing during distraction, novelty manipulations of the soothing stimuli were introduced. Because the posterior attention subnetwork is closely allied to the orienting response, it was thought that location novelty would enhance soothing during distraction. There was no theoretical reason to believe that identity novelty would do so.

Instead of presenting toys as distractors, computer images of six different animal figures were used, each accompanied by a soothing or attention-getting sound. The computer presentation allowed the identity or the location of the image to be manipulated every 3⅓ seconds, or three times within a 10-second distraction interval. For identity manipulation, one animal figure was switched to another during the trial; for location manipulation, the screen on which the figure appeared changed during the trial. Two dimensions of novelty manipulation yielded four types of trials: location novelty, identity novelty, double novelty (i.e., location and identity novelty), and double redundancy (i.e., neither location nor identity changes). Distress was induced in 3- and 6-month-old infants as described previously, followed by a series of 16 trials, 4 of each type (i.e., location novelty, identity novelty, double novelty, double redundancy).

Contrary to expectations, the study suggested involvement of the anterior attention subnetwork in the soothing-during-distraction phenomenon, whereas no evidence was found for a specific contribution by the posterior attention subnetwork. Stimulus identity novelty maintained significantly calmer behavior during the 10-second distraction durations than did stimulus identity redundancy; stimulus location novelty showed no advantage relative to stimulus location redundancy.

Five Principles of Soothing via Distraction

The series of three studies using the model system elucidated five principles concerning the interaction of attention and negative emotion in infants. First, it was seen that, without intervention, distress expression is maintained at remarkably constant levels, neither escalating nor subsiding. Second, distraction can temporarily suspend the expression of distress. In all three studies discussed previously, distraction dampened or eliminated distress expression. Third, following distraction, distress expression resumes at levels equal to those prior to distraction. It seems that distress is maintained at very particular levels of expression, regardless of whether it is being expressed. In addition to the studies described previously, this result has been obtained in studies evaluating the efficacy of pacifiers in calming infants (Campos, 1989; Gunnar, Fisch, & Malone, 1984; Smith, Fillion, & Blass, 1990). Fourth, the duration of the distraction does not affect the level of distress expression, at least for intervals of up to 1 minute. Fifth, the depth of the drop during distraction does not affect the level of distress expressed following distraction. In all three studies, there was some variability in the effectiveness of the different types of stimuli used to soothe the infants. However, the differential effectiveness never appeared to affect the return to the prior level of distress expression, although this was never directly tested.

Does Distraction Remediate Distress?

Given these principles, an important question is whether soothing by distraction actually remediates distress. The answer appears to be no. From these studies, we see that attentional distraction is capable only of blocking behavioral and perhaps some physiological manifestations of distress, but not of remediating distress. It probably also prevents the inception of further distress. The conclusion that attentional distraction does not appear to remediate distress in human infants and may serve only to block overt manifestations of distress echoes findings in the literature concerning pain management. Leventhal and colleagues (Ahles, Blanchard, & Leventhal, 1983; Leventhal, Brown, Shacham, & Engquist, 1979) found that attention to external stimuli (viewing landscape and architecture slides) accords little to no relief from pain induced by cold pressor distress following distraction, although it is effective during distraction.

Although these findings and observations suggest that distraction does not actually remediate distress, it is still possible that the infant or adult experiences relief during distraction. In addition to accounting for effects of visual and auditory distraction, and perhaps sucking on pacifiers, the notion of distraction might account for several other soothing interventions that have demonstrated efficacy. These include some forms of vestibular stimulation; somatic stimulation, such as caressing the infant or placing the infant's foot in warm water (Birns, Blank, & Bridger, 1966); and thermal stimulation (Brackbill, 1973). Although all of these forms of distraction may need to be maintained to provide relief, that they do in fact provide relief should not be ignored.

CONCLUSIONS

We began this chapter by reviewing the data on the relation between frontal EEG activation and temperament. Data suggest that infants who are easily distressed and not easily soothed display a unique pattern of frontal activation. We have speculated that this pattern of activation may reflect an inability of the infant and young child to adequately regulate his or her distress. We also speculated that some of the cognitive competencies involved in successful emotion regulation, including verbal strategies and certain forms of attention, were associated with the activation of anterior cortical regions, so that those infants and children who exhibit difficulty in distress regulation may in fact be compromised in these cognitive processes as well. In order to understand just what these cognitive processes entail, and their neural bases, we discussed the role of the developing attention subnetworks in regulating negative emotional expression. We also presented a series of experiments in which the role of attentional distraction in regulating negative emotional expression was investigated. The results of these experiments suggested that the anterior attention subnetwork is closely linked to the regulation of distress expression. This is consistent with the data linking frontal development to the regulation of negative emotional expression.

Emphasizing the role of the anterior attention subnetwork and frontal mechanisms in the regulation of distress may resolve the paradox of the role of the posterior attention subnetwork in the experience or expression of negative emotionality or both. In reviewing the role of the posterior attention subnetwork, evidence and theory were presented that this system could both make an infant more vulnerable to the distressed state, through obligatory attention to disturbing stimuli, and make the infant more prone to the soothed state, through obligatory attention to calming stimuli. Posner and Peterson (1990) proposed that, in the neurologically mature adult, the anterior attention subnetwork exerts control over the posterior attention subnetwork. Therefore, it may be that, for most infants, as they mature and as there is increased maturation of the frontal region, their ability to regulate distress increases. That is, these older infants and young children are able to regulate their negative affect as they utilize attentional strategies that are subsumed by the anterior subnetwork. Alternatively, it could be that involuntary orienting in itself leads to sensory overstimulation, and it is through anterior subnetwork maturation that sensory overload is averted. There is a sense from the data on 4-month-olds with high motor arousal and high negative affect (Calkins et al., 1995) that they are unable to look away and regulate their attention to the auditory and visual stimuli that are presented to them. These children may learn that the best strategy to deal with sensory overload that is a function of involuntary orienting is to withdraw from stimulation and avoid interaction.

The extent to which the empirical findings of Fox and colleagues and those of Rothbart and Posner and colleagues are related remains to be demonstrated. Certainly, both sets of findings demonstrate an essential role of frontal mechanisms in regulating the expression of negative emotion, but more specific links must be established. To merge these two lines of research, at least two questions must be addressed. First, to what extent does anterior subnetwork maturation account for the increased EEG activity seen in the frontal lobes that has been shown to relate to the regulation of negative emotionality? Second, if attentional distraction is a critical component of the findings of Fox and colleagues, how do the cerebral asymmetries of emotional expression relate to the neural substrates of attention?

REFERENCES
Ahles, T.A., Blanchard, E.B., & Leventhal, H. (1983). Cognitive control of pain: Attention to the sensory aspects of cold pressor stimulus. *Cognitive Therapy and Research, 7*, 159–177.

Birns, B., Blank, M., & Bridger, W.H. (1966). The effectiveness of various soothing techniques on human infants. *Psychosomatic Medicine, 28*, 316–322.

Birns, B., Blank, M., Bridger, W.H., & Escalona, S.K. (1965). Behavioral inhibition in neonates produced by auditory stimuli. *Child Development, 42*, 17–26.

Borod, J.C. (1992). Interhemispheric and intrahemispheric control of emotion: A focus on unilateral brain damage. *Journal of Consulting and Clinical Psychology, 60*, 339–348.

Brackbill, Y. (1972). Cumulative effects of continuous stimulation on arousal level in infants. *Child Development, 42*, 17–26.

Brackbill, Y. (1973). Continuous stimulation reduces arousal level: Stability of the effect over time. *Child Development, 44*, 43–46.

Brackbill, Y., Adams, G., Crowell, D.H., & Gray, M.L. (1966). Arousal level in neonates and preschool children under continuous auditory stimulation. *Journal of Experimental Child Psychology, 4*, 178–188.

Calkins, S.D., Fox, N.A., & Marshall, T.R. (1995). Behavioral and physiological antecedents of inhibition in infancy. *Child Development, 67*, 523–540.

Campos, R. (1989). Soothing pain-elicited distress in infants with swaddling and pacifiers. *Child Development, 60*, 780–792.

Clohessy, A.B., Posner, M.I., Rothbart, M.K., & Vecera, S.P. (1991). The development of inhibition of return in early infancy. *Journal of Cognitive Neuroscience, 3*, 345–350.

Cohen, R.M., Semple, W.E., Gross, M., Holcomb, H.J., Dowling, S.M., & Nordahl, T.E. (1988). Functional localization of sustained attention. *Neuropsychology and Behavioral Neurology, 1*, 3–20.

Coslett, H.B., Bowers, D., & Heilman, K.M. (1987). Reduction in cerebral activation after right hemisphere stroke. *Neurology, 37*, 957–962.

Davidson, R.J. (1992). Anterior cerebral asymmetry and the nature of emotion. *Brain and Cognition, 20*, 125–151.

Davidson, R.J., Ekman, P., Saron, C., Senulis, J., & Friesen, W.V. (1990). Approach-withdrawal and cerebral asymmetry: I. Emotion expression and brain physiology. *Journal of Personality and Social Psychology, 58*, 330–341.

Dawson, G., Grofer-Klinger, L., Panagiotides, H., Spieker, S., & Frey, K. (1992). Infants of mothers with depressive symptoms: Electroencephalographic and behavioral findings related to attachment status. *Development and Psychopathology, 4*, 67–80.

Fox, N.A. (1991). If it's not left, it's right: Electroencephalogram asymmetry and the development of emotion. *American Psychologist, 46*, 863–872.

Fox, N.A. (1994). Dynamic cerebral processes underlying emotion regulation. *Monographs of the Society for Research in Child Development, 59*(2–3), 152–166.

Fox, N.A., Bell, M.A., & Jones, N.A. (1992). Individual differences in response to stress and cerebral asymmetry. *Developmental Neuropsychology, 8*, 161–184.

Fox, N.A., & Davidson, R.J. (1984). Hemispheric substrates of affect: A developmental model. In N.A. Fox & R.J. Davidson (Eds.), *The psychobiology of affective development* (pp. 353–381). Hillsdale, NJ: Lawrence Erlbaum Associates.

Friedman, S. (1972). Habituation and recovery of visual response in the alert human newborn. *Journal of Experimental Child Psychology, 13*, 339–349.

Goldman-Rakic, P.S. (1988). Topography of cognition: Parallel distributed networks in primate association cortex. *Annual Review of Neuroscience, 11*, 137–156.

Grant, S.J., Aston-Jones, G., & Redmond, D.E. (1988). Responses of primate locus coeruleus neurons to simple and complex sensory stimuli. *Brain Research Bulletin, 21*, 401–410.

Gunnar, M.G., Fisch, R.O., & Malone, S. (1984). The effects of a pacifying stimulus on behavioral adrenocortical responses to circumcision in the newborn. *Journal of the American Academy of Child Psychiatry, 23*, 34–38.

Halsted, N. (1989). *Developmental mechanisms of soothing and orienting in infancy.* Unpublished doctoral dissertation, University of Oregon, Eugene.

Harman, C., Posner, M.I., Rothbart, M.K., & Thomas-Thrapp, L. (1994). Development of orienting to locations and objects in human infants. *Canadian Journal of Experimental Psychology, 48*, 301–318.

Harman, C., Rothbart, M.K., & Posner, M.I. (1995). *Attentional regulation of distress expression in the human infant.* Paper presented at the Biennial Meeting of the Society for Research in Child Development, Indianapolis, IN.

Heller, W. (1993). Neuropsychological mechanisms of individual differences in emotion, personality, and arousal. *Neuropsychology, 7,* 476–489.

Henriques, J.B., & Davidson, R.J. (1991). Left frontal hypoactivation in depression. *Journal of Abnormal Psychology, 99,* 22–31.

Johnson, M.H. (1990). Cortical maturation and the development of visual attention in early infancy. *Journal of Cognitive Neuroscience, 3,* 335–344.

Johnson, M.H., Posner, M.I., & Rothbart, M.K. (1991). Components of visual orienting in early infancy: Contingency learning, anticipatory looking and disengaging. *Journal of Cognitive Neuroscience, 3,* 335–344.

Jones, N.A., & Fox, N.A. (1992). Electroencephalogram asymmetry during emotionally evocative films and its relation to positive and negative affectivity. *Brain and Cognition, 20,* 280–299.

Kagan, J., Reznick, J.S., & Gibbons, J. (1989). Inhibited and uninhibited types of children. *Child Development, 60,* 838–845.

Kagan, J., Reznick, J.S., Snidman, N., Gibbons, J., & Johnson, M. (1988). Childhood derivatives of inhibition and lack of inhibition to the unfamiliar. *Child Development, 59,* 1580–1589.

Lane, R.D., & Schwartz, G.E. (1987). Induction of lateralized sympathetic input to the heart by the CNS during emotional arousal: A possible neurophysiologic trigger of sudden cardiac death. *Psychosomatic Medicine, 49,* 274–284.

Leventhal, H., Brown, D., Shacham, S., & Engquist, G. (1979). Effects of preparatory information about sensations, threat of pain, and attention on cold pressor distress. *Journal of Personality and Social Psychology, 37,* 688–714.

Palmquist, H. (1975). The effect of heart beat sound stimulation on the weight development of newborn infants. *Child Development, 46,* 292–295.

Pavlov, I.P. (1928). *Lectures on conditioned reflexes.* New York: Liveright.

Peterson, S.E., Fox, P.T., Posner, M.I., Mintun, M., & Raichle, M.E. (1988). Positron emission tomographic studies of the cortical anatomy of single word processing. *Nature, 331,* 585–589.

Posner, M.I., Inhoff, A.W., Friedrich, F.J., & Cohen, A. (1987). Isolating attentional systems: A cognitive-anatomical analysis. *Psychobiology, 15,* 107–121.

Posner, M.I., & Peterson, S.E. (1990). The attention system of the human brain. *Annual Review of Neuroscience, 13,* 25–42.

Richards, J.E., & Casey, B.J. (1991). Heart rate variability during attention phases in young infants. *Psychophysiology, 28,* 43–53.

Robinson, R.G. (1985). Lateralized behavioral and neurochemical consequences of unilateral brain injury in rats. In S.G. Glick (Ed.), *Cerebral lateralization in nonhuman species* (pp. 135–156). Orlando, FL: Academic Press.

Rothbart, M.K. (1981). Measurement of temperament in infancy. *Child Development, 52,* 569–578.

Rothbart, M.K., & Posner, M.I. (1985). Temperament and the development of self-regulation. In H. Hartlage & C.F. Telzrow (Eds.), *Neuropsychology of individual differences: A developmental perspective* (pp. 93–116). New York: Plenum.

Schiller, P.H. (1985). A model for the generation of visually guided saccadic eye movements. In D. Rose & V.G. Dobson (Eds.), *Models of the visual cortex* (pp. 62–70). Chichester, England: John Wiley & Sons.

Silberman, E.K., & Weingartner, H. (1986). Hemispheric lateralization of functions related to emotion. *Brain and Cognition, 5,* 322–335.

Smith, B.A., Fillion, T.J., & Blass, E.M. (1990). Orally mediated sources of calming in 1- to 3-day old human infants. *Developmental Psychology, 26,* 731–737.

Sokolov, E.N. (1960). Neuronal models and the orienting reflex. In M.A.B. Brazier (Ed.), *The central nervous system and behavior* (pp. 187–276). New York: Macy.

St. James-Roberts, I., & Halil, T. (1991). Infant crying patterns in the first year: Normal community and clinical findings. *Journal of Child Psychology and Psychiatry, 32,* 951–968.

Stechler, G., & Latz, E. (1966). Some observations on attention and arousal in the human infant. *Journal of the American Academy of Child Psychiatry, 5,* 517–525.

Stubbs, E.M. (1934). The effect of the duration, intensity, and pitch of sound stimuli on the responses of newborn infants. *University of Iowa Study of Child Welfare, 9*(4), 77–139.

Tennes, K., Emde, R., Kisley, A., & Metcalf, D. (1972). The stimulus barrier in early infancy: An exploration of some formulations of John Benjamin. In R.R. Holt & E. Peterfreound (Eds.), *Psychoanalysis and contemporary science* (Vol. 1, pp. 206–234). New York: Macmillan.

Thompson, R. (1994). Emotion regulation: A theme in search of definition. *Monographs of the Society for Research in Child Development, 59*(2–3), 25–52.

Tullock, J.D., Brown, B.S., Jacobs, H.L., Prugh, D.G., & Green, W.A. (1964). Normal heart beat sound and the behaviors of newborn infants: A replication study. *Psychosomatic Medicine, 26*, 661–670.

Ungerleider, L.G., & Mishkin, M. (1982). Two cortical visual systems. In D.J. Ingle, M.A. Goodale, & R.J.W. Mansfield (Eds.), *Analysis of visual behavior* (pp. 549–586). Cambridge, MA: MIT Press.

Wolff, P.H. (1966). The causes, controls, and organizations of behavior in the neonate. *Psychological Issues, 5*(Monograph 17).

Wolff, P.H. (1987). *The development of behavioral states and the development of emotion in early infancy*. Chicago: University of Chicago Press.

Yanowitz, F., Preston, J., & Abildskov, J. (1966). Functional distribution of right and left stellate innervation to the ventricles: Production of neurogenic electrocardiographic changes by unilateral alterations of sympathetic tone. *Circulation Research, 18*, 416–428.

Development of the Prefrontal Cortex: Evolution, Neurobiology, and Behavior
edited by Norman A. Krasnegor, Ph.D., G. Reid Lyon, Ph.D.,
and Patricia S. Goldman-Rakic, Ph.D.
copyright © 1997   Paul H. Brookes Publishing Co., Inc.
Baltimore • London • Toronto • Sydney

_____ *III*

NEUROPSYCHOLOGY
AND NEUROPATHOLOGY
_____ *OF PREFRONTAL CORTEX*

10

Corticolimbic Circuitry and the Development of Psychopathology During Childhood and Adolescence

Francine M. Benes

Since the mid-1980s, there has been a dramatic increase in our understanding of how altered brain mechanisms may contribute to the occurrence of adult disorders such as schizophrenia (Benes, 1995). Similar insights concerning neuropsychiatric disorders in children and adolescents have not kept pace with the advances seen in adult psychiatry. Accordingly, little is known about conditions such as autism, attention-deficit/hyperactivity disorder, mood disorder, and separation anxiety, for which only pathological investigations have been conducted. Even less, however, is understood about the role that normal brain ontogeny may play in these psychopathological states during the first 2 decades of life.

This chapter explores two basic issues concerning childhood and adolescent psychopathology. The first is which brain regions are likely candidates for playing even a partial role in emotional disorders of childhood and adolescence. In this regard, the section on the corticolimbic system describes the anatomy of the limbic system and discusses how the visceral component of emotional experience is integrated within the anterior cingulate gyrus, where selective attentional activity is also derived. Affective experience and selective attention are shown to be integrally related to motivational drives processed through the prefrontal cortex, and together these various regions comprise a complete network through which maternal nurturance, separation behaviors, and social interactiveness are mediated.

The second relevant issue that this chapter addresses is how the development of the corticolimbic system can potentially be disrupted at various stages of embryonic and postnatal life to produce different forms of psychopathology. Toward this end, there is a discussion of the differential timing of the development of different

This chapter was supported by National Institute of Mental Health Grants MH-00423 and MH-31154 and an award from the Stanley Foundation.

The author wishes to thank Patti Fitzpatrick for her help in preparing the text of the chapter and Dr. Stephen L. Vincent for his help in assembling the figures.

cortical gyri, the maturation of cortical cytoarchitecture, the time course for the in-growth of cortical and thalamic afferents, and the postnatal myelination of some key corticolimbic relays. Next, the chapter reviews the prenatal and postnatal development of neurotransmitter systems that are both intrinsic and extrinsic to the cortex. Finally, there is a discussion of how specific transmitter systems may contribute to the onset of emotional and cognitive disturbances seen in pediatric psychopathology. In this regard, consideration is given to the types of developmental perturbation that could arise at various pre- and postnatal stages and how such changes might serve as triggers for disorders of emotion and cognition in at-risk individuals.

THE CORTICOLIMBIC SYSTEM

The *Great* Limbic Lobe

Broca (1878) was the first to note that a "limbic lobe," consisting of the septal nuclei, amygdala, hippocampus, parahippocampal (entorhinal) cortex, and cingulate gyrus, appeared along the midsagittal plane of virtually all mammalian forms (Figure 10.1). Interestingly, the elaboration of this system was coincident with the appearance of audition, vocalization, maternal nurturance, and separation calls, behaviors that are phylogenetic markers for the integration of visceral responses with other cortically mediated responses (MacLean, 1985). Accordingly, the evolution of elaborate behaviors to nurture offspring has served the perpetuation of mammalian species through a corresponding increase in both the extent and the complexity of corticolimbic circuitry. Along the spectrum of mammalian forms, there has been a striking increase in the relative proportion of neocortex to Broca's limbic lobe. Figure 10.1 shows a comparison of the limbic lobe in rat, cat, and monkey brains

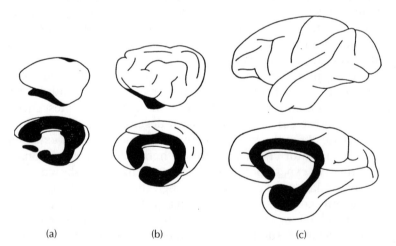

(a)   (b)   (c)

Figure 10.1.   A schematic diagram showing the appearance of the brain in different mammalian species. The brains of a rat (a), cat (b), and monkey (c) are shown in both a lateral (top) and a midsagittal (bottom) view. All three brains show a contiguous loop of limbic structures (black), including the cingulate gyrus, parahippocampal gyrus, and amygdala, that has remained remarkably similar during phylogenesis. This so-called limbic lobe is surrounded by neocortex above and laterally that has shown a progressive increase during phylogeny. (From MacLean, P.D. [1954]. Studies on limbic system [visceral brain] and their bearing on psychosomatic problems. In E. Wittkower & R. Cleghorn [Eds.], *Recent developments in psychosomatic medicine* [p. 106]. London: Pribram and Sons.)

(MacLean, 1954), and it is evident that primates show a much larger volume of neo-cortex surrounding the cingulate and parahippocampal gyri when compared with rodents and felines. In humans, this trend has culminated in the most extensive elaboration of connectivity between associative cortical regions, such as the cingulate region and the hippocampal formation, and the subcortical limbic system. Perhaps the most striking aspect of the organization of the human brain is the expanded prefrontal area that has become extensively linked through reciprocal connections with both the cingulate region and the hippocampal formation.

Integration of Emotion

Emotional expression is an attribute that first became apparent in mammals. It is probably mediated in part by primitive relays in the brainstem reticular formation, hypothalamus, amygdala, and septal nuclei. Papez (1937) was the first to postulate that the cingulate gyrus may play a central role in the integration of emotional experience with cognition because it has extensive connections not only with the limbic system but also with other associative cortical regions involved in higher cognitive functions. Consistent with this idea, autonomic responses have been altered by either stimulation or ablation of the anterior cingulate cortex. With electrical stimulation of this region in primates, visceromotor responses—such as eyelid opening, pupillary dilation, respiratory movements, cardiovascular changes, and piloerection (Anand & Dua, 1956; Kaada, Pribram, & Epstein, 1940; Smith, 1945), as well as changes in facial expression (Smith, 1945) and motor arrest (Dunsmore & Lennox, 1950; Smith, 1945), have been induced. Extensive surgical ablation of the anterior cingulate cortex, in contrast, has resulted in a decrease of emotional responsiveness (Ward, 1948) and even personality changes characterized by either inappropriate purring or growling without provocation in cats (Kennard, 1955). In humans, bilateral infarction of the cingulate gyrus has been associated with increased docility and indifference (Laplane, Degos, Baulac, & Gray, 1981) and an inability to either express or experience emotion (Damasio & Van Hoesen, 1983).

The anterior cingulate region has extensive reciprocal connections with several different cortical areas that include the prefrontal region, the presubiculum, and the inferior parietal lobe (Jones & Powell, 1970; Pandya & Kuypers, 1969; Petras, 1971; Seltzer & Pandya, 1978; Seltzer & Van Hoesen, 1979; Van Hoesen, 1982). Very important is that the anterior cingulate region also has both afferent and efferent connections with nuclear groups that mediate autonomic functions (Figure 10.2), such as the periaqueductal gray (Beckstead, 1979; Domesick, 1969; Hurley, Herbert, Moga, & Saper, 1991; Wyss & Sripanidkulchai, 1984); the nucleus solitarius; the dorsal motor nucleus of the vagus (Hurley et al., 1991; Terreberry & Neafsey, 1983, 1987; Van der Kooy, McGinty, Koda, Gerfen, & Bloom, 1982); and preganglionic sympathetic neurons in the intermediolateral cell column of the thoracic spinal cord (Hurley et al., 1991). Therefore, the anterior cingulate cortex interacts *directly* with centers that mediate both viscerosensory and visceromotor responses in the periphery, and these connections are believed to be fundamental to its role in integrating emotional responses at the cortical level (Neafsey, Terreberry, Hurley, Ruit, & Frysztak, 1992). Both ablation (Kennard, 1955; Laplane et al., 1981; Ward, 1948) and stimulation (Anand & Dua, 1956; Kaada, 1960; Kaada et al., 1940; Smith, 1945) of the anterior cingulate cortex have resulted in both autonomic and affective changes. In humans with documented seizure activity arising from the cingulate cortex (Devinsky & Luciano, 1992), emotional stimulation is a frequent precipitant

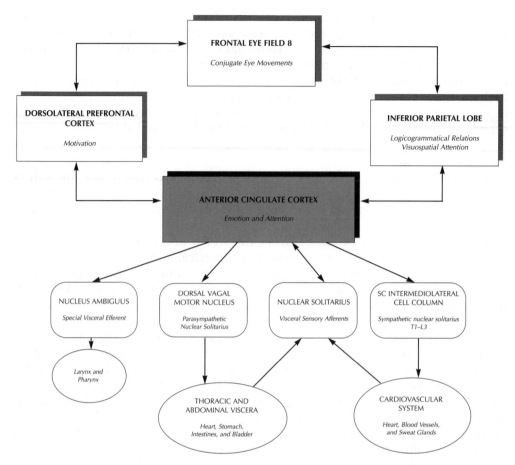

Figure 10.2.   The anterior cingulate cortex and its corticocortical, corticobulbar, and corticospinal connections involved in the integration of emotion with attentional and other cognitive responses. The anterior cingulate cortex plays a unique role in integrating the visceral component of affective experience via its extensive corticobulbar and corticospinal connections involved in autonomic processing. There are corticobulbar fibers originating in the anterior cingulate region that project to the nucleus ambiguus, the dorsal vagal motor nucleus, and the preganglionic sympathetic fibers of the intermediolateral cell column to influence, respectively, the outflow of activity to 1) special visceral efferent muscles (i.e., larynx and pharynx); 2) thoracic and abdominal viscera (i.e., the heart, esophagus, stomach, intestines, and bladder); and 3) the blood vessels and sweat glands. Extensive reciprocal connections of the anterior cingulate region with the nucleus solitarius probably influence the inflow of sensory information from all viscera of the body. The diagram also shows important cortical components of the corticolimbic system of the human brain.

The anterior cingulate cortex occupies a pivotal location in a larger network of associative cortical regions, including the dorsolateral prefrontal cortex, the inferior parietal lobe, frontal eye field 8, and the hippocampal formation (see text for details). All of these regions show extensive reciprocal connectivity and subsume a central role in the mediation of complex behaviors involving motivational (prefrontal cortex), affective, and attentional (anterior cingulate) responses. Frontal eye field 8 probably facilitates the attentional component to these responses by coordinating conjugate deviations of the eyes toward objects of interest. In humans, the inferior parietal lobe may contribute to the visuospatial component of attention as well as to logical processing.

of ictal activity (Mazars, 1970), and the majority of such patients exhibit limbically related features such as temper tantrums and fixed psychoses (Mazars, 1970).

Linkage of Emotion and Attention

Some researchers believe that the cingulate and parietal cortices may cooperate in the performance of directed attention (Mesulam, 1983). In monkeys (Glees, Cole,

Whitty, & Cairns, 1950) and cats (Kennard, 1955), bilateral lesions of the anterior cingulate cortex have been associated with neglect of surrounding objects, including cagemates. In humans with bilateral infarction of the cingulate gyrus, a lack of attentiveness to the surrounding environment has similarly been observed (Laplane et al., 1981), and a cerebral blood flow study reported that human subjects show a marked increase of activity in the anterior part of this region during performance of a Stroop attentional conflict paradigm (Pardo, Pardo, Janer, & Raichle, 1990). The neglect occurring with lesions of the cingulate cortex is thought to involve alterations in the relationship of this area with frontal eye field 8 (Belaydier & Maugierre, 1980), but this may be an indirect effect mediated via the prefrontal and inferior parietal areas. Interestingly, patients with unilateral neglect syndromes associated with lesions of the frontal or parietal regions also show some emotional disturbances, suggesting that there is "a parallelism in the integrity of attention and emotion" (Mesulam & Geschwind, 1978, p. 252).

It is noteworthy that, in monkey posterior parietal cortex, some neurons are activated by hand–eye—coordinated movements, particularly when desirable objects that can satisfy thirst or hunger are employed as targets (Mountcastle, Lynch, Georgopoulos, Sakata, & Acuna, 1975). Such motivationally driven responses are thought to require both an emotional and an attentional component (Mesulam & Geschwind, 1978). Consistent with this proposal, the inferior parietal region has extensive connections with the anterior cingulate cortex and the presubiculum (Jones & Powell, 1970; Pandya & Kuypers, 1969; Petras, 1971; Seltzer & Pandya, 1978, 1984; Seltzer & Van Hoesen, 1979; Van Hoesen, 1982), two important corticolimbic relay areas. Although Luria (1973) emphasized the role of the left (dominant) inferior parietal region in the construction of logical-grammatical relationships, he also noted unilateral neglect syndromes in patients with right-sided posterior parietal lesions. These patients not only neglect extracorporeal space on the left side but also show a peculiar inability to perceive their deficits. It now appears that an anterior attention system mediated by the anterior cingulate area plays a role in semantic processing of words and the degree of blood flow increases in this region as the number of targets increases (Posner, Peterson, Fox, & Raichle, 1990). In contrast to the contribution of the anterior system to target detection, the posterior attention system is involved in visuospatial shifts of focus (Posner & Peterson, 1990). Both systems seem to be essential to normal attention.

Motivation Requires Affect
There is also an important interaction of motivation and affect in humans, as illustrated by a rather distinctive clinical syndrome called "akinetic mutism" that occurs in patients with bilateral occlusion of the anterior cerebral arteries (Barris & Schumann, 1953; Nielsen & Jacobs, 1951) that supply the anterior cingulate cortices and other midsagittal cortical regions. Acute infarctions of this type are associated with an inability to move or speak, as well as considerable negativism. This is quite similar to the catatonic state, wherein muteness, lack of movement, and negativism are also observed. Patients with akinetic mutism who later recover describe a sudden loss of the experience of affect and a concomitant absence of the will to move (Damasio & Van Hoesen, 1983). It seems likely that the extensive reciprocal connectivity between the anterior cingulate region and the prefrontal cortex that plays a direct role in the mediation of motivational and volitional drives (Luria, 1973) probably accounts for some of the symptomatology observed in aki-

netic mutism. A similar concurrence of defects in motivation and emotional experience is commonly seen in adults with schizophrenia; this is thought to arise from a disturbance in connectivity between the dorsolateral prefrontal area and the anterior cingulate cortex (Benes, 1993).

Maternal Nurturance, Separation, and Social Interactiveness

In rodents, ablations of the cingulate gyrus are associated with a loss of maternal activities such as nursing, nest building, and retrieval of the young (Slotnick, 1967; Stamm, 1955). It has been suggested that separation calls and play activities, features observed in mammalian offspring, may have emerged in parallel with the development of the cingulate gyrus during the phylogenetic progression of reptiles into mammals (MacLean, 1985). In support of this hypothesis, vocalizations can be elicited by stimulation of the anterior cingulate region in monkeys (Ploog, 1970; Smith, 1945), whereas more extensive ablations that also include the medial subcallosal and preseptal cingulate cortices result in a complete loss of spontaneous isolation calls (MacLean, 1985). In a clinical case report, a child with documented cingulate seizures was noted to run toward her mother during ictal episodes (Geier et al., 1977), an observation suggesting that the cingulate cortex plays a role in human separation behaviors as well (MacLean, 1985). It is not known, however, whether the cingulate gyrus can be implicated in the separation anxiety seen in children.

Cingulate Cortex as Keystone in Corticolimbic Function

Based on the information presented thus far, it can readily be seen that the cingulate region is a central component in a broadly distributed network of cortical and subcortical regions that subsume functions that are altered in disorders of emotion and cognition. In addition to the connections described in the previous sections, as shown in Figure 10.2, the cingulate cortex is also connected with the dorsolateral prefrontal area, frontal eye field 8, and the inferior parietal lobe. The prefrontal and anterior cingulate cortices receive a rich supply of dopamine afferents from the midbrain ventral tegmental area (Lindvall & Bjorklund, 1984). Some of the areas indicated in Figure 10.2 are phylogenetically newer cortical regions (e.g., the dorsolateral prefrontal and inferior parietal regions) that are most extensively developed in human brain. In contrast, the hippocampal formation is phylogenetically the oldest cortical region and is believed to have first appeared in a rudimentary form in reptiles (Ulinski, 1990). The cingulate gyrus is a transitional cortex, or so-called mesocortex, that first appeared in early mammals (MacLean, 1990). The anterior portion of this gyrus provides a link between the autonomic centers controlling visceral activity and the neocortical regions represented in Figure 10.2 that are involved in motivation, attention, and logical processing.

By examining the corticolimbic regions and their interconnections represented in Figure 10.2, it can be appreciated that defective circuitry in one or several of these areas could give rise to abnormalities in the integration of emotional experience, selective attention, and other neocortically mediated functions, such as volition and cognition. Therefore, pathological processes that have an impact on one or several of these corticolimbic regions could give rise to a broad spectrum of symptoms that encompass both the emotional and the cognitive spheres.

NORMAL ONTOGENESIS OF CORTICOLIMBIC BRAIN REGIONS

With regard to psychiatric disorders of childhood and adolescence, the fact that certain psychopathological states, such as attention-deficit/hyperactivity disorder, mood disturbance, separation anxiety, and autism, appear at particular postnatal stages may imply that the onset of such disorders may be related to maturational changes in neurons and transmitters that are coincidentally occurring within the corticolimbic system. Therefore, it is pertinent to consider the time course for ontogenetic development of the corticolimbic system during pre- and postnatal life. The discussion that follows first considers gyral development in the human brain; this is followed by a description of neuronal cell genesis and migration in the neocortex. An examination of the ingrowth of afferents into the cortex and myelination of the corticolimbic system both peri- and postnatally then leads into a review of the sequential maturational changes that occur for both intrinsic and extrinsic transmitters of the cortex.

Gyral Development

The ontogenetic development of various cortical regions occurs at varying rates that, to some degree, reflect phylogeny (Table 10.1). There is a general tendency for limbic cortical areas to differentiate early in gestation. For example, at 16–19 weeks of human embryogenesis, the cingulate region can be distinguished as a gyrus; but this is well in advance of weeks 20–23, when the parahippocampal gyrus and the hippocampal formation have begun to take shape in the medial temporal area (Gilles, Shankle, & Dooling, 1983). The superior and middle frontal gyri (prefrontal regions) are not clearly delineated until 24–27 weeks of gestational age, and the angular and supramarginal gyri (inferior parietal area) are not distinguishable until 28–31 weeks in utero (Gilles et al., 1983). Paradoxically, the orbital frontal gyri, which, like the cingulate gyri, are represented in earlier mammalian forms such as rodents, are among the last to appear, making it untenable to conclude that the ontogeny of gyral patterns is a replay of vertebrate evolution.

It is noteworthy that perturbations of brain development that occur early in embryogenesis are associated with marked alterations in the normal gyral patterns of human brain. Heschl (1859) was the first to use the term *porencephaly* to describe massive disturbances of gyral formation. Today this term is employed in relation to hemispheric necrosis that arises in utero before the normal adult features of the hemispheres have developed (Barth, 1984; Norman, 1980). Most individuals who have porencephalic lesions have severe retardation and generally show extensive neurological deficits (Dekaban, 1965). As discussed in a following section, the

Table 10.1.   Embryonic development of the cortical gyri in humans

Gestational age (weeks)	Gyrus
16–19	Gyrus rectus, insula, cingulate
20–23	Parahippocampal, superior temporal
24–27	Pre- and post-rolandic, middle temporal, superior and middle frontal, occipital, cuneus, lingual
28–31	Inferior temporal, medial and lateral orbital, callosomarginal, angular, supramarginal, transverse temporal
32–35	Paracentral
36–39	Anterior and posterior orbital

Adapted from Gilles, Shankle, & Dooling (1983).

porencephalies differ dramatically from necrotic lesions induced during the perinatal period, when gyral development is complete.

Cytoarchitectural Maturation of the Cortex

Cortical ontogenesis follows a carefully timed sequence of events (Poliakov, 1965; Sidman & Rakic, 1973). Many cortical neurons are generated along the ventricular surface in the so-called ventricular zone. This area appears early and is increasingly displaced toward the surface as cells undergo several mitotic divisions and give rise to a subplate zone between them. Poliakov (1965) described five stages of cortical development in the human brain that begin with Stage I at approximately the seventh fetal week, when postmitotic cells begin to move upward. Stage V—the longest period, occurring between the 16th fetal week and the early postnatal period—involves the migration of postmitotic neuronal cells to their final destination within the cortical plate. As neurons enter the cortical plate, those destined for more superficial layers arrive later than those that occupy deeper layers and accordingly show an inside-out pattern of migration (Rakic, 1974). Studies in humans have shown that, by 7 months of gestation, Layers V and VI have attained an advanced degree of development as compared with that for Layers II and III (Marin-Padilla, 1970a; Zilles, Busching, & Schleicher, 1986). It is of interest to note that the morphological differentiation of neurons in the various laminae mirrors this migratory process, such that both large pyramidal neurons and basket cells (inhibitory interneurons) with a well-developed dendritic arborization can be distinguished in deeper layers sooner than in superficial layers (Marin-Padilla, 1970b). By 7.5 months in utero, pyramidal neurons in deeper portions of Layer III are first beginning to show an apical dendrite extending into Layer I, whereas in Layers V and VI these cells already have elaborate dendritic arborizations. During this same prenatal interval, many incoming afferent fibers are already discernible in virtually all layers of the cortex. In the months immediately prior to birth, interneurons with a basket cell appearance begin to appear in the deeper portions of Layer III, whereas in Layer II and the outer portions of Layer III they are first beginning to form. By birth, both the second and the third laminae contain pyramidal neurons, but basket cells in Layer II are largely absent (Marin-Padilla, 1970b). By 2½ months postnatally, pyramidal neurons continue to mature and show a dramatic increase in overall size, dendritic branching, and the number of dendritic spines (Michel & Garey, 1984). It is important to emphasize that Layers VI and I (the marginal zone) are the first laminae to appear and differentiate, and Layers II and III are the last to form and the latest to mature (Marin-Padilla, 1970a). At birth, Layer II in the human cortex is still quite immature (Marin-Padilla, 1970b). It is evident from this discussion that extensive and important changes in cortical maturation continue to occur perinatally, and insults during this period can potentially induce perturbations in cortical microcircuitry.

Bayer and Altman (1991) have reported that a similar inside-out progression is observed along the rostral-to-caudal extent of regions of the medial limbic cortex of rodent brain. These cortical areas (see legend to Figure 10.3) are homologous with anterior and posterior portions of the cingulate gyrus in primates and humans (Neafsey et al., 1992). As depicted in Figure 10.3, the timing of cell migration is earlier for the more rostral regions, such as the anterior cingulate cortex, than for more posterior regions, such as the retrosplenial cortex and subiculum (Bayer, 1985). This pattern reflects that described earlier for gyral development (see Table 10.1), wherein the cingulate gyrus differentiates weeks in advance of the parahippocampal gyrus and hippocampal formation, except that, in the latter instance, the progression follows a dorsal-to-ventral course. Nevertheless, this represents another example in which a normal developmental progression proceeds from the mesocortex toward the more primitive archicortex. Postnatally, the anterior cingulate region (medial prefrontal cortex) of the rat shows a progressive expansion of its cortical matrix as the neuropil surrounding neuronal cell bodies increases. As shown in Figure 10.4, this increase of neuropil occurs between postnatal day 10 (P10) and P20 of the preweanling period; this may be attributable in part to the sprouting of axon terminations from extrinsic sources (see later section on dopamine). Such changes, like those for cell migration, may follow an inside-out pattern during the first postnatal week, and it is not until P20 in the rat that this region attains a thickness similar to that of adult animals (Vincent, Pabreza, & Benes, 1995).

Based on a scant amount of data, the packing density of neurons in the human cortex may also decrease dramatically during the first year of life (Blinkov & Glezer, 1968). In the dorsolateral prefrontal cortex (Brodmann's areas 9 and 10), neuronal density may continue to decrease until 5–7 years of age, although, in Layer II of some cortical regions, this process may continue until 12–15 years of age (Blinkov & Glezer, 1968). Such changes are probably reflected in the increasing size of the human brain during the first and second decades of life (Benes, Turtle, Khan, & Farol, 1994). The fact that the neuropil within the human cortex is expanding during much of the first decade opens a broad range of possible disturbances primarily related to axodendritic connectivity in neuropil that could play a role in the onset of psychopathology during childhood. Clearly, such perturbations would be associated with more widespread changes during the first postnatal year than during later intervals, but Layer II could be more vulnerable to such disturbances (Benes, 1995).

Perinatal and Postnatal Injury and Neuropathological Changes in the Cortex

The hallmark of perinatal injury to the cortex is *ulegyria*, a narrowing of gyri at the arterial border zones that involves sclerotic changes occurring preferentially at the depths of the cortical sulci (Friede, 1989). Residual lesions include neuronal loss and gliosis. Such changes are thought to require a coincidence of catastrophic hypotension in the setting of preexisting cerebral edema. As with porencephalic lesions (see previous section), individuals who evidence such changes have severe mental disabilities (Bresler, 1899). Another pathological condition associated with perinatal injury is *pontosubicular necrosis*, in which changes in the nuclear membrane occur in neurons of the subiculum; this may extend into sector CA1, the entorhinal region and, to a lesser extent, the cingulate gyrus (Friede, 1989). Unlike ulegyria, which is associated with prolonged anoxia during early embryogenesis, pontosubicular necrosis is thought to occur in the setting of hyperoxygenation (Ahdab-Barmada, Moossy, Nemoto, & Lin, 1986).

Diffuse cortical sclerosis predominantly affecting only one hemisphere has been associated with postconvulsive–postanoxic changes (Alpers & Dear, 1939) and occurs in individuals who have experienced a disturbance of parturition. There is uniform shrinkage of the gyri and sulci, and the underlying neuronal loss and gliosis occur predominantly in the upper cortical layers (Friede, 1989). This condition is also associated with damage to the CA sectors of the hippocampal formation. In the cortex, normal gyral patterns are present despite there being widespread atrophic

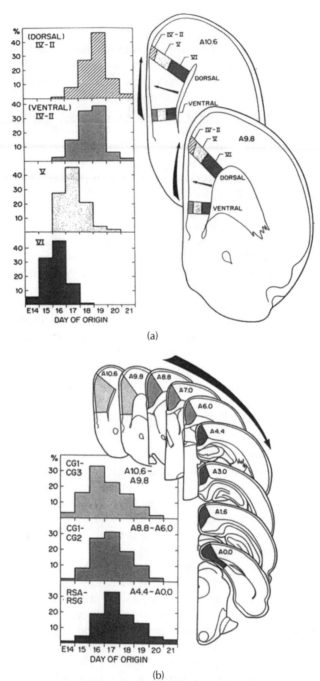

(a)

(b)

Figure 10.3.   The time of origin for neurons in the anterior cingulate areas (medial prefrontal cortex) of rat brain. (a) Neurons along the ventral-to-dorsal extent are generated earliest in the deeper laminae of the anterior cingulate cortex. The superficial layers, however, show a ventral-to-dorsal gradient for the time of origin of their neurons. (b) The time of origin for neurons of medial limbic cortex extending from the anterior cingulate (CG1–CG3) to the posterior (CG1–CG2) and retrosplenial (RSA and RSG) divisions of the region. There is an anterior-to-posterior gradient such that neurons in the anterior cingulate cortex are generated earlier than those in the retrosplenial area and the subicular portion of the hippocampal formation. (From Bayer, S.A., & Altman, I. [1991]. *Neocortical development* [pp. 193, 196]. New York: Raven Press; reprinted by permission.)

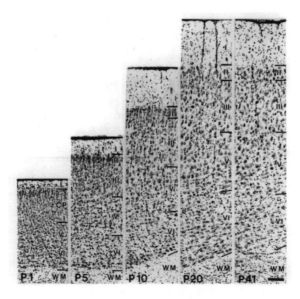

Figure 10.4. Light photomicrographs of Nissl-stained coronal section of rat anterior cingulate cortex (medial prefrontal) are at postnatal days P1, P5, P10, P20, and P41. At P1, the immature cortical plate (CP) lies between Layer I and deeper Layers V and VI. By P5, however, the cortical plate has differentiated into Layers II and III, but the density of cells in these superficial laminae is greater than that observed in the deeper layers. Between P10 and P20, the increased thickness of the cortical mantle is primarily related to the expansion of neuropil in Layers II and III. Overall, between P1 and P20, there is a gradual increase in the thickness of the cortical mantle as the packing density of neuronal cell bodies decreases. At postweanling day P41, there is no further change in the density of neurons. (WM, white matter.) Scale bar equals 100 μm. (From Vincent, S.L., Pabreza, L., & Benes, F.M. [1995]. Postnatal maturation of GABA-immunoreactive neurons of rat medial prefrontal cortex. *Journal of Comparative Neurology, 355,* 84; reprinted by permission.)

changes. Microscopically, large pyramidal cells show the greatest resistance to damage and, in severe cases, may be the only neuronal cells remaining. Layers II–IV, for the most part, show depletion of neurons, whereas the deeper laminae are usually spared (Bielschowsky, 1918; Spielmeyer, 1906). Neurological defects and seizure disorders generally are present after the initial injury at birth and may reflect a widespread occurrence of pathological changes in the basal ganglia, thalamus, pons, and subiculum (Friede, 1989).

Ingrowth of Cortical and Thalamic Afferent Inputs into the Cortex

During embryogenesis, afferent fibers from the thalamus grow toward the cortical mantle and either stop immediately beneath it or immediately begin to penetrate toward Layer IV (Wise & Jones, 1978). In rodents, the ingrowth of thalamocortical fibers is not complete until the third postnatal day, whereas commissural fibers only begin to enter the homologous cortex by Postnatal Day 5 (P5) and do not attain a mature pattern of connectivity until Postnatal Day 7 (P7) (Wise & Jones, 1978).

Generally speaking, afferent fibers seem to be present in the cortex before a mature dendritic tree is in evidence, and the formation of dendritic spines may be regulated, at least in part, by various afferent inputs (Wise, Fleshman, & Jones, 1979). The changes that occur in rat brain during Postnatal Week 1 are considered to be analogous to those that occur in primates during the prenatal period. Consistent with this, commissural fibers arising from the principal sulcus of monkey brain penetrate into the homologous cortical region of the opposite hemisphere during the late embryonic period (Goldman-Rakic, 1981).

The importance of ingrowing cortical afferents engaging in abnormal patterns of connectivity was underscored by a significant set of experiments in which the intended termination site for commissural afferents originating in the principal sulcus was extirpated (Goldman-Rakic, 1981). Under these experimental conditions, commissural fibers from the principal sulcus can alter their normal course and penetrate into a nonhomologous cortical region (Goldman-Rakic, 1981). This experiment has provided a theoretical basis for understanding how perturbations of normal brain development could result in faulty wiring patterns. It is not certain for how long during the postnatal period commissural and associative fibers can continue to form connections in primate or human brains; however, it seems plausible that the functional and perhaps even structural plasticity of such connections could persist throughout the first decade of life and possibly longer.

Based on the previous discussion, it seems reasonable to speculate that the onset of psychopathological states at a given stage of postnatal life could be related to a disturbance in the establishment of normal connectivity within certain key corticolimbic regions. Although the density of synapses seems to change in a synchronous fashion throughout the cortex of primate brain (Rakic, Bourgeois, Eckenhoff, Zecevic, & Goldman-Rakic, 1986), such synchrony does not appear to occur in human cortex (Huttenlocher, 1994). This discrepancy between findings in primate and human cortex is discussed at length in Chapters 2 and 3. It is noteworthy that there are marked differences in the time course for the maturation of specific neurotransmitter systems that must also be considered in defining critical stages of postnatal development (see following section).

Myelination of Corticolimbic Pathways

A broadly accepted marker for the functional maturation of the central nervous system is the formation of myelin sheaths around axon shafts. For some time, it has been known that various neural pathways myelinate at different stages of pre- and postnatal development; for humans, this process has long been thought to continue well after birth (Flechsig, 1920; Yakovlev & LeCours, 1967). There is a general tendency for more cephalad structures to myelinate later than those found at more caudal levels of the neuraxis and for subcortical pathways to myelinate before cortical associational paths (Yakovlev & LeCours, 1967). For example, the medial longitudinal fasciculus, a pathway that is found along the entire extent of the spinal cord and brainstem, begins myelinating at spinal levels as early as Week 20 of the gestational period, whereas the medial lemniscus, a pathway found principally in the brain stem, shows similar changes at Gestational Week 24 (Gilles et al., 1983). Within the cerebral hemispheres, the posterior limb of the internal capsule begins myelinating at Gestational Week 32, whereas the anterior limb does not show evidence of myelin formation until Week 38. Interestingly, proximal portions of the cingulum bundle do not begin to myelinate until Gestational Weeks 38–39 (Gilles et al., 1983). In comparison, some subcortical relays, such as the fornix and mammilothalamic tract, do not begin to myelinate until Weeks 44 and 48, respectively. Because the mammilothalamic tract conveys information from the mammillary body to the anterior nucleus of the thalamus, while the fornix provides an efferent outflow from the hippocampal formation to the mammillary body, these observations suggest that, at least in some cases, the time sequence for myelination of different pathways does not proceed in a direction similar to that followed during phylogenetic development. In fact, both the fornix and the mammilothalamic tract, subcortical components of the loop of Papez, myelinate 1–2 months *after* the cingulum bundle, a fiber bundle that predominantly carries associative information between the mesocortex and the archicortex. These findings clearly indicate that the progression of myelination within the corticolimbic system does not parallel the phylogenetic development of this system.

Some pathways within the corticolimbic system continue to myelinate until much later during the postnatal period (Benes, 1989; Benes et al., 1994). As demonstrated in Figure 10.5, the superior medullary lamina of the parahippocampal gyrus shows an increase of myelin staining not only during the first and second decades of life (Benes, 1989) but even during adulthood. The medial part of the superior medullary lamina, which contains fibers of the perforant pathway, is actively myelinating from birth through the first decade (Benes et al., 1994). The lateral portions of the superior medullary lamina, containing the distal portions of the cingulum bundle (Benes, 1989), seem to myelinate during the second decade and perhaps even as late as the sixth decade of postnatal life (Figure 10.6). Even though proximal portions of the cingulum bundle begin myelinating quite early (see previous discussion), the distal portions located within the parahippocampal gyrus may show a considerable delay in completing this process.

The increased myelination in the superior medullary lamina that occurs well into the postnatal period is noteworthy for two reasons. The observation of late myelination of the superior medullary lamina may present an unexpected paradox regarding human development. As proposed by Yakovlev and LeCours (1967), it has been generally held that late postnatal myelination probably occurs last in the phylogenetically most sophisticated associative neocortices, such as the prefrontal area, because this would reflect the very general tendency for brain development to parallel phylogeny. This latter idea would have been correct if the associative cortical areas showing these late postnatal changes were of the neocortical type. Instead, the area implicated in this late myelination (i.e., the cingulate cortex) is a mesocortical transitional type. Even worse, the fibers showing these changes, rather than projecting "upward" toward neocortex, may well be sending fibers downward toward even more primitive allocortex! The possibility that myelination in the cingulum bundle progresses in a *counterevolutionary* fashion is similar to the pattern described previously for gyral maturation (Gilles et al., 1983) and neuronal migration (Bayer & Altman, 1991) in the cingulate region.

With respect to childhood and adolescent psychopathology, increased myelination of two key corticolimbic links could theoretically play a direct or indirect role in the onset of symptoms during critical stages of postnatal life. Although this was originally proposed for schizophrenia (Benes, 1989; Benes et al., 1994), this idea is also tenable for childhood psychopathology because the pathways showing these

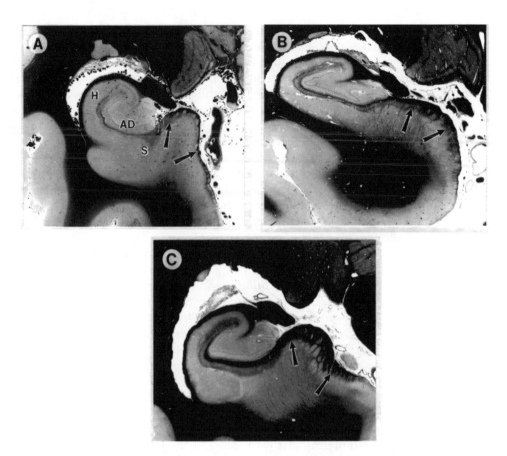

Figure 10.5.   Weigert-stained sections of the hippocampal formation from normal human brains of a 6½-year-old (A), a 17-year-old (B), and a 35-year-old (C). The area dentata (AD), hippocampus proper (H), and subiculum–presubiculum (S) are present in each of the cross-sectional profiles. Along the surface of the subiculum–presubiculum and extending along the parahippocampal gyrus lies a region called the superior medullary lamina that contains an abundance of black-staining myelin sheath material (arrows). Medially, this zone contains fibers of the perforant path; in more lateral locations, it contains distal portions of the cingulum bundle. The amount of Weigert-stained myelin material shows a progressive increase between the first and second decades of life and again later during advanced adulthood. (Adapted from Benes [1989].)

changes—the perforant path and the cingulum bundle, during the first and second decades, respectively—are likely involved in the integration of emotional experience with higher cognitive functions.

DEVELOPMENTAL CHANGES IN NEUROTRANSMITTER SYSTEMS

The functional maturation of the central nervous system must involve obligatory changes in the various neurotransmitter systems that mediate neural activity. The discussion that follows considers developmental changes of intrinsic and extrinsic cortical neurotransmitters. Although it is true that the specific timing of developmental changes in the central nervous system can vary considerably from one species to another, there are nevertheless some general principles that have been learned from studies of rodent and, to a lesser extent, primate brains regarding the possible sequence of changes that may occur in the human brain. For the purpose of the following discussion, it is useful to point out that the equivalent of adolescence

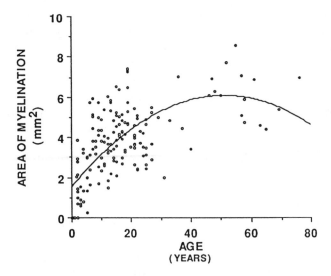

Figure 10.6.   A scatterplot graph for the area of myelination of the superior medullary lamina at different postnatal ages for human subjects. The area of myelination shows a curvilinear increase during the first 2 decades of life, but this pattern seems to continue perhaps even until the sixth decade. Using a second-order polynomial equation, the regression coefficient (r) was found to be .667. (Adapted from Benes, Turtle, Khan, & Farol [1994].)

for rats occurs roughly between Postnatal Weeks 4 and 8; by Postnatal Week 9 (P60), rats are considered to be adults. Where available, studies in the developing human brain are also described.

Intrinsic Neurotransmitters

Excitatory Cortical Transmitters   The amino acid glutamate and the closely related compound aspartate are generally considered to be the transmitters employed by pyramidal neurons of the cortex that project to both cortical and subcortical locations (Streit, 1984). Available evidence suggests that the time course for the maturation of various glutamatergic pathways may be different. For example, the corticocortical projections originating in the visual cortex of rat brain attain mature levels of glutamate *before* their corticostriatal counterparts projecting to the caudate nucleus (Johnston, 1988), another example of developmental changes occurring in a descending direction. Similarly, in the visual cortex and in the lateral geniculate nucleus, glutamate reuptake attains adult levels by P15 and P20, respectively (Kvale, Fosse, & Fonnum, 1983). Between P10 and P15, high-affinity glutamate receptor binding activity increases by 30% and is 10 times higher than it will eventually be during adulthood (Schliebs, Kullman, & Bigl, 1986). In the hippocampus, glutamate receptor binding increases up to P23 (Baudry, Arst, Oliver, & Lynch, 1981), possibly reflecting the persistence of long-term potentiation as an important component of mechanisms related to learning and memory (Johnston, 1988). The functional importance of such changes is underscored by the fact that rats monocularly deprived of visual input show a reduction of glutamate binding in the lateral geniculate nucleus, but not the visual cortex, that persists into adulthood (Schliebs et al., 1986).

Inhibitory Cortical Transmitters   γ-Aminobutyric acid (GABA) has long been considered the most important inhibitory neurotransmitter in the mammalian brain, particularly in humans. Generally speaking, the activity of the GABA reuptake mechanism seems to increase before the activity of glutamic acid decarboxylase (GAD) shows appreciable increments (Coyle & Enna, 1976). At birth, the concentration of GABA is 50% of adult levels, which are not attained until the second postnatal week. In a manner similar to cell bodies in general (Figure 10.5), the number of GABA-immunoreactive (GABA-IR) neurons present in the medial prefrontal cortex of the rat brain reaches a peak density at approximately P5 (Figure 10.7) but thereafter decreases sharply through P10–P20 as the surrounding neuropil expands (Vincent et al., 1995). GABA-IR terminals surrounding pyramidal cell bodies show a marked increase in number between P7 and P12 for the deeper layers of this region (Figure 10.8). An inside-out progression is followed as the GABA-IR terminals associated with pyramidal cells continue to increase in number in superficial laminae until the third postnatal week (Vincent et al., 1995). Similarly, the specific activity of GAD is negligible at birth, but adult levels are also attained by the third postnatal week (Johnston & Coyle, 1980).

GABA and benzodiazepine receptor binding activities do not show appreciable increases during the first postnatal week but thereafter show a sharp rise during the second week and an additional 15% increment between the second and seventh weeks (Candy & Martin, 1979). In contrast, the reuptake mechanism for GABA plateaus by the second postnatal week; but later, in the seventh week, it decreases. In the human brain, GABA receptor binding activity shows a fivefold increase during the perinatal period (Brooksbank, Atkinson, & Balasz, 1981; Diebler, Farkas-Bargeton, & Wehrle, 1979) and an additional 100% increase for several weeks thereafter (Brooksbank et al., 1981). Functional inputs are thought to regulate the maturation of the GABA system because, in the cat visual cortex, dark-rearing from birth through the sixth postnatal week results in an attenuation of GAD levels (Fosse, Heggelund, & Fonnu, 1989).

In the hippocampal formation, GABAergic neurons become postmitotic and begin migrating on Embryonic Day 14 (Amaral & Kurz, 1985; Lubbers, Wolff, &

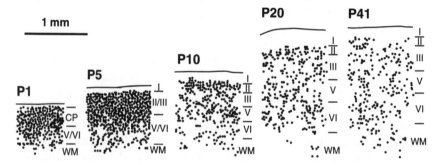

Figure 10.7.   Spatial distribution of GABA-immunoreactive (GABA-IR) cell bodies in the anterior cingulate cortex (medial prefrontal area) of rat brain at different postnatal ages. At P1, GABA-IR neurons are densely distributed through the cortical matrix, even within the cortical plate (CP). By P5, the density of GABA cells has begun to decrease in the deeper laminae as the neuropil is expanding and, by P10, it has also decreased more superficially, although Layer II still contains a relatively high density. By P20, when the thickness of the cortical mantle is equivalent to that seen in adult animals, the density of GABA-IR cell bodies has decreased throughout the cortical mantle. There are no further changes during the postweanling period (P41) and beyond. (WM, white matter.) Scale bar = 1 mm. (From Vincent, S.L., Pabreza, L., & Benes, F.M. [1995]. Postnatal maturation of GABA-immunoreactive neurons of rat medial prefrontal cortex. *Journal of Comparative Neurology, 355,* 86; reprinted by permission.)

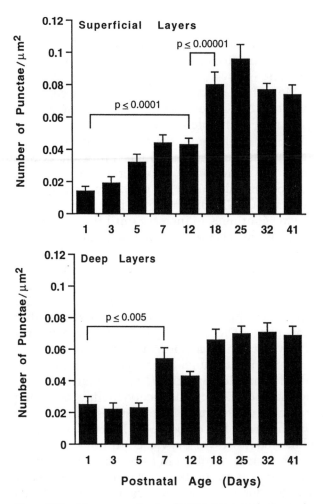

Figure 10.8.   The average density of GABA-IR terminals surrounding pyramidal neuron cell bodies in the anterior cingulate (medial prefrontal) cortex of rat brain at different postnatal ages. In the deep layers of this region (bottom), GABA-IR terminals show a sharp increase between P5 and P7 but show little change thereafter. In the superficial layers (top), however, the density of GABA-IR terminals on pyramidal neurons shows a gradual increase until P7 and later, between P12 and P18, shows a marked incremental change. The brackets connecting bars indicate that the differences observed are significant; the p values show the level at which the null hypothesis is rejected. (From Vincent, S.L., Pabreza, L., & Benes, F.M. [1995]. Postnatal maturation of GABA-immunoreactive neurons of rat medial prefrontal cortex. *Journal of Comparative Neurology, 355*, 89; reprinted by permission.)

Frotscher, 1985). Unlike the cortex, where pyramidal cells differentiate before basket cells (Marin-Padilla, 1970b), the peak of neurogenesis for GABAergic cells of the hippocampus occurs before that of other non-GABAergic neurons (Soriano, Cobas, & Fairen, 1986). GABA cell bodies are detectable as early as the third postnatal day (Rozenberg, Robain, Jardin, & Ben-Ari, 1989) but do not achieve adult levels until Postnatal Day 18 (P18) (Seress & Ribak, 1988).

Extrinsic Neurotransmitters

There are four key extrinsic neurotransmitter systems that project into the neocortex: acetylcholine, norepinephrine, serotonin, and dopamine. The postnatal development of these four afferent systems is discussed in this section.

Acetylcholine   Most of the acetylcholine found in the cortex is derived from the basal forebrain (Johnston, McKinney, & Coyle, 1979), where the nucleus basalis of Meynert gives rise to the principle cholinergic projections (Mesulam, Mufson, Levey, & Wainer, 1983). A small amount of acetylcholine may be synthesized by intrinsic cholinergic neurons (Levey, Wainer, Raye, Mufson, & Mesulam, 1984). Although the neuronal cell bodies of the cholinergic system are generated early in gestation (Bayer, 1985), they do not begin to accumulate appreciable amounts of choline acetyltransferase (ChAT) until after the first postnatal week. Thereafter the activity of this enzyme continues to increase until the sixth postnatal week (Johnston & Coyle, 1980), and this occurs in parallel with increases of muscarinic receptor binding (Coyle & Yamamura, 1976).

Not surprisingly, the ingrowth of cholinergic fibers into the cortex occurs first in the deeper layers and later in the superficial layers. In the human brain, cholinergic fibers have been observed to enter the cortex as early as Gestational Weeks 12–22 (Candy et al., 1985); however, ChAT does not attain adult levels until approximately 10 years of age (Diebler et al., 1979). In sharp contrast, muscarinic receptor binding activity in the human cortex is highest at birth and progressively diminishes during the second through sixth decades of life and possibly longer, perhaps as a result of synaptic "pruning" (Ravikumar & Sastary, 1985). Acetylcholinesterase, the enzyme that degrades acetylcholine, is found principally in interneurons in the human cortex during the first postnatal week but later shows a progressive increase in pyramidal cell bodies of Layer III, where it reaches peak levels during early adulthood (Kostovic, Skavic, & Strinovic, 1988). Because upper cortical layers are predominantly involved in associative connectivity, these latter increases of ChAT could reflect maturational changes in cognitive activity.

Norepinephrine   Noradrenergic cell bodies found in the locus ceruleus (Levitt & Moore, 1978; Lindvall, Bjorklund, & Divac, 1978) undergo their last mitotic division in a rat brain at Gestational Days 12–14 (Lauder & Bloom, 1974) and in a monkey brain at Gestational Days 27–36 (Levitt & Rakic, 1982). By birth, there is a rather extensive network of noradrenergic fibers in a rat cortex that is considerably more dense than that seen in adult animals (Coyle & Molliver, 1977). The level of tyrosine hydroxylase, the enzyme involved in the synthesis of norepinephrine and dopamine, increases steadily in the rat cortex between the first and seventh postnatal weeks (Johnston & Coyle, 1980). The level of the β-adrenergic receptor, in contrast, increases sharply between the first and second postnatal weeks before plateauing (Harden, Wolfe, Sporn, Perkins, & Molinoff, 1977). Studies in the cat have suggested that norepinephrine may play a key role in the plasticity of synaptic connections (Kasamatsu & Pettigrew, 1976). Following monocular visual deprivation, cats depleted of norepinephrine (Kasamatsu & Pettigrew, 1976) or given clonidine, a drug that inhibits the release of this transmitter (Nelson, Schwartz, & Daniels, 1975), fail to convert binocularly driven neurons to a monocularly driven pattern.

Serotonin   The timing of developmental changes in the serotonin (5-hydroxytryptamine, or 5-HT) system is similar to that observed for the noradrenergic system (Hamon & Bourgoin, 1977; Hedner & Lundberg, 1980). Serotonin-containing neurons of the raphe nuclei in the rat brain (Descarries, Beaudet, & Watkins, 1975) are first visualized between Gestational Days 13 and 17, when some of their axons have already grown toward the pyriform cortex (Wallace & Lauder, 1983). As seen with other transmitter systems in the rat brain (see next section on dopamine), 5-HT levels increase steadily between birth and the fourth postnatal week (Johnston, 1988). The synthesizing enzyme for 5-HT, tryptophan hydroxylase, is 10% of adult levels by birth, but rises to adult levels by Postnatal Day 30 (P30) (Deguchi & Barchas, 1972). During the perinatal period, high-affinity 5-HT receptor binding activity is approximately one third of that seen in adults; it does not attain adult levels until the sixth postnatal week (Uphouse & Bondy, 1981). In primates, 5-HT fibers in the cortex establish an adult pattern by Postnatal Week 6, whereas the levels of 5-HT continue to increase for an additional 2–3 weeks (Goldman-Rakic & Brown, 1982). In the human cortex, however, the density of 5-HT_2 binding sites shows a linear decline between 17 and 100 years of age; in the hippocampus, a similar but less striking change in this receptor also occurs (Marcusson, Morgan, Winblad, & Finch, 1984).

It has been suggested that timing for the ingrowth of serotonergic fibers may vary according to the degree of maturity for intrinsic circuits within a given region (Lidov & Molliver, 1982). Interestingly, at birth, the serotonin projection to the sensory cortex is found within Layers IV and VI, the two laminae predominantly involved in receiving thalamic afferents. Because the arrival of serotonin fibers precedes that of the thalamocortical afferents (Wise & Jones, 1978), it has been suggested that the serotonergic innervation to the cortex may provide a trophic influence on ingrowth of thalamic fibers, on their target neurons, or on both (D'Amato et al.,1987).

Dopamine   Dopamine cells in the ventral tegmental area and substantia nigra of the rat brain (Berger, Tassin, Blanc, Moyne, & Thierry, 1974; Thierry, Blanc, Sobel, Stinus, & Glowinski, 1973) begin to differentiate on Embryonic Day 11 (E11) and continue this process through E15 (Lauder & Bloom, 1974). Afferent dopamine fibers first arrive near the frontal cortex as early as E16 (Verney, Berger, Vigny, & Gay, 1982); however, by birth, these axons begin to penetrate into the cortical mantle and establish an abundant innervation by Postnatal Week 2 for the frontal area and Postnatal Week 3 for the cingulate region (Berger & Verney, 1984). Dopamine afferents to the prefrontal region also follow the typical inside-out progression seen for cholinergic inputs (see earlier discussion), entering the infragranular layers first and the supragranular layers last (Kalsbeek, Voorn, Buijs, Pool, & Uylings, 1988), but a full distribution of dopamine fibers is not established until adulthood (Kalsbeek et al., 1988; Verney et al., 1982). Dopamine concentrations also rise steadily until adulthood (Johnston, 1988). Dopamine receptors, in contrast, are expressed in the cortex before birth but continue to increase toward adult levels through Postnatal Day 31 (Bruinink, Lichtensteiner, & Schlumpf, 1983; Deskin, Seidler, Whitmore, & Slotkin, 1981).

Developmental Similarities Among Transmitter Systems

Some general principles concerning the development of neurotransmitter systems can be derived from the previous discussion. First, the progenitor cells responsible for the elaboration of both intrinsic and extrinsic transmitter systems in the cortex become postmitotic long before their respective neurotransmitter phenotype is expressed (Schwartz & Meinecke, 1992; Vaccarino, Schwartz, Hartigan, & Leckman, 1995). Second, at birth, virtually all neurotransmitter systems are present in the cortex, but none is yet fully matured. Third, the postnatal maturation of most transmitter systems continues beyond the weaning period and overlaps with the postweanling period, during which important changes in gonadal maturation are also occurring. Although there is a dearth of detailed information concerning the ontogenesis of transmitter systems in the cortex of the human brain, available evidence suggests that the postnatal maturation of both the cholinergic and serotonergic systems may continue throughout childhood and adolescence; in some cases, this process may persist throughout the life span of the normal individual.

Developmental Interactions Between Intrinsic and Extrinsic Cortical Transmitters

It is evident from the previous discussion that the postnatal maturation of both intrinsic and extrinsic neurotransmitter systems is extensive. At this juncture, a reasonable question to ask is whether these progressive postnatal changes may involve an increase in the degree to which some or all of these transmitter systems are interacting with one another. As shown in Figure 10.9, a 1993 study suggested that dopaminergic afferents form frequent, nonrandom appositions with both pyramidal cells and interneurons in the medial prefrontal cortex of the adult rat (Benes, Vincent, & Molloy, 1993) that progressively increase between birth and the onset of adulthood (Benes, Vincent, & Molloy, 1996). When the frequency of these contacts on nonpyramidal neurons is compared for preweanling and postweanling rats, there is a fourfold increase on nonpyramidal neurons (Figure 10.10) and pyramidal cells (not shown) in Layer VI of rat medial prefrontal cortex. In Layer II of this region, there is an eightfold increase on nonpyramidal cells during the postweanling period but no change on pyramidal cells (not shown). These findings suggest that 1) meaningful increases in the interaction of one transmitter compartment (e.g., a varicosity) with another (e.g., a cell body) probably do occur to a significant degree during the late postnatal period; 2) such changes may vary in magnitude according to cortical layer; and 3) changes of this type may occur differentially for one neuronal cell type versus another within a given cortical layer. In other words, postnatal maturational changes in the cortical neurotransmitter system may be far more complex than was heretofore suspected, and, to fully understand the implications of postnatal ontogeny, a clear delineation of how changes for a given transmitter may be reflected in alterations of specific synaptic connectivity is needed.

Critical Stages for the Development of Psychopathology

It has been recognized for some time that various mental disorders of childhood and adolescence tend to appear during certain stages of postnatal development but not others (Table 10.2). This observation suggests that normal ontogenetic changes during the early and later postnatal period could theoretically play a role in the appearance of symptoms in these various disorders (Benes, 1988, 1989; Benes et al., 1994). The nature of these putative ontogenetic changes is, at present, not well understood. As discussed previously, a variety of changes, including the elaboration of intrinsic and extrinsic connections, the myelination of key corticolimbic association paths, the maturation of specific neurotransmitter systems, and the interaction of one transmitter system with another within a given region, could all potentially contribute to the onset of a psychiatric disorder. For example, it has been suggested that myelination of the cingulum bundle (Benes et al., 1994) or perhaps even increases in the interaction of dopaminergic fibers with an impaired population of GABAergic interneurons (Benes et al., 1996) could serve as the putative trigger for the onset of symptoms during late adolescence (Benes, 1995). Corresponding

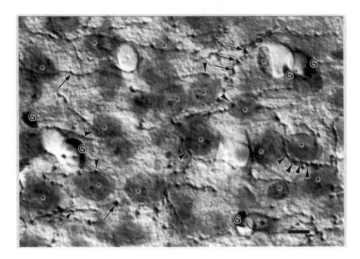

Figure 10.9.   A section of the medial prefrontal cortex from a postwean-ling rat showing dopamine-immunoreactive fibers and cresyl violet–stained neuronal cell bodies (asterisks). There are many immunoreactive varicose fibers that are coursing through the neuropil (arrows) and form-ing frequent appositions with neuronal cell bodies →. In some cases, sev-eral dopamine-containing varicosities appear to form contacts with the same neuron. Scale bar equals 10 μm.

mechanisms for the induction of childhood psychiatric disorders seem even more likely because the overall growth and maturation of the brain is much more marked during this period.

CONCLUSIONS

A neurodevelopmental approach to the study of mental illness will require that we obtain a clear understanding of how various neurotransmitter systems may be un-dergoing normal ontogenetic changes during the critical stages identified for each illness. The glutamate and GABA systems both show extensive postnatal matura-tion up to and, in some cases, including adulthood. Similarly, the dopamine system also undergoes important postnatal maturation, making it essential to know the extent to which each extrinsic transmitter system is interacting with other intrin-sic cortical elements. Each psychiatric disorder encountered in childhood and ado-lescence could conceivably involve a specific interaction of two neurotransmitter systems within key corticolimbic brain regions, such as the prefrontal area or the anterior cingulate region. Indeed, such interactions for axosomatic, axodendritic, and axoaxonic synapses between the same two transmitters may occur at different postnatal stages. The specific time course for the development of these various synaptic and junctional interactions could theoretically dictate the period during which a given illness presents. The degree to which such interactions may increase (or perhaps decrease) during postnatal life could play a role in the etiology or treat-ment response of a particular disorder at different stages of the illness, or both.

It now seems evident that our understanding of the pathophysiology of child-hood and adolescent psychopathology will have to take into account a complex in-terplay between normal developmental changes in corticolimbic regions, such as the dorsolateral prefrontal area, the anterior cingulate region, and the hippocampal

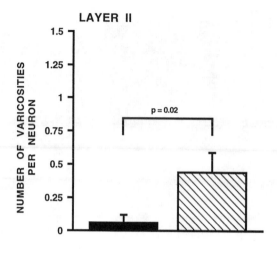

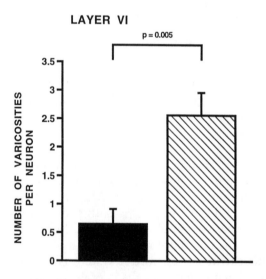

Figure 10.10.   A comparison of the number of dopamine-immunoreactive varicosities forming contacts with cell bodies of nonpyramidal neurons in Layers II (top) and VI (bottom) of rat medial prefrontal cortex from pre- and postweanling rats. During the postweanling period, nonpyramidal cells in Layer II show a fourfold increase in the number of dopamine varicosities that are in apposition with their cell bodies, whereas in Layer II there is an eightfold increase. (■, preweanling rat; ◹, postweanling rat.)

formation, and the various risk factors for these illnesses. On the one hand, it is likely that a genetic factor, an acquired insult to the brain, or both can alter the normal development of these regions, perhaps focally or perhaps even in a generalized way. On the other hand, once one of these corticolimbic regions in an individual who is at risk for a mental illness has been affected by genetic or environmental risk factors, normal ontogenetic changes, such as myelination of a key corticolimbic relay or the interaction of two important transmitter systems, may trigger the expression of the illness during critical periods of postnatal life. The inherited risk

Table 10.2. Age of onset for psychiatric disorders of childhood and adolescence

Diagnostic category	Age of onset
Autism	2–3 years
Attention-deficit/hyperactivity disorder	3 years
Separation anxiety	5–6 years
Conduct disorder	
Undersocialized type	Prepuberty
Socialized type	Postpuberty
Oppositional disorder	Late childhood–adolescence
Anorexia nervosa	Early–late adolescence
Identity disorder	Late adolescence

Source: Data from American Psychiatric Association (1994).

factor for affective disorder is probably different from that for autism or attention deficit disorder, and the types of environmental factors that influence the expression of other illnesses, such as separation anxiety and conduct disorder, may also be different.

In applying a neurodevelopmental approach to the study of childhood psychopathology, it is necessary to 1) define the unique neurobiological consequences of abnormal genes, environmental factors, or both for each of these illnesses; 2) determine how these factors alter neural circuits within the corticolimbic system; and 3) understand how these latter changes interact with other normal ontogenetic events occurring during critical periods when such an illness is apt to become manifest. The question is no longer whether postnatal ontogeny plays a role in the development of psychopathology but rather what are the changes for the various psychiatric disorders, what are the regions in which they are occurring, how do they have an impact on preexisting circuitry, and how can normal ontogeny trigger the appearance of symptoms in children who are at risk for a particular psychopathologic state?

REFERENCES

Ahdab-Barmada, M., Moossy, J., Nemoto, E.M., & Lin, M.R. (1986). Hyperoxia produces neuronal necrosis in the rat. *Journal of Neuropathology and Experimental Neurology, 45,* 233–246.

Alpers, B.J., & Dear, R.B. (1939). Hemiatrophy of the brain. *Journal of Nervous and Mental Disease, 89,* 653–671.

Amaral, D.G., & Kurz, J. (1985). The time of origin of cells demonstrating glutamic acid decarboxylase-like immunoreactivity in the hippocampal formation of the rat. *Neuroscience Letters, 59,* 33–39.

American Psychiatric Association. (1994). *Diagnostic and statistical manual of mental disorders* (4th ed.). Washington, DC: Author.

Anand, B.K., & Dua, S. (1956). Circulatory and respiratory changes induced by electrical stimulation of the limbic system (visceral brain). *Journal of Neurophysiology, 19,* 393–400.

Barris, R.W., & Schumann, H.R. (1953). Bilateral anterior cingulate gyrus lesions: Syndrome of the anterior cingulate gyri. *Journal of Neurology, 3,* 44–52.

Barth, P.G. (1984). Prenatal clastic encephalopathies. *Clinical Neurology and Neurosurgery, 86,* 65–75.

Baudry, M., Arst, D., Oliver, M., & Lynch, G. (1981). Development of glutamate binding sites and their regulation by calcium in rat hippocampus. *Developmental Brain Research, 1,* 37–38.

Bayer, S.A. (1985). Neurogenesis of the magnocellular basal telencephalic nuclei in the rat. *International Journal of Developmental Neuroscience, 3*, 229–243.

Bayer, S.A., & Altman, I. (1991). *Neocortical development.* New York: Raven Press.

Beckstead, R.M. (1979). An autoradiographic examination of cortico-cortical and subcortical projections of the mediodorsal-projection (prefrontal) cortex in the rat. *Journal of Comparative Neurology, 184*, 43–62.

Belaydier, C., & Maugierre, F. (1980). The duality of the cingulate gyrus in monkey: Neuroanatomical study and functional hypothesis. *Brain, 130*, 525–554.

Benes, F.M. (1988). Post-mortem structural analyses of schizophrenic brain: Study designs and the interpretation of data. *Psychiatric Developments, 6*, 213–226.

Benes, F.M. (1989). Myelination of cortical-hippocampal relays during late adolescence: Anatomical correlates to the onset of schizophrenia. *Schizophrenia Bulletin, 15*, 585–594.

Benes, F.M. (1993). Relationship of cingulate cortex to schizophrenia. In B.A. Vogt & M. Gabriel (Eds.), *The neurobiology of cingulate cortex and limbic thalamus* (pp. 581–605). Boston: Birkhauser.

Benes, F.M. (1995). Is there a neuroanatomic basis for schizophrenia? *Neuroscientist, 1*(2), 112–120.

Benes, F.M., Turtle, M., Khan, Y., & Farol, P. (1994). Myelination of a key relay zone in the hippocampal formation occurs in the human brain during childhood, adolescence, and adulthood. *Archives of General Psychiatry, 51*, 477–484.

Benes, F.M., Vincent, S.L., & Molloy, R. (1993). Dopamine-immunoreactive varicosities form non-random contacts with GABA-containing cell bodies. *Synapse, 15*, 285–295.

Benes, F.M., Vincent, S.L., & Molloy, R. (1996). Increased interaction of dopamine-immunoreactive varicosities with GABA cells of rat medial prefrontal cortex occurs during the postweanling period. *Synapse, 23*, 237–245.

Berger, B., Tassin, J.P., Blanc, G., Moyne, M.A., & Thierry, A.M. (1974). Histochemical confirmation for dopaminergic innervation of rat cerebral cortex after the destruction of noradrenergic ascending pathways. *Brain Research, 81*, 332–337.

Berger, B., & Verney, C. (1984). Development of the catecholamine innervation in rat neocortex: Morphological features. In L. Descarries, T.R. Reader, & H.H. Jasper (Eds.), *Monoamine innervation of cerebral cortex* (pp. 95–121). New York: Alan R. Liss.

Bielschowsky, M. (1918). Über Hemiplegie bie intakter Pyramidenbahn. *Journal of Psychology and Neurology (Leipzig), 22, Ergänzungsheft*(1), 225–266.

Blinkov, S.M., & Glezer, I.I. (1968). *The human brain in figures and tables: A quantitative handbook* (pp. 123–126). New York: Plenum.

Bresler, Dr. (1899). Klinische und pathologische-anatomische Beitrage zur Mikrogyrie. *Archiv für Psychiatrie und Nervenkraft, 31*, 566–573.

Broca, P. (1878). Anatomie comparée des circonvolutions cérébrales: Le grand lobe limbique et la scissure limbique dans la série des mammifères. *Revue d'Anthropologie, 1*, 385–498.

Brooksbank, B.W.L., Atkinson, D.J., & Balasz, R. (1981). Biochemical development of the human brain. II. Some parameters of the GABAergic system. *Developmental Neuroscience, 1*, 267–284.

Bruinink, A., Lichtensteiner, W., & Schlumpf, M. (1983). Pre- and postnatal ontogeny and characterization of dopaminergic D2, serotonergic S2, and spirodecanone binding sites in rat forebrain. *Journal of Neurochemistry, 40*, 1227–1237.

Candy, J.M., Bloxham, C.A., Thompson, J., Johnson, M., Oakley, A.E., & Edwardson, J.A. (1985). Evidence for the early prenatal development of cortical cholinergic afferents from the nucleus of Meynert in the human fetus. *Neuroscience Letters, 61*, 91–95.

Candy, J.M., & Martin, I.L. (1979). The postnatal development of the benzodiazepine receptor in the cerebral cortex and cerebellum of the rat. *Journal of Neurochemistry, 32*, 655–658.

Coyle, J.T., & Enna, S. (1976). Neurochemical aspects of the ontogenesis of GABAergic neurons in the rat brain. *Brain Research, 111*, 119–133.

Coyle, J.T., & Molliver, M. (1977). Major innervation of newborn rat cortex by monoaminergic neurons. *Science, 196*, 444–447.

Coyle, J.T., & Yamamura, H.I. (1976). Neurochemical aspects of the ontogenesis of GABAergic neurons in the rat brain. *Brain Research, 118*, 429–440.

Damasio, A.R., & Van Hoesen, G.W. (1983). Emotional disturbances associated with focal lesions of the limbic frontal lobe. In K.M. Heilman & P. Satz (Eds.), *Neuropsychology of human emotion* (pp. 85–110). New York: Guilford Press.

D'Amato, R.J., Blue, M., Largent, B., Lynch, D., Leobetter, D., Molliver, M., & Snyder, S. (1987). Ontogeny of the serotonergic projection of rat neocortex: Transient expression of a dense innervation of primary sensory areas. *Proceedings of the National Academy of Sciences of the United States of America, 84*, 4322–4326.

Deguchi, T., & Barchas, J. (1972). Regional distribution and developmental change in tryptophan hydroxylase in rat brain. *Journal of Neurochemistry, 19*, 927–929.

Dekaban, A. (1965). Large defects in cerebral hemispheres associated with cortical dysgenesis. *Journal of Neuropathology and Experimental Neurology, 24*, 512–530.

Descarries, L., Beaudet, A., & Watkins, K.C. (1975). Serotonin nerve terminals in adult rat neocortex. *Brain Research, 100*, 563–588.

Deskin, R., Seidler, F.J., Whitmore, W.L., & Slotkin, T.A. (1981). Development of noradrenergic and dopaminergic receptor systems depends on maturation of their presynaptic nerve terminals in the rat brain. *Journal of Neurochemistry, 36*, 1683–1690.

Devinsky, O., & Luciano, D. (1992). The contribution of cingulate cortex to human behavior. In B.A. Vogt & M. Gabriel (Eds.), *The neurobiology of cingulate cortex and limbic thalamus* (pp. 527–556). Boston: Birkhauser.

Diebler, M.F., Farkas-Bargeton, E., & Wehrle, R. (1979). Developmental changes of enzymes associated with energy metabolism and synthesis of some neurotransmitters in discrete areas of human neocortex. *Journal of Neurochemistry, 32*, 429–435.

Domesick, V.B. (1969). Projections from the cingulate cortex in the rat. *Brain Research, 12*, 296–320.

Dunsmore, R.H., & Lennox, M.A. (1950). Stimulation and strychnization of supracallosal anterior cingulate gyrus. *Journal of Neurophysiology, 13*, 207–213.

Flechsig, P. (1920). *Anatomie des menschlichen gehirns und ruckenmarks auf myelogenetischer gundlange.* Leipzig, Germany: G. Thieme.

Fosse, V.M., Heggelund, P., & Fonnu, F. (1989). Postnatal development of glutamatergic, GABAergic and cholinergic neurotransmitter phenotypes in the visual cortex, lateral geniculate nucleus pulvinar and superior colliculus in cats. *Journal of Neuroscience, 9*, 426–435.

Friede, R.L. (1989). Perinatal lesions of gray matter. In *Developmental Neuropathology* (pp. 82–97). Berlin: Springer-Verlag.

Geier, S., Bancaud, J., Talairach, J., Bonis, A., Szikla, G., & Enjelvin, M. (1977). The seizures of frontal lobe epilepsy. A study of clinical manifestations. *Neurology, 27*, 951–958.

Gilles, F.H., Shankle, W., & Dooling, E.C. (1983). Myelinated tracts: Growth patterns. In F.H. Gilles, A. Leviton, & E.C. Dooling (Eds.), *The developing human brain: Growth and epidemiologic neuropathology* (pp. 117–183). Boston: John Wright–PSG.

Glees, P., Cole, J., Whitty, W.M., & Cairns, H. (1950). The effects of lesions in the cingulate gyrus and adjacent areas in monkeys. *Journal of Neurology and Neurosurgery, 13*, 178–190.

Goldman-Rakic, P. (1981). Development and plasticity of primate frontal association cortex. In F.O. Smith (Ed.), *The organization of the cerebral cortex* (pp. 69–100). Cambridge, MA: MIT Press.

Goldman-Rakic, P.S., & Brown, R.M. (1982). Postnatal development of monoamine content and synthesis in the cerebral cortex of rhesus monkeys. *Developmental Brain Research, 4*, 339–349.

Hamon, M., & Bourgoin, S. (1977). Biochemical aspects of the maturation of serotonergic neurons in the rat brain. In S.R. Berenger (Ed.), *Brain: Fetal and infant* (pp. 239–261). The Hague, the Netherlands: Martinus Nijhoff.

Harden, T.K., Wolfe, B.B., Sporn, J.R., Perkins, J.P., & Molinoff, P.B. (1977). Ontogeny of beta-adrenergic receptors in rat cerebral cortex. *Brain Research, 125*, 99–108.

Hedner, T., & Lundberg, P. (1980). Serotonergic development in the postnatal rat brain. *Journal of Neural Transmission, 49*, 257–279.

Heschl, R. (1859). Gehirndefect und Hydrocephalus [Brain defect and hydrocephalus]. *Vierteljahresschrift für Praktic Heilkunde (Prague) [Quarterly Journal of Practical Medical Science], 61*, 59–74.

Hurley, K.M., Herbert, H., Moga, M.M., & Saper, C.B. (1991). Efferent projections of the infralimbic cortex of the rat. *Journal of Comparative Neurology, 308,* 249–276.

Huttenlocher, P.R. (1994). Synaptogenesis in human cerebral cortex. In G. Dawson & K.W. Fischer (Eds.), *Human behavior and the developing brain* (pp. 137–152). New York: Guilford Press.

Johnston, M.V. (1988). Biochemistry of neurotransmitters in cortical development. In A. Peter & E.G. Jones (Eds.), *Cerebral cortex* (Vol. 7, pp. 211–236). New York: Plenum.

Johnston, M.V., & Coyle, J.T. (1980). Ontogeny of neurochemical markers for noradrenergic, GABAergic and cholinergic neurons in neocortex lesioned with methylazoxymethanol acetate. *Journal of Neurochemistry, 34,* 1429–1441.

Johnston, M.V., McKinney, M., & Coyle, J.T. (1979). Evidence for a cholinergic projection to neocortex from neurons in basal forebrain. *Proceedings of the National Academy of Sciences of the United States of America, 76,* 5392–5396.

Jones, E.G., & Powell, T.P.S. (1970). An anatomical study of converging sensory pathways within the cerebral cortex of the monkey. *Brain, 93,* 793–820.

Kaada, B.R. (1960). Cingulate, posterior orbital, anterior insular and temporal pole cortex. In H.W. Magoun (Sect. Ed.), *Handbook of physiology: Section 1. Neurophysiology* (Vol. II, pp. 1345–1372). Washington, DC: American Physiological Society.

Kaada, B.R., Pribram, K.H., & Epstein, J.A. (1940). Respiratory and vascular responses in monkeys from temporal pole, insula, orbital surface and cingulate gyrus. *Journal of Neurophysiology, 12,* 347–356.

Kalsbeek, A., Voorn, P., Buijs, R.M., Pool, C.W., & Uylings, H.B. (1988). Development of the dopaminergic innervation in the prefrontal cortex of rat. *Journal of Comparative Neurology, 269,* 58–72.

Kasamatsu, T., & Pettigrew, J.W. (1976). Depletion of brain catecholamines: Failure of monocular dominance shift after monocular conclusion in kittens. *Science, 194,* 206–209.

Kennard, M.A. (1955). The cingulate gyrus in relation to consciousness. *Journal of Nervous and Mental Disorders, 121,* 34–39.

Kostovic, I., Skavic, J., & Strinovic, D. (1988). Acetylcholinesterase in the human frontal associative cortex during the period of cognitive development: Early laminar shifts and late innervation of pyramidal neurons. *Neuroscience Letters, 90,* 107–112.

Kvale, I., Fosse, V.M., & Fonnum, F. (1983). Development of neurotransmitter parameters in lateral geniculate body, superior colliculus and visual cortex of the albino rat. *Developmental Brain Research, 7,* 137–145.

Laplane, D., Degos, J.D., Baulac, M., & Gray, F. (1981). Bilateral infarction of the anterior cingulate gyri and of the fornices. *Journal of Neurological Science, 51,* 289–300.

Lauder, J.M., & Bloom, F.E. (1974). Ontogeny of monoamine neurons in the locus coeruleus, raphe nuclei and substantia nigra of the rat: I. Cell differentiation. *Journal of Comparative Neurology, 155,* 469–482.

Levey, A.I., Wainer, B.H., Raye, D.B., Mufson, E.J., & Mesulam, M.-M. (1984). Choline acetyltransferase immunoreactive neurons intrinsic to rodent cortex and distinction from acetylcholinesterase-positive neurons. *Neuroscience, 13,* 341–353.

Levitt, P., & Moore, R.Y. (1978). Noradrenaline neuron innervation of the neurocortex in the rat. *Brain Research, 139,* 219–231.

Levitt, P., & Rakic, P. (1982). The time of genesis, embryonic origin and differentiation of brainstem monoamine neurons in the rhesus monkey. *Brain Research, 4,* 35–37.

Lidov, H.G., & Molliver, M.E. (1982). An immunohistochemical study of serotonin neuron development in the rat: Ascending pathways and terminal fields. *Brain Research Bulletin, 8,* 389–430.

Lindvall, O., & Bjorklund, A. (1984). General organization of cortical monoamine system. In L. Descarries, J.R. Reader, & H.H. Jasper (Eds.), *Monoamine innervation of cerebral cortex* (pp. 9–40). New York: Alan R. Liss.

Lindvall, O., Bjorklund, A., & Divac, I. (1978). Organization of catecholamine neurons projecting to frontal cortex in the rat. *Brain Research, 142,* 1–24.

Lubbers, K., Wolff, J.R., & Frotscher, M. (1985). Neurogenesis of GABAergic neurons in the rat dentate gyrus: A combined autoradiographic and immunocytochemical study. *Neuroscience Letters, 62,* 317–322.

Luria, A.R. (1973). *The working brain* (pp. 147–160). New York: Basic Books.

MacLean, P.D. (1954). Studies on limbic system (visceral brain) and their bearing on psychosomatic problems. In E. Wittkower & R. Cleghorn (Eds.), *Recent developments in psychosomatic medicine* (p. 106). London: Pribram and Sons.

MacLean, P.D. (1985). Brain evolution relating to family, play and the separation cell. *Archives of General Psychiatry, 42*, 405–417.

MacLean, P.D. (1990). *The triune brain* (pp. 242–243). New York: Plenum.

Marcusson, J.O., Morgan, D.G., Winblad, B., & Finch, C.E. (1984). Serotonin-2 binding sites in human frontal cortex and hippocampus: Selective loss of S-2A sites with age. *Brain Research, 311*, 51–56.

Marin-Padilla, M. (1970a). Prenatal and early postnatal ontogenesis of the human motor cortex: A Golgi study: I. The sequential development of the cortical layers. *Brain Research, 23*, 167–183.

Marin-Padilla, M. (1970b). Prenatal and early postnatal ontogenesis of the human motor cortex: A Golgi study: II. The basket-pyramidal system. *Brain Research, 23*, 185–191.

Mazars, G. (1970). Criteria for identifying cingulate epilepsies. *Epilepsia, 11*, 41–47.

Mesulam, M.-M. (1983). The functional anatomy and hemispheric specialization of directed attention: The role of the parietal lobe and its commentary. *Trends in Neuroscience, 6*, 384–387.

Mesulam, M.-M., & Geschwind, N. (1978). On the possible role of neocortex and its limbic connections in the process of attention and schizophrenia: Clinical cases of inattention in man and experimental anatomy in monkey. *Journal of Psychiatric Research, 14*, 249–259.

Mesulam, M.-M., Mufson, E.J., Levey, A.I., & Wainer, B.H. (1983). Cholinergic innervation of cortex by the basal forebrain: Cytochemistry and cortical connections of the septal area, diagonal band nuclei, nucleus basalis (Substantia innominata) and hypothalamus in the rhesus monkey. *Journal of Comparative Neurology, 214*, 140–191.

Michel, A.E., & Garey, L.H. (1984). The development of dendritic spines in the human visual cortex. *Human Neurobiology, 3*, 223–227.

Mountcastle, V.B., Lynch, J.C., Georgopoulos, A., Sakata, H., & Acuna, C. (1975). Posterior parietal association cortex of the monkey: Command functions for operations within extrapersonal space. *Journal of Neurophysiology, 38*, 871–908.

Neafsey, E.J., Terreberry, R.R., Hurley, K.M., Ruit, K.G., & Frysztak, R.J. (1992). Anterior cingulate cortex in rodents: Connections, visceral control functions and implications for emotion. In B.A. Vogt & M. Gabriel (Eds.), *The neurobiology of cingulate cortex and limbic thalamus* (pp. 206–223). Boston: Birkhauser.

Nelson, S.B., Schwartz, M.A., & Daniels, J.D. (1975). Clonidine and cortical plasticity: Possible evidence for noradrenergic involvement. *Developmental Brain Research, 23*, 39–50.

Nielsen, J.M., & Jacobs, L.L. (1951). Bilateral lesions of the anterior cingulate gyri—report of a case. *Bulletin of the Los Angeles Neurological Society, 18*, 85–89.

Norman, M.G. (1980). Bilateral encephaloclastic lesions in a 26 week gestation fetus: Effect on neuroblast migration. *Canadian Journal of Neurological Sciences, 7*, 191–194.

Pandya, D.N., & Kuypers, H.G. (1969). Cortico-cortical connections in the rhesus monkey. *Brain Research, 13*, 13–36.

Papez, J.W. (1937). A proposed mechanism of emotion. *Archives of Neurological Psychiatry, 38*, 725–743.

Pardo, J.V., Pardo, P.J., Janer, K.W., & Raichle, M.E. (1990). The anterior cingulate cortex mediated processing selection in the Stroop attentional conflict paradigm. *Proceedings of the National Academy of Sciences of the United States of America, 87*, 256–259.

Petras, J.M. (1971). Connections of the parietal lobe. *Journal of Psychiatric Research, 8*, 189–201.

Ploog, D.W. (1970). Phonation, emotion, cognition with references to the brain mechanisms involved. In *Brain and mind (Ciba Foundation Series)* (pp. 79–98). Amsterdam: Exerpta Medica.

Poliakov, G.I. (1965). Development of the cerebral neocortex during the first half of intrauterine life. In S.A. Sarkisov (Ed.), *Development of the child's brain* (pp. 22–52). Leningrad: Medicina.

Posner, M.K., & Peterson, S.E. (1990). The attention system of the human brain. *Annual Review of Neuroscience, 13*, 25–42.

Posner, M.I., Peterson, S.E., Fox, P.T., & Raichle, M.E. (1990). Localization of cognitive operations in the human brain. *Science, 240*, 1627–1631.

Rakic, P. (1974). Neurons in rhesus monkey visual cortex: Systematic relation between time of origin and eventual disposition. *Science, 183,* 425–427.

Rakic, P., Bourgeois, J.-P., Eckenhoff, M.F., Zecevic, N., & Goldman-Rakic, P.S. (1986). Concurrent overproduction of synapses in diverse regions of the primate cerebral cortex. *Science, 232,* 232–235.

Ravikumar, B.V., & Sastary, P.S. (1985). Muscarinic cholinergic receptors in human fetal brain: Characterization and ontogeny of [^{3}H] quinuclidinyl benzilate binding sites in frontal cortex. *Journal of Neurochemistry, 44,* 240–246.

Rozenberg, F., Robain, O., Jardin, L., & Ben-Ari, Y. (1989). Distribution of GABAergic neurons in late fetal and early postnatal rat hippocampus. *Developmental Brain Research, 50,* 177–187.

Schliebs, R., Kullman, E., & Bigl, V. (1986). Development of glutamate binding sites in the visual structures of the rat brain: Effect of visual pattern deprivation. *Biomedica et Biophysica Acta, 45,* 4495–4506.

Schwartz, M.L., & Meinecke, D.L. (1992). Early expression of GABA-containing neurons in the prefrontal and visual cortices of rhesus monkeys. *Cerebral Cortex, 2,* 16–37.

Seltzer, B., & Pandya, D.M. (1978). Afferent cortical connections and architectonics of the superior temporal sulcus and surrounding cortex in the rhesus monkey. *Brain Research, 192,* 1–24.

Seltzer, B., & Pandya, D.M. (1984). Further observations on parietotemporal connections in the rhesus monkey. *Experimental Brain Research, 55,* 301–312.

Seltzer, B., & Van Hoesen, G.W. (1979). A direct inferior parietal lobule projection to the presubiculum in the rhesus monkey. *Brain Research, 179,* 157–161.

Seress, L., & Ribak, C.E. (1988). The development of GABAergic neurons in the rat hippocampal formation: An immunocytochemical study. *Developmental Brain Research, 44,* 197–202.

Sidman, R., & Rakic, P. (1973). Neuronal migration with special reference to developing human brain. *Brain Research, 62,* 1–35.

Slotnick, B.M. (1967). Disturbances of maternal behavior in the rat following lesions of the cingulate cortex. *Behavior, 24,* 204–236.

Smith, W.D. (1945). The functional significance of the rostral cingulate cortex as revealed by its responses of electrical excitation. *Journal of Neurophysiology, 8,* 241–255.

Soriano, E., Cobas, S.A., & Fairen, A. (1986). Asynchronism in the neurogenesis of GABAergic and non-GABAergic neurons in the mouse hippocampus. *Developmental Brain Research, 30,* 88–92.

Spielmeyer, W. (1906). Hemiplegie bei intakter pyramidenbahn (intrakortikale hemiplegie) [Hemiplegia in the setting of pyramidal tract lesions (intracortical hemiplegia)]. *Muenchen Medizinische Wochenschrift [Munich Medical Weekly Periodical], 29,* 1404–1406.

Stamm, J.S. (1955). The function of the median cerebral cortex in maternal behavior of rats. *Journal of Comparative Physiology and Psychology, 48,* 347–356.

Streit, P. (1984). Glutamate and aspartate as transmitter candidates for systems of the cerebral cortex. In E.G. Jones & A. Peters (Eds.), *Cerebral cortex* (Vol. 2, pp. 119–144). New York: Plenum.

Terreberry, R.R., & Neafsey, E.J. (1983). Rat medial frontal cortex: A visceromotor region with a direct projection to the nucleus solitarius. *Brain Research, 278,* 245–249.

Terreberry, R.R., & Neafsey, E.J. (1987). The rat medial frontal cortex projects directly to autonomic regions of the brainstem. *Brain Research Bulletin, 19,* 639–649.

Thierry, A.M., Blanc, G., Sobel, A., Stinus, L., & Glowinski, J. (1973). Dopaminergic terminals in the rat cortex. *Science, 182,* 499–501.

Ulinski, P.S. (1990). The cerebral cortex of reptiles. In E.G. Jones & A. Peters (Eds.), *Cerebral cortex: Comparative structure and evolution of cerebral cortex, Part 1* (Vol. 8A, pp. 139–215). New York: Plenum.

Uphouse, L.L., & Bondy, S.C. (1981). The maturation of cortical serotonergic binding sites. *Developmental Brain Research, 1,* 415–417.

Vaccarino, F.M., Schwartz, M.L., Hartigan, D., & Leckman, J.F. (1995). Basic fibroblast growth factor increases the number of excitatory neurons containing glutamate in the cerebral cortex. *Cerebral Cortex, 1,* 64–78.

Van der Kooy, D., McGinty, J.F., Koda, L.Y., Gerfen, C.R., & Bloom, F.E. (1982). Visceral cortex: Direct connections from prefrontal cortex to the solitary nucleus in the rat. *Neuroscience Letters, 33*, 123–127.

Van Hoesen, G.W. (1982). The parahippocampal gyrus. *Trends in Neuroscience, 5*, 345–350.

Verney, C., Berger, B.A.J., Vigny, A., & Gay, M. (1982). Development of the dopaminergic innervation of the rat cerebral cortex. A light microscopic immunocytochemical study using anti-tyrosine hydroxylase antibodies. *Developmental Brain Research, 5*, 41–52.

Vincent, S.L., Pabreza, L., & Benes, F.M. (1995). Postnatal maturation of GABA-immunoreactive neurons of rat medial prefrontal cortex. *Journal of Comparative Neurology, 355*, 81–92.

Wallace, J.A., & Lauder, J.M. (1983). Development of the serotonergic system in the rat embryo: An immunocytochemical study. *Brain Research Bulletin, 10*, 459–479.

Ward, A.A. (1948). The anterior cingulate gyrus and personality. In *The frontal lobes* (pp. 438–445). Baltimore: Williams & Wilkins.

Wise, S.P., Fleshman, J.W., & Jones, E.G. (1979). Maturation of pyramidal cell form in relation to developing afferent and efferent connections of the rat somatic sensory cortex. *Journal of Neuroscience, 4*, 1275–1297.

Wise, S.P., & Jones, E.G. (1978). Developmental studies of thalamocortical and commissural connections in the rat somatic sensory cortex. *Journal of Comparative Neurology, 178*, 187–208.

Wyss, J.M., & Sripanidkulchai, K. (1984). The topography of the mesencephalic and pontine projections from the cingulate cortex of the rat. *Brain Research, 293*, 1–15.

Yakovlev, P., & LeCours, A. (1967). The myelinogenetic cycles of regional maturation of the brain. In A. Minkowski (Ed.), *Regional development of the brain early in life* (pp. 3–70). Oxford, England: Blackwell.

Zilles, K.W.R., Busching, U., & Schleicher, A. (1986). Ontogenesis of the laminar structure in areas 17 and 18 of the human visual cortex. A quantitative study. *Anatomy and Embryology, 174*, 339–353.

Development of the Prefrontal Cortex: Evolution, Neurobiology, and Behavior
edited by Norman A. Krasnegor, Ph.D., G. Reid Lyon, Ph.D.,
and Patricia S. Goldman-Rakic, Ph.D.
copyright © 1997   Paul H. Brookes Publishing Co., Inc.
Baltimore • London • Toronto • Sydney

11

Frontal Lobe Dysfunction
Following Closed Head Injury in Children
Findings from Neuropsychology and Brain Imaging

Randall S. Scheibel and Harvey S. Levin

The relationship of quantitative brain imaging to neuropsychological test findings can help define the functions of the prefrontal brain region. Head-injured children frequently exhibit deficits in problem-solving skills, cognitive flexibility, verbal discourse, response inhibition, and other abilities that are thought to depend on the integrity of prefrontal structures. Although investigations utilizing computed tomography (CT) scans lacked the resolution to clearly identify focal lesions associated with these cognitive sequelae in head-injured children, more recent studies using magnetic resonance imaging (MRI) have confirmed that focal pathology is common following pediatric closed head injury (CHI), that lesions are often present within the frontal lobes, and that the distribution and size of frontal lesions are related to the type and severity of specific cognitive impairments. In addition, the examination of head-injured children adds the study of developmental factors to the investigation of the prefrontal region in humans. The functions of a particular brain area may change during development and the examination of a large number of children who have been injured at different ages and followed over an extensive period of time may provide some clues about how the functions of the frontal lobes change as the child matures. This chapter provides a brief review of research that has examined prefrontal brain functions in head-injured children, including a discussion of promising new techniques such as segmentation analysis and functional brain imaging. The development of better brain imaging techniques for use with children is especially important because CHI is now recognized to be a major cause of disability among the young.

This chapter was supported in part by Grant NS-21889 from the National Institutes of Health.

The authors gratefully acknowledge the assistance of Matthew A. Lilly, M.A., and Joseph Kufera, M.A., in the preparation of case material presented in this chapter. They also appreciate the assistance in manuscript preparation provided by Amy Yerkes.

INCIDENCE AND GLOBAL OUTCOME

CHI occurs in children with an incidence of 219 in 100,000 and is a major cause of death and disability in this population (Kraus, Rock, & Hemyari, 1990). As in adults, follow-up data show that cognitive impairment and behavioral disturbances are major contributors to disability after pediatric CHI (Brown, Chadwick, Shaffer, Rutter, & Traub, 1981; Rutter, 1981). The neurobehavioral sequelae of these injuries are related to the severity of impaired consciousness, as assessed by the Glasgow Coma Scale (GCS) of Teasdale and Jennett (1974). Global outcome is frequently assessed by the Glasgow Outcome Scale (GOS), developed by Jennett and Bond (1975). However, it is important to acknowledge that the GOS is primarily useful for adults, and modifications are indicated for use with children. Research into the quality of outcome in children who have sustained a CHI, including the anatomical and physiological correlates of cognitive sequelae, is at an early stage of inquiry.

PATHOPHYSIOLOGY OF HEAD INJURY

The pathophysiological mechanisms of CHI in the mature brain are thought to produce both diffuse and focal brain injury, including contusions, lacerations, and hematomas (Adams et al., 1989; Adams, Graham, Scott, Parker, & Doyle, 1980; Strich, 1961). The anterior frontal and temporal lobes, in particular, are among the most common areas of focal brain injury in adults following CHI. The proximity of the orbitofrontal and anterior temporal regions to bony protrusions and cavities contributes to their vulnerability to injury (Adams et al., 1980). Acceleration–deceleration forces can push the brain against these irregular surfaces of the skull, causing damage when local brain tissue is crushed or torn. Diffuse axonal injury is also common and is of particular significance for brain imaging because it produces shearing and stretching of axons throughout the brain (Blumbergs, Jones, & North, 1989). Although the resulting white matter damage may be difficult to detect with structural imaging techniques, MRI has documented shearing effects.

Pediatric CHI was once thought to produce predominantly diffuse brain damage and, when compared with adults, focal lesions were believed to be relatively infrequent when the injury was sustained by a child (Bruce et al., 1979; Bruce, Schut, Bruno, Wood, & Sutton, 1978). These conclusions were based primarily on the results of studies that had examined CT scans in children with acute CHI. For example, Bruce and associates (1978) found that the most common initial CT finding in head-injured children was diffuse cerebral swelling, with 18 of their 53 subjects (34%) exhibiting narrowing or obliteration of the ventricles and basal cisterns. Focal lesions were less frequent (23%), and none of the patients had evidence of brain contusions on the CT images. More recent studies with MRI indicate a far higher frequency of focal lesions (see later discussion in this chapter). In addition, the cognitive and behavior changes that occur in head-injured children also suggest that focal brain lesions are common, especially focal injury to the frontal and temporal lobes.

NEUROBEHAVIORAL SEQUELAE

Contribution of Frontal Lobe Lesions

Clinical descriptions of head-injured adults often include symptoms that are frequently observed with documented frontal lobe injury, such as poor impulse control, decreased flexibility, impaired attention, perseveration, and diminished divergent thinking (Levin & Kraus, 1994). Likewise, the behavior changes that often occur following pediatric CHI, including social disinhibition and impulsivity, suggest the presence of frontal dysfunction in this population.

Price, Daffner, Stowe, and Mesulam (1990) presented some support for the hypothesis that frontal brain dysfunction is responsible for many behavior changes that occur following pediatric CHI. They reported the case of a woman who had been unconscious for 48 hours after being struck by an automobile at the age of 4. This patient had developed normally until her injury; but, over the following year, she was said to display a variety of inappropriate and destructive behaviors, such as temper outbursts and physical aggression toward others. Additional behavior problems and psychiatric symptoms emerged as she matured, including sexual promiscuity, intermittent substance abuse, difficulty sustaining friendships, two suicide attempts, and a work history that included outbursts against co-workers and customers. When examined by Price et al. at the age of 26 years, she had just had an infant placed in foster care because of reports that she had neglected and physically abused the child. An MRI scan was performed that revealed extensive damage to the frontal lobes. Cases such as this suggest that early CHI can produce neurobehavioral sequelae that persist, or even worsen, during the years that follow the injury and that frontal lobe dysfunction contributes to behavior disorders in at least some head-injured children.

Many head-injured children exhibit deficits in planning skills and other cognitive abilities that are commonly impaired in adults with focal frontal lesions (e.g., Chapman et al., 1992; Levin, Mendelsohn, et al., 1994). However, the cognitive and behavioral manifestations of frontal brain injury are highly variable and appear to depend on the specific location of the frontal lesion (Kertesz, 1994; Stuss & Benson, 1986). Studies examining the neurobehavioral consequences of damage within various prefrontal regions have been conducted primarily with adults, but these serve as a good starting point for developing hypotheses about the effects of different lesion locations in children.

Several location-related syndromes have been described in adults with prefrontal damage, including separate syndromes associated with damage to the dorsolateral, superior medial (i.e., supplementary motor and anterior cingulate cortex), and orbital regions. Injury to the dorsolateral area has often been reported to produce impairments in executive functions (e.g., problem solving, cognitive flexibility), whereas superior medial lesions are more frequently said to be associated with akinesia, mutism, dysfluency, and reduced emotions (Benson et al., 1981; Kertesz, 1994; Milner, 1964). Orbitofrontal injury has been reported to present with an entirely different set of symptoms, including impulsivity and poor social judgment (Blumer & Benson, 1975). The concept of separate prefrontal syndromes is controversial, however, and most patients present with combinations or incomplete forms of these syndromes (Kertesz, 1994). Lateralization of frontal lesions also influences the resulting symptoms, with left-sided injury often producing a fairly global deficit in conceptual abilities and executive functions (Mattson & Levin, 1990). The cognitive dysfunction associated with left frontal brain injury may result in deficient performance on a variety of verbal and nonverbal measures (e.g., Benton, 1968; Perret, 1974; Petrides & Milner, 1982). Patients with right-sided lesions, in contrast, frequently perform well on conceptual tasks and novel problems that are primarily verbal in nature. However, these patients may exhibit severe deficits on analogous tasks that include a significant nonverbal or spatial component (Jones-Gotman & Milner, 1977).

Neurobehavioral Sequelae and Age

In addition to differences in lesion location, the study of neurobehavioral consequences of frontal injury in children is complicated by developmental factors. Many investigators have stated that the long-term effects of brain injury are milder and that recovery is faster in individuals injured at an early age (e.g., Lenneberg & Lenneberg, 1975). Consequently, the immature brain has often been said to have greater "neural plasticity," a concept supported by the relative sparing of language following focal left hemisphere damage in young children (e.g., Alajouanine & Lhermitte, 1965; Hécaen, 1976). The evidence for generally better recovery from cerebral insult in younger individuals is equivocal, however, and some cognitive abilities may be more vulnerable to the early diffuse brain injury that occurs with other disorders, such as infectious diseases and cranial irradiation (Meadows et al., 1981; St. James-Roberts, 1979). Studies of pediatric CHI also indicate a tendency for patients to exhibit more severe impairment when injured at an earlier age, including relatively greater deficits among younger patients on measures of global intellectual functioning, written language, and recognition memory (Ewing-Cobbs, Fletcher, Landry, & Levin, 1985; Levin, Eisenberg, Wigg, & Kobayashi, 1982). These findings suggest that cognitive abilities that are undergoing rapid development at the time of injury may be more vulnerable to the effects of CHI.

Some frontally mediated cognitive processes develop late in childhood, which has implications for their vulnerability to CHI. Developmental gains have been documented through adolescence on several purported tests of frontal lobe function (Levin et al., 1991; Passler, Isaac, & Hynd, 1985). CHI in older children may thus have a greater disruptive effect on these rapidly developing abilities, as compared with less severe impairment of cognitive skills that are static or have already reached mature levels. However, the relationship between age at injury and the resulting cognitive and behavior changes is complex. Findings from case studies also suggest that early frontal damage may prevent the acquisition of skills that have not yet developed (Eslinger, Grattan, Damasio, & Damasio, 1992; Grattan & Eslinger, 1992; Price et al., 1990). In one notable case report, Eslinger and associates (Eslinger et al., 1992; Grattan & Eslinger, 1992) described a woman who sustained a hemorrhagic injury to the left frontal lobe at age 7 years but later exhibited the onset of cognitive and behavior deficits during early adolescence. Similarly, nonhuman primate experiments have indicated that developmental factors can interact with lesion location to produce varying degrees and types of impairment (e.g., Goldman & Alexander, 1977). In monkeys, for example, a prefrontal insult sustained before this area becomes functionally mature may result in the apparent sparing of function followed by the delayed appearance of a deficit.

Much of what is known about the relationship between development and frontal brain injury is based on animal research, particularly experiments involving nonhuman primates. Goldman-Rakic and associates (e.g., Goldman & Alexander, 1977; Goldman & Rosvold, 1970; Goldman, Rosvold, Vest, & Galkin, 1971; Goldman-Rakic, 1987) have shown that infant monkeys who receive dorsolateral ablations do not initially exhibit impairments on the delayed response task when tested at an early age. However, their performance on repeat administration of this task in adulthood is severely impaired. There is also evidence for an interaction between lesion location and age because, unlike dorsolateral injury, orbitofrontal ablations produce deficits on the delayed response task in both infant and adult monkeys. These results have been interpreted as indicating that, in nonhuman primates, the dorsolateral cortex does not fully assume its role in spatial delay processing until relatively late in development. A similar relationship between frontal injury and developmental factors probably exists for some abilities in children; but, until recently, a detailed examination of these issues was not possible, owing to limitations associated with brain imaging technology.

NEUROIMAGING OF EARLY BRAIN INJURY

Early imaging studies had utilized the CT scan, and their results indicated that focal lesions were relatively uncommon in children with CHI (e.g., Bruce et al., 1978). CT has a number of limitations, however, and these are particularly relevant for the study of head injury in children. Radiation exposure limits the use of this technique except when clinically indicated, CT scans provide relatively poor differentiation of gray and white matter, and X-ray scatter further degrades anatomic resolution of the CT image at bony interfaces (Filipek, Kennedy, & Caviness, 1992). This latter point is especially relevant for the study of CHI because contusions and hemorrhage are most likely to occur in those brain regions that are adjacent to rough areas of the skull (Snow, Zimmerman, Gandy, & Deck, 1986).

MRI provides excellent spatial resolution of brain structure while avoiding many limitations associated with the CT scan (Filipek et al., 1992). Studies of adults who have sustained a CHI have found that MRI frequently reveals lesions that were not detected by CT scans in mild to moderate (Levin et al., 1987) and severe head injuries (Wilberger, Deeb, & Rothfus, 1987). When focal lesions are detected by both imaging techniques, the area of brain abnormality is often larger on the magnetic resonance image (Levin et al., 1987).

In children, research utilizing follow-up MRI has shown that focal lesions are far more common after CHI than was initially thought. Levin and associates (Levin et al., 1993; Mendelsohn et al., 1992) found that approximately 75% of children who sustained moderate to severe CHI had focal areas of abnormal signal on scans performed at least 3 months after injury. Many of these focal abnormalities appeared to be associated with contusions. An anterior–posterior gradient was also noted for the lesion distribution, with lesions often occurring in the frontal and anterior temporal lobes. Focal areas of abnormal signal were common within anterior frontal regions, frequently including parts of the dorsolateral cortex, orbitofrontal cortex, and frontal white matter (Levin et al., 1993; Mendelsohn et al., 1992). This pattern of injury is illustrated in Figure 11.1; it resembles the distribution of lesions found in head-injured adults (Levin et al., 1987).

NEUROIMAGING AND GLOBAL MEASURES
OF OUTCOME IN PEDIATRIC CLOSED HEAD INJURY

The presence of focal signal abnormalities on MRI is related to severity of injury and outcome following pediatric CHI. In a preliminary study, Levin and colleagues (1989) found that children with mild to moderate CHI had no focal lesions on MRI when scans were done more than 6 months after injury, whereas 8 of 11 children with severe CHI had areas of high signal intensity in the brain parenchyma when

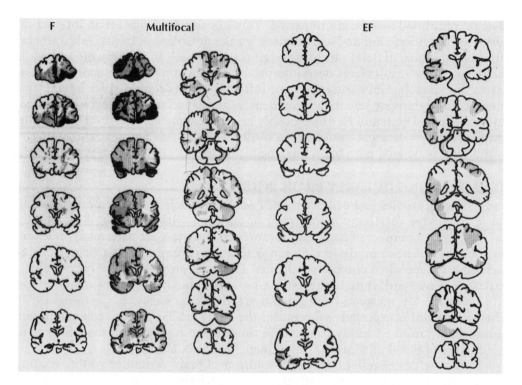

Figure 11.1   Neuroanatomical distribution of focal lesions plotted on templates developed by Damasio (1991). The overlap in the number of children with areas of abnormal signal is reflected by the degree of shading. (■ = 1 Patient, ■ = 2 Patients, ■ = 3 Patients, ■ = 4 Patients.) Coronal images are shaded for children with areas of abnormal signal confined to the frontal lobe (F) (*n* = 32), overlapping the frontal and extrafrontal areas (Multifocal) (*n* = 29), and restricted to the extrafrontal regions (EF) (*n* = 17). Note the high density of patients with abnormal signal in the orbital and inferior frontal gyri, gyrus rectus, and frontal lobe white matter. (From Levin, H.S., Mendelsohn, D., Lilly, M.A., Fletcher, J.M., Culhane, K.A., Chapman, S.B., Harward, H., Kusnerik, L., Bruce, D., & Eisenberg, H.M. [1994]. Tower of London performance in relation to magnetic resonance imaging following closed head injury in children. *Neuropsychology, 8,* 173; reprinted by permission.)

scanned at the same time interval. There is the possibility, however, that lesions associated with milder injuries may have been present during earlier stages of recovery and resolved before the 6-month follow-up. A previous study examined adolescents and adults within a few weeks of mild to moderate CHI and found that 90% of these subjects had focal abnormalities, most of which were said to involve the parenchyma of the frontal and temporal lobes (Levin et al., 1987). Focal lesions in these patients were reported to have undergone substantial resolution over the next 1–3 months. However, whether similar findings occur in children with milder head injuries awaits further investigation.

In children with moderate to severe CHI, focal areas of abnormality on MRI scans performed 3 months or more after injury are associated with greater cognitive impairment and poorer outcome. Mendelsohn and associates (1992) found that children with evidence of lesions on MRI had a poorer quality of outcome as measured by the GOS than did children without focal abnormalities. However, the sample size was small, and scores on the GOS did not differ between patients with frontal and extrafrontal lesions. Using neuropsychological tests, this same research group also found that cognitive deficits were more common in children with evidence of focal brain lesions (Levin et al., 1989), as compared with patients with normal follow-up MRI. Again, their sample size was small, and there was no consistent relationship between lesion site and the pattern of neuropsychological impairment.

PERFORMANCE ON NEUROPSYCHOLOGICAL
TESTS FOLLOWING PEDIATRIC CLOSED HEAD INJURY

Focal Brain Lesions and Cognitive Function

Studies of pediatric CHI have found that performance on neuropsychological tests is related to the location and size of focal abnormalities on MRI (e.g., Levin et al., 1993; Levin, Mendelsohn, et al., 1994). After controlling for overall injury severity in a regression analysis, as measured by the GCS, Levin and colleagues (1993) found that the total size of focal frontal lesions was related to scores on Controlled Oral Word Association (COWA) (Benton & Hamsher, 1978), a measure of verbal fluency that is thought to be sensitive to frontal lobe dysfunction (see Figure 11.2, top left). (A brief description of the tests discussed here is provided in the chapter appendix.) Performance on other putative measures of frontal lobe function, a Go–No Go task and an index of semantic clustering from the California Verbal Learning Test (CVLT) (Delis, Kramer, Kaplan, & Ober, 1987), was found to approach significance in similar regression analyses (Levin et al., 1993). Size of extrafrontal lesions, in contrast, was not related to scores on any of these cognitive measures after severity of injury was taken into consideration (Figure 11.2, top right). Consequently, there appears to be a specific relationship between frontal lesion size and cognitive deficits in executive functions that are thought to be mediated by the frontal lobes.

The effect of frontal lesions on cognitive function in pediatric CHI is also related to the laterality of focal abnormalities, as well as the specific region of frontal lobe involvement. Levin and associates (1993) explored the effects of frontal lesion laterality on a variety of neuropsychological measures. As with their examination of overall frontal lesion size, they used hierarchical multiple regression to determine whether the size of focal lesions on MRI improved the prediction of cognitive test scores after controlling for injury severity. However, for these analyses, the data were analyzed separately for right and left frontal lesions. Size of left frontal lesions incremented prediction of the number of trials to reach criterion on the Go–No Go test, as well as the percentage of conceptual-level responses obtained on the Wisconsin Card Sorting Test (WCST) (Heaton, Chelune, Talley, Kay, & Curtiss, 1993). There was also some evidence for a relationship between the size of left frontal lesions and performance on COWA. As shown in the bottom half of Figure 11.2, a different pattern of correlations was obtained with right-hemisphere lesions. The size of right frontal lesions significantly improved the prediction of scores for COWA and the percentage of clustered responses on the CVLT. The relationship between right frontal lesion size and performance on the Go–No Go test approached significance.

Additional multiple regression analyses were used by Levin and colleagues (1993) to address the role of specific frontal regions in cognitive task performance. Orbitofrontal lesion size provided a significant increment to GCS scores in the prediction of scores on COWA, whereas the examination of white matter lesions revealed nonsignificant increases for the prediction of scores on COWA, the CVLT's semantic clustering measure, and trials to criterion on the Go–No Go test. Because

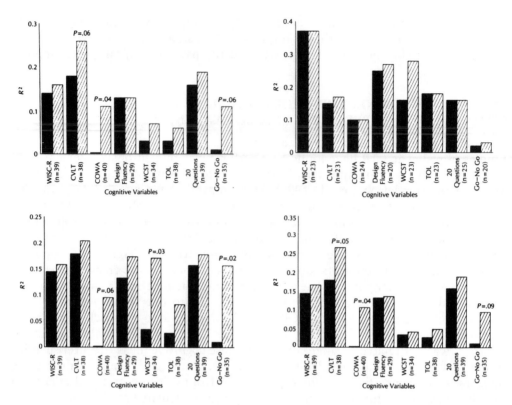

Figure 11.2.   Summary of the results of hierarchical multiple regression that evaluated the contributions of frontal (top left) and extrafrontal (top right) lesions to making incremental the variance in cognitive test scores explained by the lowest postresuscitation GCS score. The regressions were repeated to evaluate specifically the contributions of left frontal (bottom left) and right frontal (bottom right) lesions. Closed bars indicate R^2; hatched bars, incremental R^2. (WISC–R, Wechsler Intelligence Scale for Children–Revised; CVLT, California Verbal Learning Test; COWA, Controlled Oral Word Association; WCST, Wisconsin Card Sorting Test; TOL, Tower of London.) (From Levin, H.S., Culhane, K.A., Mendelsohn, D., Lilly, M.A., Bruce, D., Fletcher, J.M., Chapman, S.B., Harward, H., & Eisenberg, H.M. [1993]. Cognition in relation to magnetic resonance imaging in head-injured children and adolescents. *Archives of Neurology, 50,* 903; reprinted by permission. Copyright © 1993, American Medical Association.)

of the inadequate number of subjects with dorsolateral lesions, these researchers were unable to use regression analyses to perform a similar examination of the relationship between dorsolateral injury and neuropsychological test performance. However, the mean test scores for children with large dorsolateral lesions tended to fall below the mean performance of eight children with large extrafrontal lesions on the verbal fluency measure (i.e., COWA), the percentage of clustered responses from the CVLT, the number of trials to criterion on the Go–No Go test, and the percentage of problems solved on the first trial of the Tower of London.

The Tower of London was developed by Shallice (1982) to investigate sequential planning, a cognitive skill thought to be highly dependent on the integrity of frontal brain structures. The task is performed by rearranging beads on three vertical rods to match a model while using as few moves as possible (see Figure 11.3). This activity is believed to engage working memory to concurrently accomplish subgoals (i.e., intermediate moves) while maintaining the goal solution in memory. In a large study designed to investigate the relationship of frontal lesions to Tower of London performance, Levin and colleagues (Levin, Mendelsohn, et al., 1994) administered the task to 134 children who had sustained a CHI. The percentage of Tower of London problems solved within a limit of three trials decreased, and the number of broken rules (e.g., picking up more than one bead at a time) increased as a function of CHI severity, indicating the presence of greater impairment on this purported measure of frontal brain function in children with more severe injuries.

Levin and colleagues (Levin, Mendelsohn, et al., 1994) also examined the relationship between frontal lesion size on MRI and test scores from the Tower of London. Using hierarchical multiple regression to control for the severity of injury, the incremental multiple correlation provided by the addition of total frontal lesion size reached significance for the number of broken rules, but not for the percentage of problems solved on Trial 1 or the initial planning time (i.e., latency from the beginning of the trial until the child initiated a move). Separate regression analyses were also conducted to examine the contribution of lesions within specific frontal brain regions to deficient performance on different Tower of London measures. Size of orbitofrontal and frontal white matter lesions was observed to improve prediction for the number of broken rules, whereas the size of dorsolateral lesions incremented prediction of the number of problems solved on the first trial. Incremental squared multiple correlations provided by the addition of extrafrontal lesion size were nonsignificant for all of the cognitive measures. Consequently, these findings indicate that performance on the Tower of London is related to the severity of head injury in children, that frontal but not extrafrontal lesions make a significant contribution to impairment on the Tower of London and that injury to different regions of the frontal lobes produces different patterns of performance on the Tower of London measures. These findings are consistent with those obtained with other cognitive measures that are believed to reflect functioning of the frontal lobes, including the Go–No Go task and COWA (Levin et al., 1993).

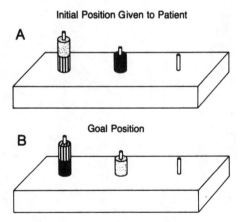

Figure 11.3. Tower of London test materials. (From Levin, H.S., Mendelsohn, D., Lilly, M.A., Fletcher, J.M., Culhane, K.A., Chapman, S.B., Harward, H., Kusnerik, L., Bruce, D., & Eisenberg, H.M. [1994]. Tower of London performance in relation to MRI following closed head injury in children. *Neuropsychology, 8,* 173; reprinted by permission.)

Tests of cognitive abilities that are thought to depend on frontal lobe function have been shown to be very sensitive to the sequelae of CHI, even in patients who have made a good recovery (Stuss et al., 1985). We examined such a case as part of a retrospective study of pediatric CHI. The boy studied was reported to have sustained a severe CHI in a fall at the age of 4. When seen for the study, at the age of 12, he was rated as having a good outcome on the GOS, and his scores were within the average to high-average range on the Vocabulary and Coding subtests from the WISC–R (Wechsler, 1974), as well as on COWA. He completed only three of six categories on the WCST, however, and problem solving on the Tower of London was impaired when compared with a group of age-matched control subjects. Magnetic resonance imaging was also performed, revealing a large lesion in the right frontal lobe (Figure 11.4). Therefore, although this child was rated as having attained a "good" recovery on the GOS, he still demonstrated deficits in problem-solving and planning skills that appear to be associated with significant frontal brain damage. There is the possibility that these cognitive impairments may have greater relevance for his daily functioning as he matures and is presented with more complex demands at home, at school, and eventually at work.

Another cognitive function that is thought to be vulnerable to frontal brain injury is verbal discourse. Studies with adults have found that discourse formulation is often disrupted in patients with frontal lesions (Alexander, Benson, & Stuss, 1989; Kaczmarck, 1984). Distinct discourse syndromes have been postulated, and the

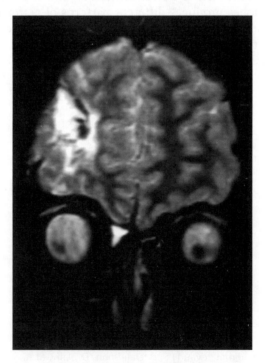

Figure 11.4. T_2-weighed coronal MRI scan performed 8 years after the patient sustained a severe closed head injury at age 4. A large lesion is disclosed within the right frontal lobe involving the white matter and the inferior and middle frontal gyri.

type of discourse impairment has been said to vary with both lesion lateralization and the specific region of frontal damage. For example, patients with left prefrontal dysfunction have been described as producing narratives that are unelaborated and sparsely detailed, whereas right prefrontal lesions have been said to result in tangential speech (Alexander et al., 1989).

The application of discourse analysis to the study of head-injured patients, including children, has indicated impaired discourse in many of these individuals (Chapman et al., 1992; Chapman, Levin, Wanek, Weyrauch, & Kufera, in press; Dennis & Barnes, 1990). Chapman et al. (in press) found that children who had sustained a severe CHI exhibited decreased performance on several measures of information structure, including a reduction in the amount of information provided and impairments in the structure and content of their narratives. A set of regression analyses failed to document a relationship between discourse performance and the size of left or right frontal lesions as visualized by MRI. There were also no significant correlations between these discourse measures and total lesion volume for the entire right or left hemisphere. The sample size for this study was small, however, and examination of individual cases with frontal damage suggested that discourse impairments were especially severe with left-sided lesions, provided the CHI occurred after age 5. A similar pattern was not observed when the injury occurred at a younger age. Further investigation is needed to elucidate the relationship of discourse deficits to frontal lesions in children.

Developmental Issues: Age and Cognitive Dysfunction

Additional evidence for a relationship between the severity of cognitive dysfunction and the child's age is provided by the Tower of London study (Levin, Mendelsohn, et al., 1994). Subjects used in this investigation were divided into two groups based on their age at the time of assessment, with one group consisting of children between the ages of 6 and 10 and another including those between 11 and 16 years of age. On the Tower of London test, the number of rules that were broken was noted to increase markedly as a function of injury severity in the younger children but not in the older group. Consistent with their impression of more marked effects of CHI in the 6- to 10-year-olds, these researchers found that the interaction of age with injury severity was significant. A similar interaction was noted by Levin and colleagues (1993) for the Similarities subtest from the WISC–R, with young head-injured children displaying the greatest level of impairment on that measure. In addition, they found that the interaction between age and injury severity approached significance for two other subtests from the WISC–R, Vocabulary and Picture Completion. However, a similar interaction was not found for several purported measures of frontal lobe function, such as COWA, design fluency, and the number of categories from the WCST.

Some cognitive abilities may mature so late in development that an interaction between age and injury severity might not be apparent unless a broad range of ages is examined. For example, planning and problem-solving skills have been found to undergo developmental changes until at least the age of 15 (e.g., Levin et al., 1991). The failure to find greater impairment on many of these tests among children between the ages of 6 and 10, as compared with a group of 11- to 16-year-olds (Levin et al.,1993), may therefore reflect the continuing development of frontally mediated abilities in both age groups. In contrast, cognitive skills associated with performance on subtests from the WISC–R may have been undergoing faster development among the youngest patients, and this may be the reason why Levin et al. (1993) found disproportionately greater impairment on WISC–R subtests in their younger group.

Other cognitive skills that mature very early in development may not be especially vulnerable to injury unless the insult occurs at a very young age. Delayed alternation and several related tasks are thought to rely on cognitive functions that emerge during early stages of human development (Diamond, 1991). Performance gains for delayed response and the $\overline{AB}$ task, both of which are similar to the delayed alternation test, have been demonstrated in human infants (Diamond, 1985; Diamond & Doar, 1989). However, equivalent developmental changes in delayed alternation performance have not been found in children over the age of 7 years (Levin et al., 1991). This contrasts with the developmental gains found on more complex tests that are also believed to be especially dependent on frontal lobe function, including measures of verbal and design fluency, verbal memory, planning skills, and problem solving. Normal children have been found to exhibit improvement on these tests through late childhood and, in some cases, further advances have been shown to continue into adolescence (Levin et al., 1991).

Children who have sustained a CHI often exhibit severe deficits on tests of planning and problem-solving skills, such as the Tower of London and WCST (Levin et al., 1993; Levin, Mendelsohn, et al., 1994). However, Levin, Culhane, et al. (1994) found that impairments were not present on the delayed alternation test in a large group of head-injured children between the ages of 5 and 15 years. This difference in sensitivity to the effects of CHI may reflect the emergence of separate frontally mediated cognitive abilities at different stages of development. The assessment of children injured at an earlier age, when cognitive abilities associated with the delayed alternation test are undergoing rapid changes, may reveal impairments on that task. Additional research is needed to examine these developmental issues, as well as the relationship between age and the specific region of the frontal lobe that is damaged. As in nonhuman primates, the type of cognitive deficit exhibited in humans with frontal injury may depend on a variety of factors, including task parameters, the age of the patient at assessment, the age at injury, and the location of focal lesions within the frontal lobes.

DIFFUSE DAMAGE FOLLOWING
PEDIATRIC CLOSED HEAD INJURY

Although contusions and other focal lesions are common following head injury, Levin et al. (1993) found that 25% of children who sustained moderate to severe injuries had no evidence of focal cerebral lesions on MRI. Many of these children with diffuse CHI continue to exhibit cognitive deficits, which raises the question of frontal dysfunction. Consequently, there is the possibility that the continuing cognitive impairment found in these patients is associated with diffuse damage to the frontal lobes, including tissue loss secondary to diffuse axonal injury, multifocal ischemic necrosis, and the posttraumatic release of excitatory neurotoxins (Faden, Demediuk, Panter, & Vink, 1989; Graham et al., 1989).

Diffuse brain injury sometimes results in ventricular enlargement, lesions within the corpus callosum, and other changes that can be visualized at long-term follow-up with structural brain imaging (Mendelsohn et al., 1992; Wilson et al., 1988). In many other cases, however, the changes that accompany diffuse brain damage may be too subtle to be consistently detected by gross findings on MRI. Recent advances in MRI technology and the development of software to segment MRIs may permit the quantification of subtle changes associated with this diffuse injury.

Berryhill and associates (1995) examined MRI scans from children who had sustained a CHI and were without evidence of focal frontal lesions on brain imaging. Using segmentation methods with magnetic resonance images, they calculated the percent volume of gray matter, white matter, and cerebrospinal fluid within prefrontal areas. When compared with children with mild CHI, patients with severe head injuries were found to have decreased gray matter tissue volume and larger cerebrospinal fluid space within the entire prefrontal area. A nonsignificant trend toward lower prefrontal white matter volume was also found among the severely injured children.

Additional analyses were conducted to determine whether specific areas of the prefrontal region are especially vulnerable to diffuse tissue loss following severe CHI. Examining gray matter volumes within specific prefrontal areas, Berryhill et al. (1995) obtained evidence for tissue loss in the orbitofrontal and dorsolateral prefrontal regions of severely injured children, a distribution similar to the pattern of focal injury in head-injured children with lesions (Levin et al., 1993). However, Berryhill et al. did not examine brain areas outside the frontal lobe. Therefore, it is not known whether the volumetric changes they observed are specific for prefrontal regions or are associated with diffuse tissue loss involving the entire brain. There is also the possibility that other brain areas may share a special vulnerability to diffuse tissue loss following severe pediatric CHI, including regions of the temporal lobe that are known to be frequent sites of damage in patients with focal injury.

DIRECTIONS FOR FUTURE RESEARCH

Research is needed to examine whether the diffuse tissue loss observed by Berryhill and associates (1995) is greatest among frontal brain regions. In addition, it would be useful to know whether declines in prefrontal tissue volume are associated with particular cognitive impairments. In the Berryhill et al. study, for example, 64% of severely injured subjects without focal frontal lesions had moderate disabilities after an average postinjury interval that exceeded 3 years. Information about the specific cognitive deficits found in these children may provide insights into the nature of their disability, as well as some clues about the relationship between cognitive dysfunction and diffuse brain pathology. It is possible that symptoms associated with diffuse frontal pathology differ from those produced by focal frontal lesions.

Another promising area for future research involves the application of functional brain imaging techniques to the study of pediatric CHI. Findings from research with adult survivors of CHI indicate a dissociation between structural lesions, as visualized on MRI, and metabolic abnormalities revealed by positron emission tomography (PET) and single-proton emission tomography (SPECT) (e.g., Prayer et al., 1993). The number and distribution of brain abnormalities indicated by these structural and functional imaging techniques has been shown to differ (Humayun et al., 1989; Newton et al., 1992). Moreover, there is some preliminary evidence that perfusion or metabolic abnormalities, or both, revealed by functional imaging techniques may relate well to the cognitive sequelae of CHI, including performance on neuropsychological measures (e.g., Ichise et al., 1994).

Figure 11.5 (see p. xxxiv) shows SPECT and MRI scans performed 5 months after a 10-year-old child sustained a CHI (Newton et al., 1992). Although MRI disclosed no structural lesion of the left hemisphere, SPECT revealed a focal area of decreased blood flow within the left parietal region. This finding was interpreted as consistent with reports that the child had experienced difficulties with reading since the head injury. Functional brain imaging techniques may therefore be especially useful in situations in which patients exhibit deficits despite normal results on structural brain imaging or in cases in which the observed symptoms are inconsistent with the location of lesions visualized on conventional MRI scans. Newer MRI methods should also permit the examination of functional brain images while avoiding the radiation exposure that occurs with PET and SPECT.

Functional MRI (fMRI) techniques have been developed that detect regional metabolic changes associated with sensory stimulation (Binder et al., 1994) and performance of cognitive tasks (Shaywitz, Shaywitz, et al., 1995). Detection of the effects of regional changes in blood flow and oxygen balance in tissues is possible because the oxygenation state of hemoglobin influences the magnetization decay time (T_2) of brain tissue water. The intensity of the tissue magnetic resonance signal therefore increases as a function of decreases in the concentration of deoxyhemoglobin. Utilization of fMRI facilitates studying recovery from brain injury in children because this procedure is noninvasive and involves no radiation burden. Disadvantages of fMRI include a signal-to-noise ratio less robust than PET, the claustrophobic reaction in some children to insertion into a scanning unit, and long scanning sessions, which can exceed 1 hour.

In view of the vulnerability of the prefrontal region to structural brain lesions after CHI in children (Levin et al., 1993), cognitive tasks that produce a frontal activation could potentially be used to investigate reorganization of function. Because fMRI is a recently developed technique for human studies, the published work is essentially confined to normal adults. Semantic processing tasks have been used extensively to produce frontal lobe activations with PET and fMRI (Petersen, Fox, Posner, Mintum, & Raichle, 1988; Posner, Petersen, Fox, & Raichle, 1988; Shaywitz, Shaywitz, et al., 1995). However, there is inconsistency across PET activation studies concerning the concurrent activation of temporal and parietal regions of the brain during semantic processing (Demonet et al., 1992; Petersen et al., 1988). This variation in patterns of activation across studies may reflect differences in the task conditions.

Semantic processing tasks have involved the individual generating a verb (e.g., flies) in response to auditory or visual presentation of a noun (e.g., bird); generating exemplars of a category (e.g., *robin* or *sparrow* in response to presentation of the word *bird*); or deciding whether two words are drawn from the same category or different categories. Figure 11.6 displays the inferior frontal, superior frontal, and temporal lobe activations reported for semantic processing using the verb-generation task with visual presentation of nouns to normal subjects by Shaywitz and colleagues (Shaywitz, Pugh, et al., 1995). These investigators also found that a phonological comparison task in the same subjects produced bilateral activation of the inferior frontal and temporal regions in women, whereas the activation was primarily restricted to the left hemisphere in men.

Brain mapping, which involves investigating the pattern of task-specific activations in various neuroanatomical regions, raises methodological issues for fMRI and PET, including the appropriate control tasks and the statistical method for comparing the brain activation produced by the experimental versus control tasks. To control for sensory stimulation associated with a semantic processing task,

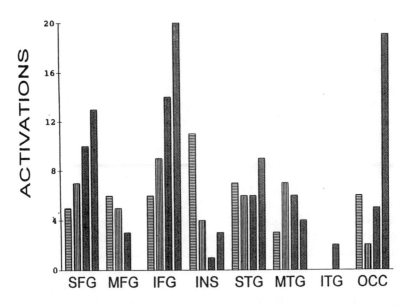

Figure 11.6.   Brain activations in regions of interest from fMRI. Total number of activations over all subjects are shown along the ordinate for eight regions: superior frontal gyrus (SFG), middle frontal gyrus (MFG), inferior frontal gyrus (IFG), insula (INS), superior temporal gyrus (STG), middle temporal gyrus (MTG), inferior temporal gyrus (ITG), and occipital cortex (OCC). Results are shown for left and right hemispheres (L, R) resulting from phonologic (PHON) and semantic (SEM) activations. (▤ = PHON L, ▥ = PHON R, ▨ = SEM L, ▨ = SEM R.) (From Shaywitz, B.A., Pugh, K.R., Constable, R.T., Shaywitz, S.E., Bronen, R.T., Fulbright, R.K., Shankweiler, D.P., Katz, L., Fletcher, J.M., Skudlarski, P., & Gore, J.C. [1995]. Localization of semantic processing using functional magnetic resonance imaging. *Human Brain Mapping, 2*, 154. Copyright © 1995 by John Wiley & Sons, Inc. Reprinted by permission of Wiley-Liss Inc., a subsidiary of John Wiley & Sons, Inc.)

Petersen et al. (1988) had subjects repeat nouns that were presented aurally or visually. As pointed out by Shaywitz and associates (Shaywitz, Pugh, et al., 1995), noun repetition differs from the semantic processing task in a number of respects, including the lack of a self-generative response and the confinement to a single class of words as contrasted with the crossover from nouns to verbs in the experimental task. To more closely approximate the generic task demands of semantic processing, Shaywitz, Pugh, et al. (1995) used a generative form of rhyming (i.e., phonological processing) as a comparison task (e.g., generate words that rhyme with *cat*). Other methodological issues include the use of covert responding, which mitigates movement artifact but precludes measurement of cognitive performance during the scan and thus raises a question of the subject's engagement in the task. In a study in which normal adults pressed a response bulb to indicate that pairs of visually displayed stimuli (e.g., rhymes, patterns of upper- and lower-case consonants, pairs of words that came from the same or different categories) had similar or different items, Shaywitz and colleagues (Shaywitz, Shaywitz, et al., 1995) found evidence that semantic processing activated both the inferior frontal and temporal regions bilaterally. An alternative strategy is to employ a foot pedal response, which mitigates movement artifact while providing a performance measure.

A detailed discussion of statistical methods for identifying task-specific, neuroanatomical regions of activation is beyond the scope of this chapter. However, it is appropriate to mention two major approaches, the region of interest method and statistical probability mapping. The region of interest method entails an a priori selection of anatomically defined regions for comparison of the activation produced by the experimental and control conditions. In contrast, statistical probability mapping empirically identifies regions that exhibit significant differences in activation under the experimental and control conditions.

In summary, fMRI challenges the creativity and methodological rigor of investigators while offering the potential for elucidating mechanisms of recovery and development after brain injury in children. This technique could also be used to evaluate the effects of interventions, both in the acute stage and in the course of rehabilitation, on reorganization of function.

CONCLUSIONS

The neurobehavioral sequelae of pediatric CHI are often consistent with the presence of frontal lobe dysfunction. Not until the 1990s, however, has technology permitted a detailed examination of the relationship between lesion characteristics and the cognitive sequelae of CHI. Investigations using MRI to study head-injured children have found that focal brain pathology is common, that lesions are often present within the frontal lobes, and that the size and distribution of these frontal lesions are related to the severity of specific cognitive impairments.

Studies of head-injured children have shown that these patients often experience difficulties with problem-solving skills, cognitive flexibility, verbal discourse, and response inhibition. Some preliminary hypotheses can also be advanced regarding the interaction of these cognitive impairments with lesion location and developmental factors. For example, scores on COWA and semantic clustering from the CVLT are related to the size of right frontal lesions after controlling for overall severity of the head injury (Levin et al., 1993). Such findings suggest that the right frontal lobe makes a special contribution to the organization of verbal information in children, especially in view of the fact that categorization skills are thought to be important for both the initial learning and the retrieval of verbal material. These conclusions should be considered tentative, however, because they are based on exploratory analyses conducted with relatively small samples.

Another cognitive skill that has been examined in head-injured children is problem solving. The significant relationship between a problem-solving measure from the Tower of London test and the size of dorsolateral lesions, but not orbitofrontal lesions (Levin, Mendelsohn, et al., 1994), is consistent with reports that executive functions depend on the integrity of the dorsolateral frontal cortex (Kertesz, 1994). Orbitofrontal and white matter lesions, in contrast, were found to be related to the number of broken rules on the Tower of London test. The tendency to break rules on the Tower of London test may be secondary to impulsivity and behavioral disinhibition of the type reported in adults with orbitofrontal damage (Kertesz, 1994); but the nature of this rule-breaking behavior has not been explored, and it may be due to an attention deficit or other cognitive impairment. Levin and associates (Levin, Mendelsohn, et al., 1994) also presented some preliminary data suggesting that rule breaking on the Tower of London test is disproportionately severe in younger children. Again, more studies are needed to confirm and extend these findings because they are based on exploratory analyses.

Research using new brain imaging techniques, such as fMRI, has the potential to make substantial contributions to the study of head-injured children. These methods may provide explanations for the cognitive dysfunction that often persists following diffuse CHI, even in the absence of obvious abnormalities on structural MRI. Functional brain imaging techniques can also reveal changes over time in the regional pattern of metabolism and cerebral blood flow. Serial examination of these patterns may provide insights into mechanisms of recovery from injury, including the possible reorganization of brain function. Head injury is common in children, and the use of functional imaging with this population may characterize brain activity associated with lesions, recovery, and maturation. When used in combination with neuropsychological test results, these data will greatly expand the study of brain–behavior relationships in children.

REFERENCES

Adams, J.H., Doyle, D., Ford, I., Gennarelli, T.A., Graham, D.I., & McLellan, D.R. (1989). Diffuse axonal injury in head injury: Definition, diagnosis, and grading. *Histopathology, 15*, 49–59.

Adams, J.H., Graham, D.I., Scott, G., Parker, L.S., & Doyle, D. (1980). Brain damage in fatal non-missile head injury. *Journal of Clinical Pathology, 33*, 1132–1145.

Alajouanine, T., & Lhermitte, F. (1965). Acquired aphasia in children. *Brain, 88*, 653–662.

Alexander, M.P., Benson, D.F., & Stuss, D.T. (1989). Frontal lobes and language. *Brain and Language, 37*, 656–691.

Benson, D.F., Stuss, D.T., Naeser, M.A., Weir, W.C., Kaplan, E.F., & Levine, H. (1981). The long-term effects of prefrontal leukotomy. *Archives of Neurology, 38*, 165–169.

Benton, A.L. (1968). Differential behavioral effects in frontal lobe disease. *Neuropsychologia, 6*, 53–60.

Benton, A.L., & Hamsher, K. deS. (1978). *Multilingual aphasia examination.* Iowa City, IA: AHA Associates.

Berryhill, P., Lilly, M.A., Levin, H.S., Hillman, G., Mendelsohn, D., Brunder, D.G., Fletcher, J.M., Kufera, J., Kent, T.A., Yeakley, J., Bruce, D., & Eisenberg, H.M. (1995). Frontal lobe changes after severe diffuse closed head injury in children: A volumetric study of magnetic resonance imaging. *Neurosurgery, 37*, 392–400.

Binder, J.R., Rao, S.M., Hammeke, T.A., Yetkin, F.Z., Jesmanowicz, A., Bandettini, P.A., Wong, E.C., Estkowski, L.D., Goldstein, M.D., Haughton, V.M., & Hyde, J.S. (1994). Functional magnetic resonance imaging of human auditory cortex. *Annals of Neurology, 35*, 662–672.

Blumbergs, P., Jones, N., & North, J. (1989). Diffuse axonal injury in head trauma. *Journal of Neurology, Neurosurgery, and Psychiatry, 52*, 938–941.

Blumer, D., & Benson, D.F. (1975). Personality changes with frontal and temporal lobe lesions. In D.F. Benson & D. Blumer (Eds.), *Psychiatric aspects of neurological disease* (pp. 151–170). New York: Grune & Stratton.

Brown, G., Chadwick, O., Shaffer, D., Rutter, M., & Traub, M. (1981). A prospective study of children with head injuries: III. Psychiatric sequelae. *Psychological Medicine, 11*, 63–78.

Bruce, D.A., Raphaely, R.C., Goldberg, A.I., Zimmerman, R.A., Bilaniuk, L.T., Schut, L., & Kuhl, D.E. (1979). Pathophysiology, treatment and outcome following severe head injury in children. *Child's Brain, 5*, 174–191.

Bruce, D.A., Schut, L., Bruno, L.A., Wood, J.H., & Sutton, L.N. (1978). Outcome following severe head injuries in children. *Journal of Neurosurgery, 48*, 679–688.

Chapman, S.B., Culhane, K.A., Levin, H.S., Harward, H., Mendelsohn, D., Ewing-Cobbs, L., Fletcher, J.M., & Bruce, D. (1992). Narrative discourse after closed head injury in children and adolescents. *Brain and Language, 43*, 42–65.

Chapman, S.B., Levin, H.S., Wanek, A., Weyrauch, J., & Kufera, J. (in press). Discourse after closed head injury in young children. *Brain and Language.*

Damasio, H.C. (1991). Neuroanatomy of frontal lobe in vivo: A comment on methodology. In H.S. Levin, H.M. Eisenberg, & A.L. Benton (Eds.), *Frontal lobe function and dysfunction* (pp. 92–121). New York: Oxford University Press.

Delis, D.C., Kramer, J.H., Kaplan, E., & Ober, B.A. (1987). *California Verbal Learning Test–research edition.* New York: Psychological Corporation.

Demonet, J.F., Chollet, F., Ramsey, S., Cardebat, D., Nespoulous, J.L., Wise, R., Rascol, A., & Frackowiak, R. (1992). The anatomy of phonological and semantic processing in normal subjects. *Brain, 115*, 1753–1768.

Dennis, M., & Barnes, M.A. (1990). Knowing the meaning, getting the point, bridging the gap, and carrying the message: Aspects of discourse following closed head injury in childhood and adolescence. *Brain and Language, 39*, 428–446.

Diamond, A. (1985). Development of the ability to use recall to guide action, as indicated by infants' performance on AB. *Child Development, 56*, 868–883.

Diamond, A. (1991). Guidelines for the study of brain–behavior relationships during development. In H.S. Levin, H.M. Eisenberg, & A.L. Benton (Eds.), *Frontal lobe function and dysfunction* (pp. 339–378). New York: Oxford University Press.

Diamond, A., & Doar, B. (1989). The performance of human infants on a measure of frontal cortex function, the delayed response task. *Developmental Psychobiology, 22*, 272–294.

Drewe, E.A. (1975). Go–no go learning after frontal lobe lesions in humans. *Cortex, 11*, 8–16.

Eslinger, P.J., Grattan, L.M., Damasio, H., & Damasio, A.R. (1992). Developmental consequences of childhood frontal lobe damage. *Archives of Neurology, 49*, 764–769.

Ewing-Cobbs, L., Fletcher, J.M., Landry, S.H., & Levin, H.S. (1985). Language disorders after pediatric head injury. In J.K. Darby (Ed.), *Speech and language evaluation in neurology: Childhood disorders* (pp. 97–111). San Diego, CA: Grune & Stratton.

Faden, A.I., Demediuk, P., Panter, S., & Vink, R. (1989). The role of excitatory amino acids and NMDA receptors in traumatic brain injury. *Science, 244*, 798–800.

Filipek, P.A., Kennedy, D.N., & Caviness, V.S. (1992). Neuroimaging in child neuropsychology. In I. Rapin & S.J. Segalowitz (Eds.), *Handbook of neuropsychology: Vol. 6. Child neuropsychology* (pp. 301–329). New York: Elsevier Science Publishers.

Goldman, P.S., & Alexander, G.E. (1977). Maturation of prefrontal cortex in the monkey revealed by focal reversible cryogenic depression. *Nature, 267*, 613–615.

Goldman, P.S., & Rosvold, H.E. (1970). Localization of function within the dorsolateral prefrontal cortex of the rhesus monkey. *Experimental Neurology, 27*, 291–304.

Goldman, P.S., Rosvold, H.E., Vest, B., & Galkin, T.W. (1971). Analysis of the delayed alternation deficit produced by dorsolateral prefrontal lesions in the rhesus monkey. *Journal of Comparative and Physiological Psychology, 77*, 212–220.

Goldman-Rakic, P.S. (1987). Development of cortical circuitry and cognitive function. *Child Development, 58*, 601–622.

Graham, D.I., Ford, I., Adams, J.H., Doyle, D., Lawrence, A.E., McLellan, D.R., & Ng, H.K. (1989). Fatal head injury in children. *Journal of Clinical Pathology, 42*, 18–22.

Grattan, L.M., & Eslinger, P.J. (1992). Long-term psychological consequences of childhood frontal lobe lesion in patient DT. *Brain and Cognition, 20*, 185–195.

Heaton, R.K., Chelune, G.H., Talley, J.L., Kay, G.G., & Curtiss, G. (1993). *Wisconsin Card Sorting Test*. Odessa, FL: Psychological Assessment Resources.

Hécaen, H. (1976). Acquired aphasia in children and the ontogenesis of hemispheric functional specialization. *Brain and Language, 3*, 114–134.

Humayun, M.S., Presty, S.K., Lafrance, N.D., Holcomb, H.H., Loats, H., Long, D.M., Wagner, H.N., & Gordon, B. (1989). Local glucose abnormalities in mild closed head injured patients with cognitive impairments. *Nuclear Medicine Communications, 10*, 335–344.

Ichise, M., Chung, D.-G., Wang, P., Wortzman, G., Gray, B.G., & Franks, W. (1994). Technetium-99m-HMPAO SPECT, CT and MRI in the evaluation of patients with chronic traumatic brain injury: A correlation with neuropsychological performance. *Journal of Nuclear Medicine, 35*, 217–226.

Jennett, B., & Bond, M. (1975). Assessment of outcome after severe brain damage. *Lancet, 1*, 480–487.

Jones-Gotman, M., & Milner, B. (1977). Design fluency: The invention of nonsense drawings after focal cortical lesions. *Neuropsychologia, 15*, 653–674.

Kaczmarck, B.L.J. (1984). Neurolinguistic analysis of verbal utterances in patients with focal lesions of the frontal lobes. *Brain and Language, 21*, 52–58.

Kertesz, A. (1994). Frontal lesions and function. In A. Kertesz (Ed.), *Localization and neuroimaging in neuropsychology* (pp. 567–598). New York: Academic Press.

Kraus, J.F., Rock, A., & Hemyari, P. (1990). Brain injuries among infants, children, adolescents, and young adults. *American Journal of Diseases of Children, 144*, 684–691.

Lenneberg, E.H., & Lenneberg, E. (1975). *Foundations of language development: A multidisciplinary approach*. New York: Academic Press.

Levin, H.S., Amparo, E.G., Eisenberg, H.M., Miner, M.E., High, W.M., Ewing-Cobbs, L., Fletcher, J.M., & Guinto, F.C. (1989). Magnetic resonance imaging after closed head injury in children. *Neurosurgery, 24,* 223–227.

Levin, H.S., Amparo, E., Eisenberg, H.M., Williams, D.H., High, W.M., McArdle, C.B., & Weiner, R.L. (1987). Magnetic resonance imaging and computerized tomography in relation to the neurobehavioral sequelae of mild and moderate head injuries. *Journal of Neurosurgery, 66,* 706–713.

Levin, H.S., Culhane, K.A., Fletcher, J.M., Mendelsohn, D.B., Lilly, M.A., Harward, H., Chapman, S.B., Bruce, D.A., Bertolino-Kusnerik, L., & Eisenberg, H.M. (1994). Dissociation between delayed alternation and memory after pediatric head injury: Relationship to MRI findings. *Journal of Child Neurology, 9,* 81–89.

Levin, H.S., Culhane, K.A., Hartman, J., Evankovich, K., Mattson, A.J., Harward, H., Ringholtz, G., Ewing-Cobbs, L., & Fletcher, J.M. (1991). Developmental changes in performance on tests of purported frontal lobe functioning. *Developmental Neuropsychology, 7,* 377–395.

Levin, H.S., Culhane, K.A., Mendelsohn, D., Lilly, M.A., Bruce, D., Fletcher, J.M., Chapman, S.B., Harward, H., & Eisenberg, H. (1993). Cognition in relation to magnetic resonance imaging in head-injured children and adolescents. *Archives of Neurology, 50,* 897–905.

Levin, H.S., Eisenberg, H.M., Wigg, N.R., & Kobayashi, K. (1982). Memory and intellectual ability after head injury in children and adolescents. *Neurosurgery, 11,* 668–673.

Levin, H., & Kraus, M.F. (1994). The frontal lobes and traumatic brain injury. *Journal of Neuropsychiatry, 6,* 443–454.

Levin, H.S., Mendelsohn, D., Lilly, M.A., Fletcher, J.M., Culhane, K.A., Chapman, S.B., Harward, H., Kusnerik, L., Bruce, D., & Eisenberg, H.M. (1994). Tower of London performance in relation to magnetic resonance imaging following closed head injury in children. *Neuropsychology, 8,* 171–179.

Mattson, A.J., & Levin, H.S. (1990). Frontal lobe dysfunction following closed head injury: A review of the literature. *Journal of Nervous and Mental Disease, 178,* 282–291.

Meadows, A.T., Massari, D.J., Fergusson, J., Gordon, J., Littman, P., & Moss, K. (1981). Declines in IQ scores and cognitive dysfunction in children with acute lymphocytic leukaemia treated with cranial irradiation. *Lancet, 2,* 1015–1018.

Mendelsohn, D., Levin, H.S., Bruce, D., Lilly, M., Harward, H., Culhane, K.A., & Eisenberg, H.M. (1992). Late MRI after head injury in children: Relationship to clinical features and outcome. *Child's Nervous System, 8,* 445–452.

Milner, B. (1964). Some effects of frontal lobectomy in man. In J.M. Warren & K. Akert (Eds.), *The frontal granular cortex and behavior* (pp. 313–314). New York: McGraw-Hill.

Newton, M.R., Greenwood, R.J., Britton, K.E., Charlesworth, M., Nimmon, C.C., Carroll, M.J., & Dolke, G. (1992). A study comparing SPECT with CT and MRI after closed head injury. *Journal of Neurology, Neurosurgery, and Psychiatry, 55,* 92–94.

Passler, M.A., Isaac, W., & Hynd, G.W. (1985). Neuropsychological development of behavior attributed to frontal lobe functioning in children. *Developmental Neuropsychology, 1,* 349–370.

Perret, E. (1974). The left frontal lobe of man and the suppression of habitual responses in verbal categorical behavior. *Neuropsychologia, 12,* 323–330.

Petersen, S.E., Fox, P.T., Posner, M.I., Mintum, M., & Raichle, M.E. (1988). Positron emission tomographic studies of the cortical anatomy of single-word processing. *Nature, 331,* 585–589.

Petrides, M., & Milner, B. (1982). Deficits on subject-ordered tasks after frontal- and temporal-lobe lesions in man. *Neuropsychologia, 20,* 249–262.

Posner, M.I., Petersen, S.E., Fox, P.T., & Raichle, M.E. (1988). Localization of cognitive operations in the human brain. *Science, 240,* 1627–1631.

Prayer, L., Wimberger, D., Oder, W., Kramer, J., Schindler, E., Podreka, I., & Imhof, H. (1993). Cranial MR imaging and cerebral ^{99m}Tc HM-PAO-SPECT in patients with subacute or chronic severe closed head injury and normal CT examinations. *Acta Radiologica, 34,* 593–599.

Price, B.H., Daffner, K.R., Stowe, R.M., & Mesulam, M.M. (1990). The comportmental learning disabilities of early frontal lobe damage. *Brain, 113,* 1383–1393.

Rutter, M. (1981). Psychological sequelae of brain damage in children. *American Journal of Psychiatry, 138*, 1533–1544.

Shallice, T. (1982). Specific impairments in planning. *Philosophical Transactions of the Royal Society of London, 289*, 199–209.

Shaywitz, B.A., Pugh, K.R., Constable, R.T., Shaywitz, S.E., Bronen, R.T., Fulbright, R.K., Shankweiler, D.P., Katz, L., Fletcher, J.M., Skudlarski, P., & Gore, J.C. (1995). Localization of semantic processing using functional magnetic resonance imaging. *Human Brain Mapping, 2*, 149–158.

Shaywitz, B.A., Shaywitz, S.E., Pugh, K.R., Constable, R.T., Skudlarski, P., Fulbright, R.K., Bronen, R.A., Fletcher, J.M., Shankweiler, D.P., Katz, L., & Gore, J.C. (1995). Sex differences in the functional organization of the brain for language. *Nature, 373*, 607–608.

Snow, R.B., Zimmerman, R.D., Gandy, S.E., & Deck, M.D.F. (1986). Comparison of magnetic resonance imaging and computed tomography in the evaluation of head injury. *Neurosurgery, 18*, 45–52.

St. James-Roberts, I. (1979). Neurological plasticity, recovery from brain insult, and child development. In H.W. Reese & L.P. Lipsitt (Eds.), *Advances in child development and behavior* (pp. 253–319). New York: Academic Press.

Strich, S.J. (1961). Shearing of nerve fibers as a cause of brain damage due to head injury: A pathological study of twenty cases. *Lancet, 2*, 443–448.

Stuss, D.T., & Benson, D.F. (1986). *The frontal lobes*. New York: Raven Press.

Stuss, D.T., Ely, P., Hugenholtz, H., Richard, M.T., LaRochelle, S., Poirier, C.A., & Bell, I. (1985). Subtle neuropsychological deficits in patients with good recovery after closed head injury. *Neurosurgery, 17*, 41–47.

Teasdale, G., & Jennett, B. (1974). Assessment of coma and impaired consciousness: A practical scale. *Lancet, 2*, 81–84.

Wechsler, D. (1974). *Weschler Intelligence Scale for Children–Revised*. New York: Psychological Corp.

Wilberger, J.E., Deeb, Z., & Rothfus, W. (1987). Magnetic resonance imaging in cases of severe head injury. *Neurosurgery, 20*, 571–576.

Wilson, J.T.L., Wiedmann, K.D., Hadley, D.M., Condon, B., Teasdale, G., & Brooks, D.N. (1988). Early and late magnetic resonance imaging and neuropsychological outcome after head injury. *Journal of Neurology, Neurosurgery, and Psychiatry, 51*, 391–396.

Appendix: Test Glossary

A$\overline{B}$

The A$\overline{B}$ is a test adapted from experimental tasks used in behavioral research with nonhuman primates (Diamond, 1991). At the beginning of the test, the subject is seated between two identical hiding wells. The examiner holds up an object of interest to the subject, and, as the subject watches, the object is placed into one of the two wells. Both hiding wells are then covered simultaneously, and a brief delay of 0–10 seconds is imposed during which the subject is prevented from removing, moving toward, or looking at the well covers. After the delay, the subject is allowed to reach for the well, and, in the case of a correct response, the subject is permitted to retrieve the object as a reward. On the next and subsequent trials, the object is placed in the same well until the subject is correct to a specified criterion, usually two correct responses; then the reward is hidden in the other well, and the procedure is repeated.

California Verbal Learning Test (CVLT)

The CVLT is designed to assess the recall and recognition of word lists over a number of trials, as well as the associated memory strategies, processes, and errors (Delis, Kramer, Kaplan, & Ober, 1987). Each of the 16 words in each CVLT list belongs to one of four categories of "shopping list" items: names of fruits, herbs and spices, articles of clothing, and tools. The semantic clustering index indicates the degree to which words from the same category are listed consecutively during the subject's free recall.

Controlled Oral Word Association (COWA)

Several different types of verbal fluency tests are in use, but COWA is one of the most popular. It consists of three word-naming trials during which the subject is given 1 minute to name words that start with a specified letter of the alphabet (Benton & Hamsher, 1978). The score is calculated by adding the number of words produced for each trial.

Delayed Alternation

Delayed alternation is a simple problem-solving test utilizing an apparatus that consists of two drawers and a curtain that hangs between the subject and the examiner to hide the drawers from the subject's view (Levin et al., 1991). On each trial, a coin is hidden in one of the drawers, and the subject selects the drawer that is thought to hold the coin. If the choice is correct, the examiner places a coin in the opposite drawer on the next trial; if incorrect, the coin is left on the same side on subsequent trials until the subject makes the correct choice. The task is discontinued when the subject correctly identifies 12 alternations of the coin, and both the number of errors and number of trials to criterion are scored.

Delayed Response

This test is identical to the $A\overline{B}$ test described earlier, except that the hiding location of the reward is varied randomly according to a predetermined schedule (Diamond, 1991).

Design Fluency

The design fluency test is a nonverbal analogue of the various word fluency tests that requires the creation of drawings that do not represent objects or nameable abstract forms (Jones-Gotman & Milner, 1977). The subject is initially given 3 minutes to produce different drawings that do not violate these rules. Afterward, the task is repeated with an additional restriction limiting each design to only four straight or curved lines. Scores are often reported for the total number of correct drawings, as well as the number of perseverative and nonperseverative errors.

Glasgow Coma Scale (GCS)

The GCS was developed to describe altered states of consciousness associated with brain injury (Teasdale & Jennett, 1974). The total GCS score ranges from 3 to 15 points and is based on the sum of three scales that independently assess different components of wakefulness: the type of stimulus required to induce eye opening, the subject's best motor response, and the best verbal response. According to commonly applied criteria, *coma* is defined as the absence of eye opening, an inability to obey commands, and the failure to produce recognizable words. This definition corresponds to a GCS score of 8 or less.

Glasgow Outcome Scale (GOS)

The GOS is a rating scale that classifies outcome into one of five categories: death, persistent vegetative state, severe disability, moderate disability, and good recovery (Jennett & Bond, 1975). Although originally developed for use with adults, the GOS criteria are sometimes modified for use with children.

Go–No Go

The Go–No Go test is a computerized test of problem solving and inhibitory control (Drewe, 1975). The subject is seated at the display and is instructed to press a computer key when presented with a red light (Go) and to withhold the response when presented with a blue light (No Go). The test continues until the subject performs 10 consecutive correct responses, with the score consisting of the number of trials required to reach this criterion.

Tower of London

Developed to study sequential planning, the Tower of London test requires the subject to rearrange colored beads on vertical rods to match a model (Shallice, 1982). Scores obtained from the Tower of London test often include the total percentage of problems solved, the percentage of problems solved within the first three trials, the number of broken rules (e.g., attempting to move more than one bead at a time), and latency from the beginning of the trial until the first move is initiated (i.e., "planning time").

Wechsler Intelligence Scale for Children–Revised (WISC–R)

The WISC–R is a standardized intelligence test that covers an age range from 6 years to 16 years, 11 months (Wechsler, 1974). In addition to providing a Full-Scale intelligence quotient (IQ), the 14 subtests on the WISC–R are divided into two groups that are used to derive separate Verbal and Performance IQ scores. The Vocabulary and Similarities subtests are on the Verbal Scale. Items on the Vocabulary subtest assess the ability to generate word definitions, and the Similarities subtest is a measure of verbal concept formation that requires the subject to explain what each of a pair of words has in common. The Picture Completion subtest is part of the Performance Scale; it assesses the subject's ability to identify the missing part in each of a series of drawings. The Coding subtest, also on the Performance Scale, requires the rapid transcription of symbols.

Wisconsin Card Sorting Test (WCST)

The WCST is a test of problem solving and set shifting that requires the subject to match cards on which are printed drawings of one to four colored geometric shapes (Heaton, Chelune, Talley, Kay, & Curtiss, 1993). The cards can be matched on each of three different stimulus characteristics, however, and the subject must use feedback from the examiner (i.e., whether the cards are matched correctly) to determine whether the current matching principle is based on the color, shape, or number of drawings on the cards. The matching principle is changed every time the subject completes a run of 10 consecutive correct sorts. A variety of measures can be calculated from the WCST, but the number of perseverative errors and the number of categories achieved are most widely used. The number of categories achieved reflects the subject's ability to consistently sort to a single matching principle for a run of 10 cards.

Development of the Prefrontal Cortex: Evolution, Neurobiology, and Behavior
edited by Norman A. Krasnegor, Ph.D., G. Reid Lyon, Ph.D.,
and Patricia S. Goldman-Rakic, Ph.D.
copyright © 1997   Paul H. Brookes Publishing Co., Inc.
Baltimore • London • Toronto • Sydney

12

Dimensions of Executive Functions in Normal and Abnormal Development

Bruce F. Pennington _____

There is increasing interest within the field of developmental neuropsychology in using the functions of the prefrontal cortex (PFC) to understand many aspects of both normal and abnormal development. This work has considerable promise, but it is important to bear in mind that much of it rests on a "frontal metaphor" that involves finding a similarity between the behavioral symptoms or cognitive test performances, or both, of some group of individuals, either at a particular developmental stage or with a given behavioral disorder, and the behavioral symptoms or cognitive test performances, or both, of humans or other animals with acquired frontal lesions. I use the term *metaphor* because an analogy rather than a homology is involved; we rarely know that actual structural or neurochemical differences in the PFC underlie the behavioral similarity. In this chapter, I consider conceptual and empirical issues that must be dealt with in order for the frontal metaphor to fulfill its promise.

Next, I briefly consider three examples of the promise of the frontal metaphor for explaining a wide range of developmental phenomena. Dempster (1992) argued that prefrontally mediated inhibitory processes play a major role in cognitive development in both youth and age. Duncan (1995) argued that prefrontally mediated goal management underlies both dual task performance and fluid intelligence; he presented evidence that 1) normal adults with lower fluid intelligence exhibit considerable goal neglect in a simple dual task, and 2) adults with focal frontal lesions also exhibit goal neglect on this dual task and have fluid intelligence scores consid-

This chapter was supported by National Institute of Child Health and Human Development Grants P50 HD27802 (Differential Diagnosis in Learning Disabilities) and P30 HD04024 (Center Grant for Research in Mental Retardation) and National Institute of Mental Health grants 5 K02 MH00419 (RSA) (Genotype and Phenotype Analyses of Familial Dyslexia), 5 R37 MH38820 (MERIT) (The Linguistic Phenotype in Familial Dyslexia), and R01 MH45916 (The Neurocognitive, Emotional and Physical Phenotype of Fragile X Females).

The author extends thanks to Chris Aman, Loisa Bennetto, and Rob Roberts for sharing some of the data presented here.

erably lower than would be predicted by their scores on more crystallized IQ measures, such as the Wechsler Adult Intelligence Scale–Revised (Wechsler, 1981). Pennington (1994b) argued that the working memory function of the PFC begins to provide an integrated account of cognitive differences, whether developmental or individual, or normal or abnormal.

Each of these authors is essentially using a frontal metaphor to integrate cognitive phenomena ordinarily studied by separate research traditions. Therefore, the frontal metaphor is potentially quite powerful because it promises to explain both developmental and individual cognitive differences across the life span with a common theoretical framework based in neuroscience. Achieving such a unified account in psychology would be a major accomplishment because our field generally lacks universal theories such as those found in physics, and earlier attempts to provide such theories in psychology have been mostly disappointing. Neuroscience may change that because it holds the promise of integrating psychology with both biology and the rest of science.

In this chapter, I try to make a small step toward the goal of providing a unified account of cognitive differences by 1) examining the scope and limits of the frontal metaphor in developmental neuropsychology, 2) providing some data on dimensions of executive functions in normal and abnormal development, and 3) discussing implications for future research.

SCOPE AND LIMITS OF THE FRONTAL METAPHOR

As discussed, the scope of application of the frontal metaphor is quite broad; it has been applied to the behavior of normal young children and normal older adults; individuals with lower but still normal IQ scores; and individuals with a number of different developmental disorders, including attention-deficit/hyperactivity disorder (ADHD), conduct disorder, autism, Tourette syndrome, schizophrenia, fragile X syndrome, and early-treated phenylketonuria (PKU). I would argue that only in the case of the last disorder, early-treated PKU, do we have strong evidence for an underlying neurological mechanism in PFC that causes the observed cognitive deficit. For the other populations listed, there is at best correlative neurological evidence or none at all.

A broad scope of application of the frontal metaphor is partly justified by the diversity of behaviors and cognitive tests found to be impaired after frontal lesions. Briefly, several distinct frontal syndromes are now commonly recognized corresponding to lesions in different parts of the PFC. Three of these most prominently affect social behavior, although the traditional social-versus-cognitive distinction is particularly misleading in the case of PFC functions. Medial lesions are associated with a syndrome of *akinetic mutism*, in which there is a profound deficit in the initiation of speech and other spontaneous behavior, apparently resulting from a defect in the experience and expression of emotion rather than from an aphasia or motor deficit. Individuals with this syndrome appear to lack affect and motivation and, in fact, apparently experience little of either, based on their postrecovery reports. They can, however, repeat speech and perform actions on command (Damasio & Van Hoesen, 1983). Overlapping somewhat with this syndrome is an *apathetic* (Fuster, 1989), or *pseudodepressed* (Stuss & Benson, 1986), *syndrome* in which there is reduced awareness, lack of initiative, unconcern, and blunting of emotional responses. This syndrome is produced by either medial lesions or lesions to the anterior convexity, frontal poles, or both. Orbital lesions are associated with a *euphoric syndrome* (Fuster, 1989), or *pseudopsychopathic syndrome* (Stuss & Benson, 1986), in which there is sporadic hypomania, childish humor or facetiousness, disinhibition of sexual and eating behavior, lack of concern for others, and disregard for ethical principles. Fuster (1989) categorized the more cognitive effects of PFC lesions into 1) disorders of attention and perception; 2) disorders of motility, including hypokinesis and hyperkinesis; and 3) disorders of temporal integration. These cognitive effects are associated with (but not restricted to) dorsolateral lesions.

In sum, this list of frontal syndromes makes it amply clear that the scope of the frontal metaphor provides analogies for several distinct behavioral pathologies. In terms of the developmental disorders listed previously, the pseudopsychopathic syndrome provides a fairly close analogy for conduct disorder, akinetic mutism and the apathetic syndrome provide some similarities to autism, and hyperkinesis and disorders of attention provide an analogy for ADHD. The main analogy for Tourette syndrome is the deficit in inhibition observed after some frontal lesions.

In terms of tests of frontal or executive functions, the list is also quite broad and includes measures that are quite heterogeneous in their surface characteristics (Table 12.1). As can be seen, not all of these measures have been validated empirically as being prefrontal. Although this table provides some provisional categories of executive functions, these are mainly heuristic and need further empirical validation, some of which is provided later in this chapter.

As already discussed, the value of this frontal metaphor is the promise that it holds of integration both across different areas of psychology and with neuroscience. Research based on this metaphor has already led to a clearer delineation of the neuropsychological phenotype in the various developmental disorders listed earlier, as well as in some of the normal populations to which it has been applied. This metaphor contains the promise that the primary cognitive cause of the distinctive symptoms in each of these populations can be identified and that this identification may help guide the search for the underlying brain mechanisms.

For this promise to be realized, however, we must recognize clearly some of the limitations of this metaphor as currently used and remedy those limitations with future theoretical and empirical work. In particular, there are six limitations, each of which can be thought of as a constraint that an adequate theoretical and empirical account of the role of executive functions in normal and abnormal development must satisfy. Addressing these limitations will help to refine the frontal metaphor and ultimately test its validity.

Unconstrained Metaphor
The list of behaviors and cognitive tests (Table 12.1) affected by PFC lesions is so broad that one can object that the frontal metaphor can be applied to practically any special population. To address this limitation, we need a better and more articulated theoretical characterization of the functions of the PFC. How many functions are there? Are they all executive functions? How do they interrelate? How localized are they? Besides answering these questions, this theoretical account will need to be computational and avoid the homunculus, which is a prominent weakness of the executive metaphor in the term *executive functions*. As Hebb (1939, 1945) recognized a long time ago, vague and purely metaphorical constructs such as "abstract attitude" or "power of synthesis" will not do. Most of our current theoretical constructs for describing the functions of the PFC suffer from the same problem.

Table 12.1.   Executive function measures

Measures	Basis[a]	Source
Set shifting		
Wisconsin Card Sorting Test	E, T	Milner (1963)
Trail Making Test, Part B	T, not E	Reitan (1958)
Contingency Naming Test	T	Taylor (1988)
Necker Cube	T	Gorenstein, Mammato, and Sandy (1989)
Intradimensional, extradimensional shift	T, E	Hughes, Russell, and Robbins (1994)
Planning		
Porteus mazes	E	Mettler (1952)
Cork out of burette	T, E	Klosowska (1976)
Tower of London	T, E	Shallice (1988)
Tower of Hanoi	T, E	Welsh, Pennington, Ozonoff, Rouse, and McCabe (1990)
Working memory		
Delayed Response	E, T	Goldman-Rakic (1987)
Delayed Alternation	E, T	Goldman-Rakic (1987)
Delayed Response Alternation	T, E	Weinberger, Berman, Gold, and Goldberg (1994)
Self-ordered pointing	T, E	Petrides and Milner (1982)
Sentence Span	T	Siegel and Ryan (1989)
Counting Span	T	Siegel and Ryan (1989)
Mental Counters	T	Larson and Sacuzzo (1989)
Sequential Matching Memory Test	T	Gorenstein et al. (1989)
Sequential Memory Test	T	Gorenstein et al. (1989)
Contextual memory		
Temporal order memory	T, E	Milner, Corsi, and Leonard (1991)
Source memory	T, E	Schacter (1987)
Inhibition		
Stroop test	E, T	Cohen and Servan-Schreiber (1992)
Go–No Go	T	Shue and Douglas (1992)
CPT AX	E, T	Cohen and Servan-Schreiber (1992)
Stopping task	T	Logan, Cowan, and Davis (1984)
Negative Priming task	T	Tipper (1985)
Antisaccade task	T, E	Guitton, Buchtel, and Douglas (1985)
Conflicting motor response	T	Shue and Douglas (1992)
Matching Familiar Figures Test (MFFT)	T	Kagan, Rosman, Day, Albert, and Phillips (1964)
Fluency		
Thurstone Word Fluency Test	T, E	Milner (1964)
Design fluency	T, E	Jones-Gotman and Milner (1977)

[a] "Basis" means the reason the task is considered to be an executive function task. Here T represents a theoretical and E an empirical study of prefrontal lesions or, more rarely, of prefrontal metabolism in normal adults. If T precedes E, then the task was first developed to test a theory of prefrontal function and then validated empirically. If E precedes T, the test was discovered to be sensitive to prefrontal lesions and then analyzed theoretically (usually in a computational model).

However, there has been some progress at providing a computational account of performance on some executive function tasks (e.g., Cohen & Servan-Schreiber, 1992; Kimberg & Farah, 1993). The seminal work of Goldman-Rakic (1987; see also

Chapter 2) and this modeling work have led to a clearer understanding that at least two cognitive processes, working memory and inhibition, underlie most behaviors and tasks associated with the PFC (Pennington, 1994b; Pennington, Bennetto, McAleer, & Roberts, 1996; Roberts, Hager, & Heron, 1994). It is already clear that different forms of inhibition must be recognized (Dempster & Brainerd, 1995), and some PFC researchers, such as Goldman-Rakic (1987; see also Chapter 2), argue for multiple working memory systems within the PFC.

Discriminant Validity Problem

Closely related to the problem of the broadness of the prefrontal metaphor is the discriminant validity problem, the impossibility that exactly the same executive deficit can be primary in all of the special populations to which the frontal metaphor has been applied. This problem and possible solutions to it are discussed at length in Pennington and Ozonoff (1996), which reviews studies of executive functions in four developmental psychopathologies: ADHD, conduct disorder, autism, and Tourette syndrome. That review makes it clear that the consistency, severity, and profile of executive function deficits vary across these four disorders, so the discriminant validity problem is not as acute as commonly supposed (e.g., Bishop, 1993). Specifically, consistent executive function deficits are found only in autism and ADHD, not in conduct disorder (without ADHD) or Tourette syndrome. Across autism and ADHD, there are clear differences in both the severity and the profile of executive function deficits observed; I present some data later that show these differences. Therefore, although executive function deficits may be found in many special populations, the severity and nature of those deficits are expected to vary across populations, as are the specific neural mechanisms underlying those deficits. Obviously, empirical progress in defining these differences will interact with theoretical progress in providing a more articulated and computational account of the functions of the PFC.

Effects of Early Focal PFC Lesions

Although the existing database is fairly small and may suffer from ascertainment biases, we already know that early focal lesions to the PFC have not been reported as causing some of the developmental disorders to which the frontal metaphor has been applied (see Pennington & Ozonoff, 1996; see also Chapter 14). Specifically, there is no report of such lesions causing autism, schizophrenia, or Tourette syndrome. In contrast, conduct-disordered behavior is a prominent sequela to such lesions, as are deficits on various executive function tasks. Studies of larger samples of children with early focal PFC lesions will be very fruitful for testing the role of the PFC in development. To account for the executive function deficits observed in populations with autism or schizophrenia, there may be lesions in neural systems closely connected to the PFC, such as the basal ganglia, or even diffuse lesions. Again, better specification of the effects of such extrafrontal lesions is required to rescue the frontal metaphor from becoming vacuous.

Direction of Effects

The executive function deficits identified in the various populations may not be primary (i.e., the proximal cognitive cause of the behaviors that distinguish a given population) but may instead be secondary to or correlated with some other primary cognitive cause. For instance, the primary deficit in autism might be in some social skill that produces social avoidance. Social avoidance in turn would lead to fewer social interactions. I would argue that social interactions provide unremitting practice in several executive functions. Reduced practice in turn would lead to worse executive function performance. Similar arguments could be advanced for the executive function deficits found in other populations.

Therefore, the basic issue is that the finding of executive function deficits in the various populations listed earlier is nearly always based on cross-sectional studies and, hence, has only correlational status. For some populations, we generally lack methods for testing causality. Longitudinal studies are always difficult to conduct and are particularly difficult in rare populations, such as children with autism. Even in studies of children with early focal lesions to the PFC, the data are only correlational, because we usually lack cognitive test results from before the lesion. Even with previous testing, it is difficult to completely exclude other causes for the apparent behavioral effects of the PFC lesion. A better understanding of neurobiological mechanisms can help remedy this problem because it can allow us to test dose–response relations and even sometimes manipulate the relevant neurobiological parameter. The classic example here is early-treated PKU, in which a relation between executive function deficits and dopamine depletion caused by elevated phenylalanine levels has been demonstrated (Diamond, Ciaramitaro, Donner, Djali, & Robinson, 1994). ADHD, because it responds to medications that affect dopamine transport, is also amenable to this strategy.

Heterogeneity
There are very likely neurological as well as cognitive subtypes within each of the populations to which the frontal metaphor has been applied. The deficits in some of these subtypes may be truly nonfrontal, both neurologically and cognitively. Others may be characterized by a combination of frontal and nonfrontal problems. Such heterogeneity, of course, will contribute to conflicting results across studies.

Nonfocal Lesions
The neurological mechanism in some or even in many of these populations may not be a focal one. Instead, it may be a diffuse structural or metabolic difference in brain development. Adult patients with diffuse lesions also fit the frontal metaphor. We do not understand whether this is because a diffuse lesion often includes the PFC or because disrupting the connectivity of the *whole* brain mimics some of the effects of a focal PFC lesion, or both. In our efforts to understand normal and abnormal development, it is important not to become too fixated on localizationist hypotheses, because variations in brain development are rarely localized. The rarity of localized changes in early brain development is both a problem and a promise because the findings from developmental neuropsychology may help us rethink a modular, localizationist view of how the brain works (Pennington, 1994a.)

DIMENSIONS OF EXECUTIVE FUNCTIONS
In this section, two empirical approaches are used to identify dimensions of executive functions: 1) factor analysis of a battery of executive function measures in an essentially normal population and 2) an examination of severity and profile differences in executive function performance across several abnormal populations. If the two methods converge on similar dimensions, then we can be more sure of the validity of the dimensions identified, although further experimental analysis would be needed to identify which cognitive components really define the empirically based dimensions.

Factor Analyses

In one program at the Colorado Learning Disability Research Center, we have administered measures of executive function, ADHD, and other psychiatric diagnoses to two large samples of twins, one in which at least one member of the twin pair has reading disability (RD sample) and one in which neither member of the twin pair has reading disability (control sample). The goal of this program is to use neuropsychological and behavior genetic analyses to understand the causal basis of the observed comorbidity between reading disability and several psychiatric disorders, including ADHD. For present purposes, we are merely interested in the factor structure of the executive function battery in these large samples. Because the factor structures were similar in both the RD and control samples and because children with reading disability for the most part do not have marked executive function problems, I present results from these two samples combined.

Subject Characteristics   In the RD sample, there were 80 monozygotic (MZ) pairs and 104 dizygotic (DZ) pairs; in the control sample, there were 40 MZ pairs and 45 DZ pairs. Table 12.2 presents data for three groups of individuals: 1) members of pairs both of whom had reading disability (RD), 2) co-twins of probands with reading disability who did not themselves have reading disability (Co-twins), and 3) control twins without reading disability (Control). As can be seen, these three groups were similar in age and sex ratio but different in Wechsler full-scale IQ (FSIQ) and reading skill (DISCR; see note *b* of Table 2 for explanation). RD individuals were lowest, Co-twins were next lowest, and Controls were highest on both

Table 12.2.   Twin study demographic variables by reading diagnosis

Measure	RD	Co-twins	Control
N	230	137	170
Zygosity			
MZ	116	43	80
DZ	114	94	90
Gender			
M	145	69	96
F	115	69	78
Age	10.75 (2.1)	10.91 (2.4)	10.95 (2.1)
FSIQ[a]	98.01 (10.3)	104.6 (10.6)	112.6 (10.4)***
			3 > 1,2; 2 > 1
DISCR[b]	−1.16 (.85)	.84 (.68)	1.26 (.85)***
			3 > 1,2; 2 > 1
EF 1[c]	−0.23 (1.05)	−.04 (.83)	.39 (.93)***
			3 > 1,2
EF 2[c]	−0.18 (.96)	−0.001 (1.1)	.28 (.95)***
			3 > 1,2

[a]Wechsler full-scale IQ.

[b]A weighted composite of the Reading Recognition, Reading Comprehension, and Spelling scores on the Peabody Individual Achievement Test that provided maximal separation between children with and without a history of reading problems in an earlier study.

[c]Executive function factor scores.

***$p < .001$.

variables, although the magnitude of the differences were greater for DISCR than for FSIQ. There was a difference of about .5 standard deviation (SD) in FSIQ both between RDs and Co-twins and between Co-twins and Controls. For DISCR, there was also a difference of about .5 SD between Co-twins and Controls, but RDs were a full 2 SD below Co-twins and about 2.5 SD below Controls. Therefore, the RD proband difference in DISCR greatly exceeded their difference in FSIQ.

Factor Analyses of Executive Function Batteries   For the entire data set, results of four executive function measures were available, the contingent version of the Continuous Performance Test, known as CPT AX; the Stopping task (Logan, Cowan, & Davis, 1984); the Wisconsin Card Sorting Test (WCST; Heaton, Chelune, Talley, Kay, & Curtiss, 1993); and the Contingency Naming Test (CNT; Taylor, 1988). The WCST is a measure of concept formation and set shifting, and the CPT AX is a classic measure of sustained attention. The Stopping task is an experimental measure of voluntary motor inhibition; subjects are given varying amounts of time (relative to their own reaction time) to inhibit an already programmed motor response. The CNT is a Strooplike task that does not require reading; subjects name either the color or the shape of a figure depending on contingency rules of varying complexity. The task requires set shifting because the subject must ignore cues based on an earlier rule to perform successfully.

We analyzed the one variable from each test that had proven maximally discriminating of clinical groups from controls in previous research. We used false alarms from the CPT AX, percent correct rejections from the Stopping task, percent perseverative responses from the WCST, and total errors and self-corrections on part B of the CNT. Each variable was tested for deviations from normality and log-transformed if necessary. A principal components factor analysis with varimax rotation was then performed. As can be seen in Table 12.3, two factors emerged that together accounted for 63% of the variance. The CPT AX and the Stopping task loaded on the first factor, which we labeled "Inhibition," and the WCST and the CNT loaded on the second factor, which we labeled "Set Shifting."

For a subset of subjects (n = 145), an additional four executive function measures were given, including two working memory measures, Sentence Span and Counting Span, as well as the Stroop Test and the Trail Making Test (time on Part B minus time on Part A). The Trail Making Test (Reitan, 1958) requires the subject to draw connecting lines between randomly arrayed dots in the correct order, either a simple numerical sequence (in Part A) or an alternating numerical and alphabetical sequence (in Part B). The latter two measures were added because some previous studies reviewed earlier had found them to be sensitive to ADHD; the former

Table 12.3.   Factor analysis of executive function measures in whole sample[a]

	Factor 1 (Inhibition)	Factor 2 (Set Shifting)
CPT AX	.824	−.111
Stopping task	.716	.268
WCST	−.124	.835
CNT	.304	.653

[a]These two factors accounted for 62.7% of the variance in a principal components factor analysis with varimax rotation.

two measures were added because we wished to tap other dimensions of executive function. In this factor analysis, we also included several discriminant measures: Digit Span, the Wechsler and Raven IQ tests, and our reading measure (DISCR). A principal components factor analysis with varimax rotation was performed.

As shown in Table 12.4, four factors emerged, accounting for 59% of the variance. The results from the larger analysis (Table 12.3) were maintained; once again, the Stopping task and CPT AX loaded on a separate Inhibition factor, and the WCST and the CNT loaded on a second factor, Set Shifting or Cognitive Flexibility, which also includes the two IQ measures and the Stroop. Therefore, the Inhibition factor appears to be relatively independent of IQ, but the Set Shifting factor does not. Indeed, Set Shifting is related to a classic measure of fluid intelligence (Raven's Matrices), consistent with the work of Duncan (1995) and others relating executive function to fluid intelligence. One additional dimension of executive function was identified in this analysis, a Working Memory factor on which all three span tasks loaded. Finally, the Trail Making Test loaded on the same factor as the DISCR reading measure (Trails/DISCR). In sum, these factor analyses indicate that we have succeeded in measuring at least three distinguishable dimensions of executive function, which we have labeled Inhibition, Set Shifting, and Working Memory. I later examine which of these dimensions of executive function is related to ADHD, autism, and fragile X syndrome in women.

The overall finding that executive function batteries administered to normal children do not have a unitary factor structure replicates the results of other studies (Levin, Eisenberg, & Benton, 1991; Welsh, Pennington, & Groisser, 1991). Therefore, these results provide empirical validation of the hypothesis that there are distinguishable dimensions of executive function. The current results are also consistent with the theoretical analyses discussed earlier in distinguishing working memory and inhibition as somewhat separate dimensions of executive function, although it is a mistake to consider them as independent cognitive processes, because manipulating working memory load affects the ability to inhibit (Roberts et al., 1994). These results also indicate that the relation between fluid intelligence

Table 12.4. Factor analysis of executive function measures in subsample ($n = 145$)[a]

	Factor 1 (Working Memory)	Factor 2 (Set Shifting)	Factor 3 (Trails/DISCR)	Factor 4 (Inhibition)
Sentence span	.79	.13	−.05	−.15
Counting span	.75	.25	−.05	−.14
Digit span	.70	.09	.34	.15
WCST	−.11	−.74	.25	.00
Raven's Matrices	.14	.70	.28	−.03
FSIQ	.18	.65	.37	−.07
CNT	−.32	−.63	.11	.26
Stroop	−.08	.35	.20	.15
Trail (B−A) Making	.05	−.05	−.77	.10
DISCR	.47	.16	.62	−.13
CPT AX	.00	−.16	−.10	.87
Stopping task	.43	−.20	.12	−.53

[a]These four factors accounted for 59% of the variance in a principal components factor analysis with varimax rotation.

(measured here by the Raven's Matrices) and dimensions of executive function is not uniform, but instead is stronger for the dimension we have labeled Set Shifting, or Cognitive Flexibility, on which the WCST and CNT load.

Of course, labeling a factor is not the same thing as identifying an underlying cognitive component; that is the weakness of factor analysis. Experimental analyses are needed to uncover which underlying cognitive components actually differentiate these dimensions. Another validity test for the dimensions found here is to see if they are dissociable in populations with abnormal executive function development; I next present data bearing on this question.

Comparisons Across Disorders

This section presents data from our studies for two molar executive function tasks, the WCST and the Tower of Hanoi, as well as two measures of verbal working memory (Sentence Span and Counting Span) and a measure of voluntary motor inhibition (the Stopping task) across three disorders: ADHD, autism, and fragile X syndrome in women. Unfortunately, in our studies, we do not have results for all measures on all groups. However, data are available from other studies to complete the critical contrasts. These measures (except for the Tower of Hanoi) span the three factors identified in the factor analyses just presented. The Tower of Hanoi loaded on a distinct factor in two earlier factor analyses of executive function tests (Levin et al., 1991; Welsh et al., 1991), so, by extrapolation, we could argue that four executive function dimensions are included here: Planning, Set Shifting, Working Memory, and Inhibition. Therefore, we can examine both severity and profile differences in the executive function impairments in each disorder. The characteristics of the samples are given in Table 12.5. For all but the Tower of Hanoi comparison in women with fragile X syndrome, the experimental and control groups were matched on IQ.

For the WCST (number of perseverative responses), there were clear severity differences across the three groups (Figure 12.1). Individuals with autism were most impaired relative to controls; individuals with ADHD were the least impaired, and women with fragile X were intermediate. The results for ADHD and autism are similar to those found in a meta-analysis of all published studies of executive function measures in those two groups (Pennington & Ozonoff, 1996).

In that meta-analysis, 8 of 10 studies found significant differences on the WCST between the group with autism and controls (most of whom were IQ-matched); the mean effect size (d) was 1.06, which qualifies as a "large effect" (Cohen, 1992). This result means that individuals with autism perform on average 1 SD below IQ expectation on the WCST. Their average number of perseverative responses (about 60; see Figure 12.1) means that, as a group, they were perseverating on nearly half of the 128 trials in this measure. This is a remarkable degree of cognitive inflexibility, which is also found on other measures that have been given to this group, including experimental measures that better isolate the component of cognitive flexibility (Hughes, Russell, & Robbins, 1994; Ozonoff, Strayer, McMahon, & Filloux, 1994).

In contrast, only 4 of 10 studies found a significant difference between the ADHD group and controls on the WCST; the mean effect size was only .45. Therefore, in contrast to autism, cognitive inflexibility is not the principal executive function deficit in ADHD.

For the Tower of Hanoi, a measure of planning, significant differences were found for all three groups considered here (Figure 12.2). However, there were once

Table 12.5.   Characteristics of groups with developmental disorders

Study	N	Age	SD	IQ	SD	Measures[a]
ADHD (non-RD)						
Pennington, Groisser, and Welsh (1993)						
Experimental	16	8.7	(1.0)	103.3	(17.7)	WCST, TOH
Control	23	8.8	(0.9)	111.7	(10.9)	
Aman, Roberts, and Pennington (1997)						
Experimental	22	12.1	(1.2)	110.5	(8.2)	TOH,
Control	22	12.1	(1.2)	110.0	(7.3)	Stopping
Women with fragile X syndrome						
Experimental	7	30.0	(7.3)	79.1	(6.4)	WCST,
Control	5	32.4	(2.6)	84.4	(4.7)	Stopping, WM
Experimental	15	28.9	(6.6)	85.1	(11.0)	TOH
Control	107	32.7	(6.8)	104.2	(12.5)	
High-functioning autism						
Bennetto, Pennington, and Rogers (1996)						
Experimental	19	16.0	(3.3)	88.9	(11.1)	WCST,
Control	19	15.2	(2.6)	91.7	(12.1)	TOH, WM

[a]TOH, Tower of Hanoi; WM, working memory measures (Sentence Span and Counting Span).

again clear severity differences, with the group with autism again being most impaired.

Problems in voluntary motor inhibition in ADHD are documented in Figure 12.3, which depicts results on the Stopping task devised by Logan and co-workers (1984). As described earlier, this is an experimental measure of the ability to inhibit an already programmed motor response. Logan and colleagues have found that children with ADHD have deficits on this task (Schachar & Logan, 1990; Schachar, Tannock, & Logan, 1993) that are eliminated by stimulant medication (Tannock, Schachar, Carr, Chajczyk, & Logan, 1989). In a study by Aman, Roberts, and Pennington (1997), children with ADHD were tested first on and then off stimulant medication. There were no group differences when the ADHD group was on medication; off medication, however, they were significantly worse than both their earlier performance and the controls at both times (who performed similarly at each time). The graph in Figure 12.3 depicts Time 2 data for both groups. The medication sensitivity of the inhibition deficit across studies demonstrates some evidence for its primacy in ADHD because it provides a link between this deficit and the neurobiological mechanisms in ADHD.

Perhaps even more interesting is the *lack* of differences between women with fragile X syndrome and IQ-matched controls on this task. Across the tasks presented thus far, the profile of executive function deficits is different in individuals with fragile X syndrome and ADHD; subjects in the former group were more impaired on the WCST and less impaired on the Stopping task than those in the latter group. A similar contrast is found between autism and ADHD. Ozonoff and Strayer (in press) found that subjects with autism were not different from IQ-matched con-

Wisconsin Card Sorting Test

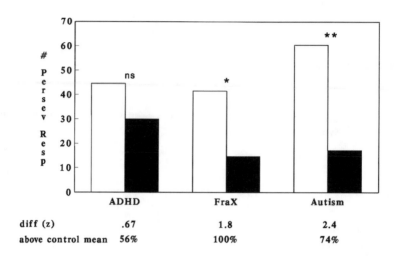

Figure 12.1.   Subject performance on Wisconsin Card Sorting Test. (Diff [z] calculation is the mean of the experimental group minus the mean of the control group divided by the standard deviation of the control group. For example, the ADHD group was .67 SD worse than control mean. Solid bar = control, open bar = experimental; Persev Resp, perseverative responses; FraX, fragile X syndrome; *, $p < .05$; **, $p < .01$.)

trols on two measures of different aspects of inhibition, the Stopping task and the Negative Priming task, a measure of involuntary cognitive inhibition (Tipper, 1985). Interestingly, the Negative Priming task has been found to be sensitive to inhibition deficits in both normal aging and schizophrenia (for a review, see May, Kane, & Hasher, 1995). Recall that subjects with autism were much more impaired than children with ADHD on the WCST and the Tower of Hanoi. Therefore, across these two pairs of groups—children with ADHD and women with fragile X syndrome, and children with ADHD and those with autism—there is evidence for *opposite* profiles of executive function impairments. The profile thus far in ADHD includes deficits in inhibition and planning, but not in cognitive flexibility. The profile thus far in autism and women with fragile X syndrome includes deficits in cognitive flexibility and planning, but not in inhibition.

On the fourth dimension of executive function, working memory, there are also profile differences. Figures 12.4 and 12.5 present data for both subjects with autism and those with fragile X syndrome compared with IQ-matched controls on the two verbal working memory measures, Sentence Span and Counting Span, respectively. Both groups exhibited deficits on both tasks. Unfortunately, we do not have data from our lab from subjects with ADHD on these measures. However, Siegel and Ryan (1989) compared two age groups (7–8 years and 9–10 years) of children with ADHD with normal controls on both of these working memory tasks. The only group difference found was that younger children with ADHD performed worse than controls on the Sentence Span task. Therefore, deficits in verbal working memory do not appear to be a prominent feature of ADHD. Once again, we

Tower of Hanoi

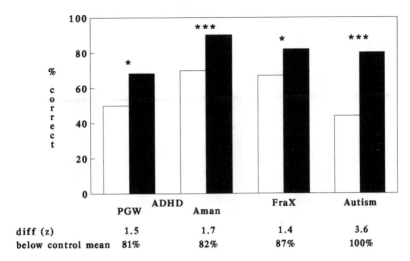

Figure 12.2.   Subject performance on Tower of Hanoi. (Solid bar = control, open bar = experimental.) (*, $p < .05$; ***, $p < .001$.) (PGW, study by Pennington, Grossier, and Welsh [1993]; Aman, study by Aman, Roberts, and Pennington [in press].)

have evidence for opposite profiles of executive function deficits. Individuals with autism and women with fragile X syndrome have deficits in verbal working memory, but children with ADHD do not.

CONCLUSIONS

We have identified at least three dimensions of executive function—verbal working memory, cognitive flexibility or set shifting, and motor inhibition—that appear to possess some validity in both normal and abnormal populations. Of these three dimensions, motor inhibition is the best defined experimentally, and cognitive flexibility the least. Undoubtedly, tasks such as the WCST and the Tower of Hanoi have multiple cognitive components; moreover, we should be wary of reifying a construct such as cognitive flexibility or set shifting. Although the two working memory tasks are experimental tasks based on a theoretical account of working memory, one that emphasizes resource sharing between concurrent storage and processing tasks, this theoretical account must be empirically validated. As we have seen from the factor analysis presented earlier, these two tasks share variance with a standard verbal short-term memory task, Digit Span, which validates their storage component. However, the amount of their variance that is due either to their processing component or, more important, to resource sharing has not been validated empirically.

For the Counting Span, Towse and Hitch (1995) have noted that task difficulty is confounded with counting time. The longer the subject's counting time, the longer the span over which items must be retained in memory. Hence, developmental (and individual) differences in Counting Span may be due simply to memory decay operating across different retention intervals (caused by differences in

Stopping Task

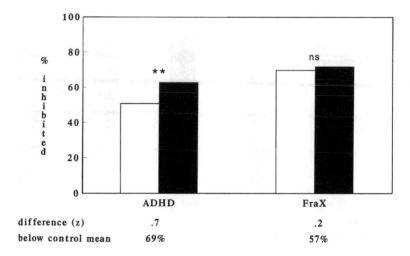

difference (z)	.7	.2
below control mean	69%	57%

Figure 12.3.   Subject performance on Stopping task. (Solid bar = control, open bar = experimental; **, $p < .01$.)

counting time), rather than differences in resource sharing. When they tested this hypothesis experimentally in children 6–11 years of age, Towse and Hitch found counting time effects but no load effects, consistent with the memory decay hypothesis. Simply put, the presence of concurrent tasks does not guarantee that a

Sentence Span

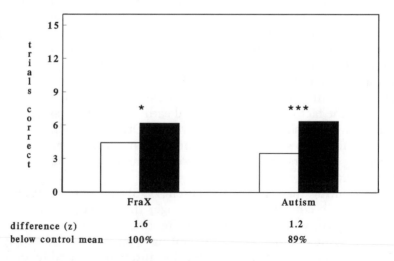

difference (z)	1.6	1.2
below control mean	100%	89%

Figure 12.4.   Subject performance on Sentence Span. (Solid bar = control, open bar = experimental.) (*, $p < .05$; ***, $p < .001$.)

Counting Span

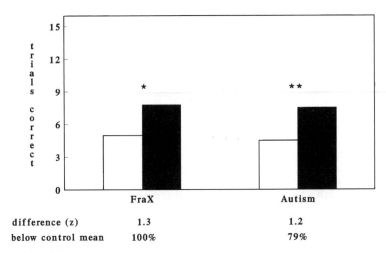

Figure 12.5.   Subject performance on Counting Span. (Solid bar = control, open bar = experimental; *, $p < .05$; **, $p < .01$.)

major or even minor source of variance in the task will be due to executive processes such as resource sharing; that assumption must be tested empirically.

The results presented here are encouraging with respect to the discriminant validity problem; they indicate that both the severity and the profile of executive function deficits vary across populations. Further work is needed, both to define the executive function deficit(s) in each population and to tie them causally to the neurobiological mechanisms operating in each. In this way, the frontal metaphor can 1) become more precise and articulated, 2) move from being an analogy to being a homology for at least some populations, and 3) fulfill its promise for providing an integrated understanding of cognitive differences.

REFERENCES

Aman, D.J., Roberts, R.J., & Pennington, B.F. (1997). *A neuropsychological examination of the underlying deficit in ADHD: The frontal lobe versus right parietal lobe theories.* Manuscript submitted for publication.

Bennetto, L., Pennington, B.F., & Rogers, S.J. (1996). Intact and impaired memory functions in autism. *Child Development, 67,* 1816–1835.

Bishop, D.V.M. (1993). Annotation: Autism, executive functions and theory of mind: A neuropsychological perspective. *Journal of Child Psychology and Psychiatry, 34,* 279–293.

Cohen, J. (1992). A power primer. *Psychological Bulletin, 112,* 155–159.

Cohen, J.D., & Servan-Schreiber, D. (1992). Context, cortex, and dopamine: A connectionist approach to behavior and biology in schizophrenia. *Psychological Review, 99,* 45–77.

Damasio, A.R., & Van Hoesen, G.W. (1983). Emotional disturbances associated with focal lesions of the limbic frontal lobe. In K.M. Heilman & P. Satz (Eds.), *Neuropsychology of human emotion* (pp. 85–110). New York: Guilford Press.

Dempster, F.N. (1992). The rise and fall of the inhibitory mechanism: Toward a unified theory of cognitive development and aging. *Developmental Review, 12,* 45–75.

Dempster, F.N., & Brainerd, C.J. (1995). *Interference and inhibition in cognition.* New York: Academic Press.

Diamond, A., Ciaramitaro, V., Donner, E., Djali, S., & Robinson, M. (1994). An animal model of early-treated PKU. *Journal of Neuroscience, 14,* 3072–3082.

Duncan, J. (1995). Attention, intelligence, and the frontal lobes. In M.S. Gazzaniga (Ed.), *The cognitive neurosciences* (pp. 721–733). Cambridge, MA: MIT Press.

Fuster, J.M. (1989). *The prefrontal cortex: Anatomy, physiology and neuropsychology of the frontal lobe* (2nd ed.). New York: Raven Press.

Goldman-Rakic, P.S. (1987). Circuitry of primate prefrontal cortex and regulation of behavior by representational memory. In F. Plum (Vol. Ed.), *Handbook of physiology: Sect. 1. The nervous system: Vol. V. Higher functions of the brain* (pp. 373–417). Bethesda, MD: American Physiological Society.

Gorenstein, E.E., Mammato, C.A., & Sandy, J.M. (1989). Performance of inattentive-overactive children on selected measures of prefrontal-type function. *Journal of Clinical Psychology, 45*, 619–632.

Guitton, D., Buchtel, H.A., & Douglas, R.M. (1985). Frontal lobe lesions in man cause difficulties in suppressing reflexive glances and in generating goal-directed saccades. *Experimental Brain Research, 58*, 455–472.

Heaton, R.K., Chelune, G.J., Talley, J.L., Kay, G.G., & Curtiss, G. (1993). *Wisconsin Card Sorting Test: Revised and updated.* Odessa, FL: Psychological Assessment Resources.

Hebb, D.O. (1939). Intelligence in man after large removals of cerebral tissue: Report of four left frontal lobe cases. *Journal of General Psychology, 21*, 73–87.

Hebb, D.O. (1945). Man's frontal lobes: A critical review. *Archives of Neurology and Psychology, 54*, 10–24.

Hughes, C., Russell, J., & Robbins, T.W. (1994). Evidence for executive dysfunction in autism. *Neuropsychologia, 32*, 477–492.

Jones-Gotman, M., & Milner, B. (1977). Design fluency: The invention of nonsense drawings after focal cortical lesions. *Neuropsychologia, 15*, 653–674.

Kagan, J., Rosman, B.L., Day, L., Albert, J., & Phillips, W. (1964). Information processing in the child: Significance of analytic and reflective attitudes. *Psychological Monographs, 78*(No. 578).

Kimberg, D.Y., & Farah, M.J. (1993). A unified account of cognitive impairments following frontal lobe damage: The role of working memory in complex, organized behavior. *Journal of Experimental Psychology: General, 122*, 411–420.

Klosowska, D. (1976). Relation between ability to program actions and location of brain damage. *Polish Psychological Bulletin, 7*, 245–255.

Larson, G.E., & Sacuzzo, D.P. (1989). Cognitive correlates of general intelligence: Toward a process theory of g. *Intelligence, 13*, 5–31.

Levin, H.S., Eisenberg, H.M., & Benton, A.L. (1991). *Frontal lobe function and dysfunction.* New York: Oxford University Press.

Logan, G.D., Cowan, W.B., & Davis, K.A. (1984). On the ability to inhibit simple and choice reaction time responses: A model and a method. *Journal of Experimental Psychology: Human Perception and Performance, 10*, 276–291.

May, C.P., Kane, M.J., & Hasher, L. (1995). Determinants of negative priming. *Psychological Bulletin, 118*, 35–54.

Mettler, F.A. (1952). *Psychosurgical problems.* New York: Blakiston.

Milner, B. (1963). Effects of different brain lesions on card-sorting. *Archives of Neurology, 9*, 90–100.

Milner, B. (1964). Some effects of frontal lobectomy in man. In J. Warren & K. Akert (Eds.), *The frontal granular cortex and behavior* (pp. 75–89). New York: McGraw-Hill.

Milner, B., Corsi, P., & Leonard, G. (1991). Frontal-lobe contribution to recency judgements. *Neuropsychologia, 29*, 601–618.

Ozonoff, S., & Strayer, D.L. (in press). Inhibitory function in nonretarded children with autism. *Journal of Autism and Developmental Disorders.*

Ozonoff, S., Strayer, D.L., McMahon, W.M., & Filloux, F. (1994). Executive function abilities in autism: An information processing approach. *Journal of Child Psychology and Psychiatry, 35*, 1015–1031.

Pennington, B.F. (1994a). Genetics of learning disabilities. *Journal of Child Neurology, 10*(Suppl.), S69–S76.

Pennington, B.F. (1994b). The working memory function of the prefrontal cortices: Implications for developmental and individual differences in cognition. In M.M. Haith, J. Benson, R. Roberts, & B.F. Pennington (Eds.), *The development of future oriented processes* (pp. 243–289). Chicago: University of Chicago Press.

Pennington, B.F., Bennetto, L., McAleer, O.K., & Roberts, R.J., Jr. (1996). Executive functions and working memory: Theoretical and measurement issues. In G.R. Lyon & N.A. Krasnegor (Eds.), *Attention, memory, and executive function* (pp. 327–348). Baltimore: Paul H. Brookes Publishing Co.

Pennington, B.F., Groisser, D., & Welsh, M.C. (1993). Contrasting cognitive deficits in attention deficit hyperactivity disorder versus reading disability. *Developmental Psychology, 29,* 511–523.

Pennington, B.F. & Ozonoff, S. (1996). Annotation: Executive functions and developmental psychopathologies. *Journal of Child Psychology and Psychiatry, 37,* 51–87.

Petrides, M., & Milner, B. (1982). Deficits on subject-ordered tasks after frontal- and temporal-lobe lesions in man. *Neuropsychologia, 20,* 249–262.

Reitan, R.M. (1958). Validity of the Trail Making Test as an indicator of organic brain damage. *Perceptual and Motor Skills, 8,* 271–276.

Roberts, R.J., Hager, L., & Heron, C. (1994). Prefrontal cognitive processes: Working memory and inhibition in the Antisaccade task. *Journal of Experimental Psychology: General, 123,* 374–393.

Schachar, R., & Logan, G.D. (1990). Impulsivity and inhibitory control in normal development and childhood psychopathology. *Developmental Psychology, 26,* 710–720.

Schachar, R.J., Tannock, R., & Logan, G. (1993). Inhibitory control, impulsiveness, and attention deficit hyperactivity disorder. *Clinical Psychology Review, 13,* 721–739.

Schacter, D.L. (1987). Memory, amnesia, and frontal lobe dysfunction. *Psychobiology, 15,* 21–36.

Shallice, T. (1988). *From neuropsychology to mental structure.* Cambridge, England: Cambridge University Press.

Shue, K.L., & Douglas, V.I. (1992). Attention deficit hyperactivity disorder and the frontal lobe syndrome. *Brain and Cognition, 20,* 104–124.

Siegel, L.S., & Ryan, E.B. (1989). The development of working memory in normally achieving and subtypes of learning disabled children. *Child Development, 60,* 973–980.

Stuss, D.T., & Benson, D.F. (1986). *The frontal lobes.* New York: Raven Press.

Tannock, R., Schachar, R.J., Carr, R.P., Chajczyk, D., & Logan, G.D. (1989). Effects of methylphenidate on inhibitory control in hyperactive children. *Journal of Abnormal Child Psychology, 17,* 473–491.

Taylor, H.G. (1988). Learning disabilities. In E.J. Mash & L.G. Terdal (Eds.), *Behavioral assessment of childhood disorders* (2nd ed., pp. 402–450). New York: Guilford Press.

Tipper, S.P. (1985). The negative priming effect: Inhibitory priming by ignored objects. *Quarterly Journal of Experimental Psychology, 37,* 571–590.

Towse, J.N., & Hitch, G.J. (1995). Is there a relationship between task demand and storage space in tests of working memory capacity? *Quarterly Journal of Experimental Psychology, 48,* 108–124.

Wechsler, D. (1981). *Wechsler Adult Intelligence Scale–Revised.* New York: The Psychological Corporation.

Weinberger, D.R., Berman, K.F., Gold, J., & Goldberg, T. (1994). Neural mechanisms of future-oriented processes: In vivo physiological studies of humans. In M.M. Haith, J.B. Benson, R.J. Roberts, & B.F. Pennington (Eds.), *The development of future-oriented processes* (pp. 221–242). Chicago: University of Chicago Press.

Welsh, M.C., Pennington, B.F., & Groisser, D.B. (1991). A normative-developmental study of executive function: A window on prefrontal function in children? *Developmental Neuropsychology, 7,* 131–149.

Welsh, M.C., Pennington, B.F., Ozonoff, S., Rouse, B., & McCabe, E.R.B. (1990). Neuropsychology of early-treated phenylketonuria: Specific executive function deficits. *Child Development, 61,* 1697–1713.

Development of the Prefrontal Cortex: Evolution, Neurobiology, and Behavior
edited by Norman A. Krasnegor, Ph.D., G. Reid Lyon, Ph.D.,
and Patricia S. Goldman-Rakic, Ph.D.
copyright © 1997   Paul H. Brookes Publishing Co., Inc.
Baltimore • London • Toronto • Sydney

13

Prefrontal–Subcortical Circuits in Developmental Disorders

Martha Bridge Denckla and Allan L. Reiss ⎯⎯⎯⎯⎯⎯⎯⎯⎯⎯⎯⎯⎯⎯

Whereas the anatomical existence of pathways linking prefrontal and subcortical regions have been known for some time, the specific role of these circuits in human cognition and behavior have begun to be elucidated only in the 1990s. In this chapter, we draw on established neurological theory, information derived from the analysis of well-defined neurological syndromes, and findings from our research center and from other investigators to begin to assemble a more cohesive picture of the contribution of prefrontal–subcortical systems to cognitive dysfunction in developmental disorders. We begin by defining the cognitive domain thought to be most affected by dysfunction of prefrontal–subcortical circuits. Conceptual issues and problems inherent in attempting to separate prefrontal from subcortical components of neurological dysfunction are then discussed. Finally, research findings in two common neurobehavioral conditions, attention-deficit/hyperactivity disorder (ADHD) and Tourette syndrome (TS), are used to illustrate the potential role of prefrontal–subcortical circuits in developmental disorders.

EXECUTIVE FUNCTION

To elucidate brain–behavior relationships involving the dorsolateral prefrontal cortex (PFC) in developmental disorders, the most robust strategies utilize tasks, modeled upon those found in studies of adults with acquired lesions, that belong in the neuropsychological domain of executive function. *Executive function* refers to a cognitive module consisting of effector output elements involving inhibition, working memory, and organizational strategies necessary to prepare a response.

This chapter was supported by Grants HD25806, NS35359, and MH01142 from the National Institutes of Health.

The authors wish to acknowledge Pamela D. Yerby and Carol Taylor for their help in the preparation of this manuscript.

Pennington (see Chapter 12) has pointed out the difficulty with developmental neuropsychology's relatively recent discovery of the importance of executive function: Too many developmental disorders have been declared to exhibit selective deficits in executive function. Clearly, as Pennington points out, different components of executive function must contribute to such clinically different disorders as autism and ADHD. Furthermore, ADHD is a clinically defined entity that harbors much heterogeneity (Shaywitz, Fletcher, & Shaywitz, 1995; Voeller, 1991).

SEPARATION AND INTEGRATION OF SUBCORTICAL AND PREFRONTAL COMPONENTS OF NEUROLOGICAL DYSFUNCTION

The central purpose of this chapter is to review the prefrontal–subcortical circuitry necessary for executive function, with particular emphasis on evidence that certain developmental disorders may arise from anomalies predominantly at the subcortical rather than the prefrontal level. At the outset, it must be admitted that, because the prefrontal–subcortical circuit subserving executive function acts as an integrated and synergistic system, it is only with difficulty that one can document distinctions between the effects of the cortical level and those attributable to its subcortical partners (Figure 13.1). For example, whether there is a specifically subcortical dementia has been a focus of controversy; a volume (Cummings, 1990) and an article (Mega & Cummings, 1994) devoted to the construct of a subcortical dementia do not even insist literally upon excluding frontal lobe pathology from the list of lesions producing "the syndrome of subcortical dementia." As a matter of fact, among the alternative names proposed for subcortical dementia are *frontal-subcortical dementia* and *frontal systems dementia*.

The principal characteristics of subcortical dementia straddle neurology and psychiatry, including the cognitive feature that is most distinctively subcortical,

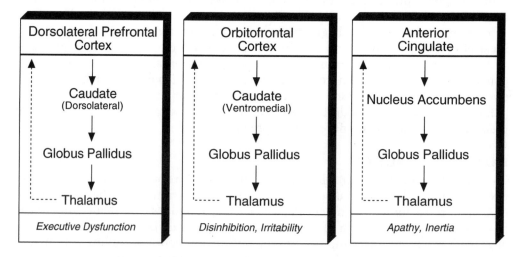

Figure 13.1   Three parallel frontostriatal circuits underlying executive dysfunction and emotion. Frontal components are illustrated at the top level of each circuit, and subcortical elements are shown in the middle segment. Symptom complexes associated with dysfunction of each circuit are shown in the bottom segment of the three boxes. Note that there is spatial convergence of each of the pathways through the globus pallidus. Not shown are motor and oculomotor circuits, which are also in parallel to those illustrated. (Adapted from Cummings [1993].)

cognitive slowing, the formal term for which is *bradyphrenia*. Often overshadowed or masked by extrapyramidal motoric difficulties (e.g., bradykinesia, dyskinesia), subcortical dementia consists of impairment in fundamental, content-nonspecific operations that cut across the instrumentalities of language, perception, and memory modules.

Luria (1973) envisaged the subcortical structures (he called these the *basal compartment*, using an adjective somewhat unintentionally overlapping with the anatomical term *basal ganglia*) as suppliers of cerebral tone. The frontal compartment contributed analysis, integration, and modulation of all perceptions and memories. Both the basal and the frontal compartments enjoyed a reciprocal relationship and a partnership in regulation of the posterior cortical (i.e., language, perception, memory) compartment (Luria, 1973). From this Lurian perspective, given the subtleties of clinical differences between diseases that afflict predominantly the frontal or the subcortical levels of the reciprocal circuits, it is possible to envisage what is still speculative: a distinctive neurobehavioral profile for each level.

It is possible that the study of certain developmental disorders, especially with longitudinal analysis, may make it possible to delineate a distinctive subcortical contribution to human cognition; development may clarify an earlier tonic preparatory state implied by Luria's basal compartment. Later in development there may arise the more elaborate executive functions (e.g., strategies, organized searches, self-monitoring) that can easily be subsumed under the term *metacognition*. In fact, it is the emerging purpose of some researchers to keep executive function from floating up to the lofty aspects of cognition, where it is in danger of coalescing with the "G" of intelligence or encountering what Pennington (see Chapter 12) calls "the homunculus problem" (i.e., some component of cognition that runs all other cognition). Emphasis upon the subcortical platform of executive function, keeping in mind the zone of interface or overlap between motor function and cognition, may be especially useful in tracing the executive function of developmental disorders back to its ontogenetic roots.

Grounds for emphasizing the subcortical anatomical associations and the basal (fundamental) neuropsychological aspects of executive function arise from 1) magnetic resonance imaging (MRI) and cerebral blood flow data, 2) several lines of research concerning neuropsychological or cognitive deficits seen with ADHD, and 3) some research concerning the neuropsychology of TS. Some data sets contribute to two categories (i.e., both 1 and 2 or 1 and 3) but are presented separately for the sake of clarity.

NEUROIMAGING STUDIES AND BASAL GANGLIA ANOMALIES

Early functional imaging studies of children with ADHD, using xenon-133 single-photon emission computerized tomography, revealed low blood flow in the caudate nucleus, reduced more on the right than on the left (Lou, Henriksen, Bruhn, Borner, & Nielsen, 1989). Blood flow, like any physiological method of study, may reflect secondary remote effects of an anatomically connected primary site. Accordingly, structural imaging is necessary to examine directly whether there are striatal anomalies underlying the hypothesized abnormal blood flow.

An initial MRI study of children with ADHD showed reduced size (as derived from a single slice area) of the left caudate nucleus (Hynd et al., 1993). In a subsequent MRI study conducted by a different research group, reduced size (i.e., volume) of the right caudate nucleus in children with ADHD was reported (Castellanos et al., 1994). In findings from our research center, the primary anatomical site of outflow from the striatum, the globus pallidus, was found to be smaller than normal on the left side in yet another group of children with ADHD (Aylward et al., 1996). The right–left conflict among these studies may be a function of the operational method for defining the subcortical regions of interest (e.g., area in Hynd et al. versus volume analysis in the other two studies) as well as ADHD subtype representation, which appeared to be substantially different across studies. In the Castellanos et al. (1994) volumetric study, all children studied were characterized as showing "prominent motor restlessness and impulsivity" (p. 2), and more than half of them were comorbid for either oppositional defiant or conduct disorder. In the Aylward et al. (1996) study, which used similar methods (Rasband, 1993) for computerized volumetric analysis, the small group of children with ADHD was one free of comorbid externalizing disorders and far more inattentive than either impulsive or hyperactive. This latter group was gender, age, and IQ matched to a previously reported TS group that was comorbid for ADHD (discussed later in this chapter).

Other structural MRI studies focused upon ADHD have further contributed speculation as to the pathogeneses of the disorder. Two volumetric studies appeared in 1994 focusing on the corpus callosum in groups of children with ADHD. In one study, anterior callosal regions (rostrum and rostral body) were smaller in children with ADHD and correlated in the pathophysiologically relevant direction with teacher and parent ratings of hyperactivity and impulsivity (Giedd et al., 1994). In the other study, it was the posterior callosum (splenium) that was abnormally small in the ADHD group (Semrud-Clikeman et al., 1994). This anterior–posterior contradiction between two apparently carefully done studies highlights the potential problem of heterogeneity within groups diagnosed with ADHD and of overlapping diagnoses comorbid with ADHD. Conceptually, the apparent contradiction between a frontal and a parietal localization for the pathophysiology of ADHD is equal in importance to the conflict between right and left basal ganglia, although an explanation for the left–right issue is at present less difficult to propose, as has been stated. (It is beyond the scope of this chapter to discuss theories of attention and the possible parietal relationship to learning disability of the language-based type; either of these could suggest why parietal anomalies may enter the picture for some subgroup of ADHD.)

Tourette syndrome, when coexisting with ADHD, is associated with reversed asymmetry of the basal ganglia; on further fractionation of the groups along lines of ADHD comorbidity (TS/ADHD), it emerges that the TS/ADHD group accounts for the asymmetry shift by virtue of a smaller left globus pallidus (Singer et al., 1993). It was this finding that prompted the matching of an ADHD (no TS) group and thus confirmed the smaller left globus pallidus associated with ADHD (Aylward et al., 1996). Magnetic resonance imaging studies of adults with TS have not investigated the ADHD comorbidity relationship but do demonstrate the same altered left–right asymmetry (Peterson et al., 1993). Because TS and its associated neuropsychiatric features are under suspicion of underlying causation grounded in the intricate dopaminergic circuitry of the basal ganglia, the "company kept" by ADHD again thrusts that subcortical issue into a prominent position that is at least moderately supported by structural neuroimaging data.

ATTENTION-DEFICIT/HYPERACTIVITY
DISORDER AND PARKINSON DISEASE

One of the most intriguing clues about the pathophysiology of ADHD (or at least one subtype of ADHD) comes from the history of those conditions believed to be ancestors of the concept. After the great pandemic of the second decade of the 20th century, Von Economo's encephalitis (known popularly as sleeping sickness), some adults who recovered were left with residual parkinsonism. It is widely known that this was a severe form of Parkinson disease and, of further interest, sometimes accompanied by obsessions, compulsions, or tics. Less widely known is that some children who awoke from the sleeping sickness developed severe disturbances of deportment; although they had no mental disabilities, they were wild and willful children, referred to as incorrigibles (Bender, 1942; Hohman, 1922). Medical historians who read the descriptions of the postencephalitic incorrigible children find in them a striking similarity to hyperactive or impulsive behaviors. Thus the postencephalitic sequelae of sleeping sickness provide a surprising link between adult parkinsonism and childhood hyperactivity or impulsivity. As is the case with the high comorbidity of ADHD with TS, these postencephalitic data converge upon the basal ganglia.

More recent evidence exists that the methylphenyltetrahydropyridine (MPTP) model for Parkinson disease may reaffirm in primates that subtle differences in how that toxin affects the caudate may result in a different clinical mixture of cognitive and motor deficits. Chronic low-dose MPTP administration, although it does not cause motor deficit, causes monkeys to exhibit cognitive deficits usually described as prefrontal in type (Roeltgen & Schneider, 1991). These monkeys are also restless, irritable, and poorly focused on prefrontal executive tasks (Roeltgen & Schneider, 1991). The researchers who have done the MPTP studies point out that dopamine and norepinephrine metabolism is disrupted by the toxin, thus increasing the relevance of the behavioral findings to ADHD, in which these catecholamines have long been the focus of interest. Although the MPTP research suggests that dysfunction of the caudate end of the frontocaudate axis can simulate ADHD-like deficits in primates, it also inspired investigators to construct for children with ADHD a clinical research test designed to tap the caudate role as a sensory filter and gate for motor actions (D. Roeltgen, personal communication, May 1995). This task, of potential applicability to clinical practice, consists of a simple sensorimotor tracking challenge. Instructed to keep the eyes closed, the child is asked to keep an index finger (placed before eyes are closed) on the vertical palm of the dorsiflexed hand of the examiner, who, with extended arm, is moving the hand according to a preset pattern (capital alphabet letters) at an amplitude covering the head-to-waist vertical dimension of the child. The child is not told that a specific set of forms (letters) are mapping the movement, but is instructed to move in sustained contact with the examiner's moving hand. This is a task failed by children with ADHD and patients with Parkinson disease, who lose contact with the palm of the examiner (D. Roeltgen, personal communication, May 1995).

HETEREOGENEITY IN THE COGNITIVE,
BEHAVIORAL, AND NEUROLOGICAL CONCEPTUALIZATION
OF ATTENTION-DEFICIT/HYPERACTIVITY DISORDER

Investigation of the information-processing characteristics of children with ADHD has called into question the very construct of attention as central to the disorder named *attention deficit*. Remarkably, experimental cognitive psychologists, based upon exhaustive meta-analysis of the literature as well as their own systematic research programs, have concluded that output motor factors and activation of the subject are the loci of both the deficits and the effectiveness of stimulant medication in the disorder called ADHD (Sergeant & van der Meere, 1990). These researchers have carried out a systematic program of research on unmedicated subjects with ADHD; they have published evidence that in ADHD there is no disturbance in the aspects of attention referred to as freedom from distractibility, shifting, sustaining, or dividing. Furthermore, Sergeant and van der Meere found no reliable evidence for deficits in the encoding or central processing of stimuli (i.e., stimulus search and decision). Rather, it was in the response selection, motor programming, and motor adjustment stages that reliable and robust deficits were demonstrable in children with ADHD. This block of processes close to the output side of the information-processing chain is linked with the energetic activation system. Thus, many so-called attention tasks are heavily dependent upon the ability to preset motor systems prior to incoming information or to adjust motor controls as information arrives. All of this research has been carried out on ADHD as defined in the *Diagnostic and Statistical Manual of Mental Disorders, Third Edition–Revised* (American Psychiatric Association, 1987) and has yet to be reformulated in terms of subtypes (with and without significant ratings of hyperactivity or impulsivity). It is possible that the information-processing profile of the preponderantly inattentive type will not conform to that established for children with full-syndrome ADHD as motor output or activation deficit.

Based on available cognitive psychology data, the behavioral neurologist, using different terminology, would recognize the ADHD deficit profile as belonging to the *intention* rather than attention category, based on concepts of a top-down (intentional) and a bottom-up (attentional) analysis of the phenomenology of neglect. A distributed system underlying neglect includes the reticular formation; thalamus; mesencephalon; striatum; and parietal, dorsolateral frontal, and mesial frontal cortices (Heilman, Voeller, & Nadeau, 1991). Sometimes the intention pathway is linked with motor activation or executive aspects of attention. The vocabulary is not uniform even within neurology (much less if one crosses disciplines to various divisions of psychology), but the action-oriented nature of intention and its affiliation with parallel circuits of overt motor effector systems is unmistakable. The striatum appears to have a physiological role in gating sensation into motor "when" and "how" (Heilman, 1994; Heilman et al., 1991). As a consequence of a "when" deficit, inputs that should trigger action may fail to do so, and inputs that should not be acted upon do trigger action (i.e., defective response inhibition). The "how" programs are involved in praxis and higher order organization. Parallel frontal–striatal circuits involved in response preparation and response inhibition are anatomically convergent at the more closely packed globus pallidus level, where motor control, cognitive control, and emotional control may all be conjointly affected by a smaller lesion, structural or biochemical. The syndrome of ADHD in its full or combined manifestations, which are motoric, cognitive, and social-emotional, is not difficult to imagine as a consequence of anomalous structure or chemistry of the basal ganglia. Individual behavioral components belonging to subtypes of ADHD may be more distinctly frontal; an example is that motor restlessness (i.e., hyperactivity of the fidgety, nonexploratory, adventitious type) may be due to deficient prefrontal mesocortical dopamine rather than striatal dopamine (Heilman et al., 1991). Left or right lateralized differences in anatomical substrate, at either the PFC or the basal ganglia level, may equally well underlie the heterogeneity subsumed under the ADHD diagnosis, as has been noted when MRI evidence was under discussion.

NEUROPSYCHOLOGICAL PROFILES OF CHILDREN WITH ATTENTION-DEFICIT/HYPERACTIVITY DISORDER AND TOURETTE SYNDROME IN THE PRESENCE OF ABOVE-AVERAGE INTELLIGENCE

In the research program conducted at the Kennedy Krieger Institute/Johns Hopkins University, we have been fortunate in recruiting groups of pure ADHD and pure TS research subjects and finding (after recruitment, not as an inclusion criterion) that both of these groups were of high-average (mean IQ of 117) intelligence. (Details about these subjects and explanations of what is meant by pure can be found in the two primary references for this entire section: Reader, Harris, Schuerholz, and Denckla [1994] and Schuerholz, Baumgardner, Singer, Reiss, and Denckla, 1996.) The purpose of the research was to find academic learning disabilities, which might involve reading, arithmetic, or written expression, and to seek a neuropsychological process deficit profile explanatory of any learning disability found. Thirty percent of the ADHD group had some learning disability, whereas no learning disability was found among children with TS. Twenty percent of the ADHD group exhibited choreiform movements, whereas fully one third of those with Tourette syndrome did so. Choreiform movements, which are irregular lapses of posture holding of the hands, fingers, or both, are thought to be minor versions of the involuntary movements called chorea. Therefore, choreiform-positive status is invoked as a possible localizing sign implicating the basal ganglia. Analysis of TS choreiform-positive subgroups with respect to reaction time revealed that those without choreiform movements were the slowest members of those groups. Most surprising was that the TS group, which had no learning disabilities and was motorically speedy, was impaired on letter word fluency, whereas this particular executive dysfunction was not found in the ADHD group. Analyses still in progress in our research program reveal another slowing—difficulty in rapid naming among those ADHD subjects who are also acquiring reading skills at an unexpectedly poor rate for their IQ level.

The letter word fluency deficit in the pure TS group was their only higher level executive failure found across a sampling of executive tasks that included Wisconsin Card Sorting Test (Heaton, Chelune, Talley, Kay, & Curtiss, 1993) variables, memorization and memory strategies, and organizationally oriented scores on copy and recall of the Rey-Osterrieth complex figure. Based on clinical experience with ADHD and the widely held view that tics in TS represent failures of inhibition, the research team expected to find that attention and executive function would suffer secondary to inhibitory deficits so that, for each syndrome, poor response inhibition would carry much of the explanatory weight. What was found was surprising: Slowed reaction time and excessive variability thereof (in the absence of commission error excess) on a Go–No Go (Drewe, 1975) continuous performance test was characteristic of both pure groups; these slow and variable reaction times were worse among those with ADHD. Among the admittedly heterogeneous bright ADHD group, a minority were disinhibited in that set maintenance on the WCST

(Heaton et al., 1993) was a variable on which they were deficient. Timed motor co-ordination (Denckla, 1985) revealed slowing with ADHD but not with TS. As a group, the children with TS showed slowing relative to a normal control group, but that was less severe than the reaction time slowing of the ADHD group. The distinctive TS-related slowing (*not* characteristic of the ADHD group) was on output-per-minute for letter word fluency (Milner, 1964). Because semantic word fluency and rapid automatized naming (Denckla, 1974) were not slowed in the TS group, the most conservative interpretation of the striking letter word fluency deficit would be that it reflects a left frontal deficit. As is the case with patients in the early stages of Huntington disease, our children with TS performed simply with sparse output punctuated by long silences but without rule breaks or perseverations (Schuerholz et al., 1996).

Although clearly this is a speculation that calls for further research investigation, the hypothesis that is suggested by the poor timed output in children with TS is that cognitive slowing (for choice or decision making) may be important in understanding of TS as a disorder of the basal ganglia. How indecisiveness may relate to obsessive-compulsive tendencies with TS is yet another intriguing aspect of this subcortical focus. Clinically, patients with pure TS (and without clinically diagnosed obsessive-compulsive disorder) have presented themselves as suffering from academic underachievement resulting from inability to finish homework or tests in the time allotted. It is clinically impressive to interview and examine bright youngsters with TS who, aside from tics, suffer most from their slowness of pace and low productivity. There is also a subgroup of children presenting clinically with ADHD who are bright but hypokinetic and slow, although they have additional problems of disorganization and nonstrategic study skills.

PREFRONTAL CORTEX, BASAL GANGLIA, IQ, AND BRAIN MATURATION

The groups seen in our research studies and clinics clearly fall in the nonretarded range of cognitive function. In fact, the research groups described previously were above average (mean IQ score of 117 for both the ADHD and the TS groups). The children with TS were of higher IQ than would have been predicted from their mid-parental IQ score (Schuerholz et al., 1996). This assumes some localization interest in that another involuntary movement disorder (dystonia musculorum deformans) is also associated with upward deviation in IQ score (higher IQ score in those affected than in unaffected family members). From the perspective of a volume devoted to the PFC, however, in which this chapter represents an attempt to argue for a subcortical rather than a PFC origin for some syndromes, there is yet another point to be taken. This point was brought up by Diamond (1994a), during a National Institutes of Health workshop. Based upon published work documenting the impact of frontal lesions on IQ score in adults (Stuss & Benson, 1986), Diamond (1994a) suggested a further connection between the PFC and IQ score. Although noting low-normal IQ scores in the developmental context of imperfectly but acceptably controlled phenylketonuria, Diamond (1994b) suggested that a neurochemically dysfunctional PFC (e.g., when elevated phenylalanine causes lower dopamine) would preclude IQ score rising above the 25th percentile (90 or so).

It is possible to integrate Diamond's remarks about phenylketonuria with the TS and ADHD data summarized earlier. We speculate that the combination of above-average intelligence with motor signs referable to the basal ganglia (e.g., tics or choreiform movements) and slowing on some cognitive tasks (choice reaction time being the most replicable across groups) may permit the inference that, in these groups of children, an intact PFC allows above-average IQ score and is not the source of executive dysfunction. Furthermore, it is possible that an intact PFC may account for the good prognosis in a sizable proportion of young children with ADHD or TS, many of whom appear to outgrow their diagnoses by adult life. Although well-planned longitudinal investigations following forward the groups with basal ganglia markers are necessary to confirm such a hypothesis, it is interesting to speculate that overgrowing (i.e., cortex maturing to dominate subcortical partners) may underlie outgrowing (i.e., diminished clinical signs and symptoms in adult life). There is a precedent for such a pathway because children with the mildest form of cerebral palsy, known as ataxic and attributable to cerebellar insult or anomaly, often appear to be motorically normal after puberty.

CONCLUSIONS

Careful design of experimental cognitive tasks in future studies may help to elucidate and validate the concept of subcortical executive function. For example, Eslinger and Grattan (1993) have already succeeded in illustrating a neuroanatomical distinction between different aspects of cognitive flexibility (reactive and generative). With the availability of functional MRI, it may soon be possible to transfer such well-worked-out dissociations between aspects of executive function into differential activation tasks. Tasks that differentiate between activation of brain regions required for stimulus processing in a single cognitive domain (e.g., visuospatial) versus multimodality modulation (i.e., executive function) will be particularly revealing in this regard (D'Esposito et al., 1995).

In summary, there are clues, existing in the literature, in research data, and in clinical experience, that point to the possibility of a subcortical origin for certain developmental disabilities not involving retardation. From a cognitive neuroscientist's perspective, this possibility is particularly intriguing because the elucidation of subcortical etiologies for developmental disability will likely lead to a more precise understanding of the pathways involved in human behavioral and cognitive function, as well as dysfunction. It is also probable that methods leading to more accurate neuroanatomical localization (PFC versus subcortical) of cognitive or behavioral dysfunction will facilitate the development of a more valid diagnostic nomenclature, as well as more effective strategies for remediation. Although making PFC–subcortical behavioral distinctions will no doubt be an exceedingly difficult endeavor (Mega & Cummings, 1994), there are several methodological approaches from which one can initiate the process. For example, studies ongoing in our research center accentuate more homogeneous genetic and neurobiological groups with learning and developmental disabilities to decrease the potentially deleterious effect of etiological heterogeneity on experimental outcome (Baumgardner, Green, & Reiss, 1994). In addition to those described in this chapter, groups under study in our center include individuals with fragile X syndrome, Turner syndrome, and neurofibromatosis-1.

REFERENCES

American Psychiatric Association. (1987). *Diagnostic and statistical manual of mental disorders* (3rd ed., Rev.). Washington, DC: Author.

Aylward, E.H., Reiss, A.L., Reader, M.J., Singer, H.S., Brown, J.E., Abrams, M., & Denckla, M.B. (1996). Basal ganglia volumes in children with attention deficit hyperactivity disorder. *Journal of Child Neurology, 11*, 112–115.

Baumgardner, T.L., Green, K.E., & Reiss, A.L. (1994). A behavioral neurogenetics approach to developmental disabilities: Gene-brain-behavior associations. *Current Opinion in Neurology, 7*, 172–178.

Bender, L. (1942). Postencephalitic behavior disorders in childhood. In J.B. Neal (Ed.), *Encephalitis: A clinical study* (pp. 363–384). New York: Grune & Stratton.

Castellanos, F.X., Giedds, J.N., Eckburg, P., Marsh, W.L., Vaituzis, C.V., Kaysen, D., Hamburger, S.D., & Rapoport, J.L. (1994). Quantitative morphology of the caudate nucleus in attention deficit hyperactivity disorder. *American Journal of Psychiatry, 151*, 1791–1796.

Cummings, J.L. (Ed.). (1990). *Subcortical dementia*. New York: Oxford University Press.

Cummings, J.L. (1993). Frontal-subcortical circuits and human behavior. *Archives of Neurology, 50*, 873–880.

Denckla, M.B. (1974). Rapid "automatized" naming of pictured objects, colors, letters and numbers by normal children. *Cortex, 10*, 186–202.

Denckla, M.B. (1985). Revised neurological examination for subtle signs (PANESS). *Psychopharmacological Bulletin, 21*, 773–800.

D'Esposito, M., Detre, J.A., Alsop, D.C., Shin, R.K., Atlas, S., & Grossman, M. (1995). The neural basis of the central executive system of working memory. *Nature, 378*, 279–281.

Diamond A. (1994a, September). *PFC: Evolution, neurobiology and behavioral development.* Workshop presentation at NIH Conference on Development of the Prefrontal Cortex, Bethesda, MD.

Diamond, A. (1994b). Phenylalanine levels of 6-l0mg/dl may not be as benign as once thought. *Acta Paediatrica Scandinavica Supplement, 407*, 89–91.

Drewe, E.A. (1975). Go–no go learning after frontal lobe leisions in humans. *Cortex, 11*, 8–16.

Eslinger, P.J., & Grattan, L.M. (1993). Frontal lobe and frontal-striatal substrates for different forms of human cognitive flexibility. *Neuropsychologia, 31*, 17–28.

Giedd, J.N., Castellanos, F.X., Casey, B.J., Kozuch, P., King, A.C., Hamburger, S.D., & Rapoport, J.L. (1994). Quantitative morphology of the corpus callosum in attention deficit hyperactivity disorder. *American Journal of Psychiatry, 151*, 665–669.

Heaton, R.K., Chelune, G.J., Talley, J.L., Kay, G.G., & Curtiss, G. (1993). *Wisconsin Card Sorting Test: Revised and updated*. Odessa, FL: Psychological Assessment Resources.

Heilman, K.M. (1994, January). *"Praxis."* Presented at NIH Conference on Attention, Memory, and Executive Function, Bethesda, MD.

Heilman, K.M., Voeller, K.K.S., & Nadeau, S.E. (1991). A possible pathophysiologic substrate of attention deficit hyperactivity disorder. *Journal of Child Neurology, 6*(Suppl.), S76–S81.

Hohman, L.B. (1922). Postencephalitic behavior disorders in children. *Johns Hopkins Hospital Bulletin, 380*, 372–375.

Hynd, G.W., Hern, K.L., Novey, E.S., Eliopoulos, D., Marshall, R., Gonzalez, J.J., & Voeller, K.K.S. (1993). Attention deficit hyperactivity disorder and asymmetry of the caudate nucleus. *Journal of Child Neurology, 8*, 339–347.

Lou, H.C., Henriksen, L., Bruhn, P., Borner, H., & Nielsen, J.B. (1989). Striatal dysfunction in attention deficit and hyperkinetic disorder. *Archives of Neurology, 46*, 48–52.

Luria, A.R. (1973). *The working brain*. New York: Basic Books.

Mega, M.S., & Cummings, J.L. (1994). Frontal subcortical circuits in neuropsychiatric disorders. *Journal of Neuropsychiatry and Clinical Neurosciences, 6*, 358–370.

Milner, B. (1964). Some effects of frontal lobectomy in man. In J. Warren & K. Akert (Eds.), *The frontal granular cortex and behavior*. New York: McGraw-Hill.

Peterson, B.S., Riddle, M.A., Cohen, D.J., Katz, L.D., Smith, J.C., Hardin, M.T., & Leckman, J.F. (1993). Reduced basal ganglia volumes in Tourette's syndrome using 3-dimensional reconstruction techniques from magnetic resonance images. *Neurology, 43*, 941–949.

Rasband, W. (1993). *NIH image manual*. Bethesda, MD: National Institutes of Health.

Reader, M.J., Harris, E.L., Schuerholz, L.J., & Denckla, M.B. (1994). Attention deficit hyperactivity disorder and executive dysfunction. *Developmental Neuropsychology, 10*, 493–512.

Roeltgen, D.P., & Schneider, J.S. (1991). Chronic low-dose MPTP in nonhuman primates: A possible model for attention deficit disorder. *Journal of Child Neurology, 6*(Suppl.), S80–S87.

Schuerholz, L.J., Baumgardner, T.L., Singer, H.S., Reiss, A.L., & Denckla, M.B. (1996). Neuropsychological status of children with Tourette syndrome with and without attention deficit hyperactivity disorder. *Neurology, 46*, 958–965.

Semrud-Clikeman, M., Filipek, P.A., Biederman, J., Steingard, R., Kennedy, D., Renshaw, P., & Bekken, K. (1994). Attention deficit hyperactivity disorder: Magnetic resonance imaging morphometric analysis of the corpus callosum. *Journal of the American Academy of Child Psychiatry, 33*, 875–881.

Sergeant, J.A., & van der Meere, J.J. (1990). Convergence of approaches in localising the hyperactivity deficit. In B.B. Lahey & A.E Kazdin (Eds.), *Advancements in clinical child psychology* (Vol. 13, pp. 207–245). New York: Plenum.

Shaywitz, B.A., Fletcher, J.M., & Shaywitz, S.E. (1995). Defining and classifying learning disabilities and attention deficit hyperactivity disorder. *Journal of Child Neurology, 10*(Suppl. 1), S50–S61.

Singer, H.S., Reiss, A.L., Brown, J.E., Aylward, E.H., Shih, B., Chee, E., Harris, E.L., Reader, M.J., Chase, G.A., Bryan, N., & Denckla, M.B. (1993). Volumetric MRI changes in basal ganglia of children with Tourette syndrome. *Neurology, 43*, 950–956 .

Stuss, D.T., & Benson, D.F. (1986). *The frontal lobes.* New York: Raven Press.

Voeller, K.K.S. (1991). Toward a neurobiologic nosology of attention deficit hyperactivity disorder. *Journal of Child Neurology, 6*(Suppl.), S2–S8.

Development of the Prefrontal Cortex: Evolution, Neurobiology, and Behavior
edited by Norman A. Krasnegor, Ph.D., G. Reid Lyon, Ph.D.,
and Patricia S. Goldman-Rakic, Ph.D.
copyright © 1997   Paul H. Brookes Publishing Co., Inc.
Baltimore • London • Toronto • Sydney

14

Cognitive and Social Development
in Children with Prefrontal Cortex Lesions

Paul J. Eslinger,
Kathleen R. Biddle, and Lynn M. Grattan

Among the greatest challenges to cognitive neuroscience is the study of how
the developing brain mediates the cognitive, behavioral, and social-emotional
processes of maturation and adaptation. One may view the brain, of course, as
developing throughout the entire life span because neural modifications are continually necessary for successful adaptation in a complex, changing environment.
There is, however, a unique series of events within the early years of life that provide the neurobiological and neuropsychological foundations for learning, cognition, and long-term behavioral adaptation. These events are the fundamental building blocks for independent thought and action, self-regulation of behavior, moral
maturity, vocational achievement, and social responsibility. In these domains, the
role of the prefrontal cortex may be considered paramount and unlike any other
brain area. Such a prominent role has been supported by anatomical and physiological studies indicating that the prefrontal cortex is in a unique position to monitor,
integrate, and influence the neural activity of diverse cortical and subcortical regions through feedforward and feedback pathways devoted to body systems, perceptions of the environment, and access to stored knowledge as well as to the motor
system for actions of initiation, inhibition, and modification of responding. There
is also strong evidence from neurobehavioral studies of frontal lobe damage to associate this anatomical region with many aspects of social behavior, self-regulation,
and what have been termed *executive control processes* such as planning, goal formulation, flexibility of responding, and delay of responding until appropriate circumstances. The neurobehavioral approach to development of the prefrontal cortex
is the focus of this chapter. Specifically, we first review several of the main con-

This chapter was supported in part by a National Institutes of Health fellowship award to Kathleen
R. Biddle through Tufts University.

We thank Tricia Spitler for her able assistance with manuscript preparation and Arthur Benton for
his insightful comments about patient JP and other clinical cases.

cepts and observations that are available from extant cases of early prefrontal cortex lesions in humans. Second, we discuss methodological issues for such research, particularly the importance of prospective studies of anatomically well-defined early lesion cases. Third, we summarize our current studies of two cases of childhood prefrontal cortex lesion, emphasizing anatomical, cognitive, and social measures and their interrelationships. Finally, we offer suggestions for further research in this area.

PRIOR STUDIES OF CHILDHOOD FRONTAL LOBE LESION

The behavioral effects and profile of recovery from cerebral lesions incurred during childhood are different from those incurred during adulthood (Benton, 1985; Grattan & Eslinger, 1991; Teuber & Rudel, 1962). Generally, investigators emphasize three distinctions: 1) that childhood cerebral lesions cause less severe impairments immediately after the event, 2) that a greater recovery of function occurs after childhood cerebral lesions, and 3) that certain impairments after childhood cerebral lesions may not appear until later in development. However, few studies have addressed these comparisons directly, especially for prefrontal cortex lesions, and provided adequate explanation for the differences. There are also minimal data upon which to specify the development and differentiation of brain– behavior relationships at different ages during infancy, childhood, and adolescence and their implications for enhanced or diminished recovery of function. Hence, stating whether it is better to have a frontal lobe lesion early or late does not define the issues very well. Instead, contemporary research centers around the following topics:

- Identifying the neurobiological events that are occurring at various phases of development of the prefrontal cortex and its interconnecting pathways
- Determining the time course for differentiation of component cognitive and behavioral processes mediated by the prefrontal cortex
- Determining how component processes become linked to neural networks
- Delineating the neuropsychological effects of various alterations in prefrontal cortex development
- Elucidating what neurobiological events underlie recovery of function after early prefrontal cortex damage and what role environmental factors and experience have in recovery
- Empirically defining the influence of early prefrontal cortex lesion on adjustment and adaptation throughout the remaining life span as a potential model of certain neurodevelopmental disorders

The paucity of knowledge in the human literature is attributable in part to the low base rate of childhood diseases that produce restricted prefrontal cortex damage, together with limitations of brain imaging techniques for precisely detecting and characterizing neurodevelopmental alterations, and the historically few experimental behavioral paradigms for assessing processes mediated by the frontal lobe in children. Studies of nonhuman primates have been the major source for generating empirical brain–behavior relationships involving the frontal lobe. This includes the various parameters of normal development and the patterns of recovery from early prefrontal lobe damage (e.g., Diamond & Goldman-Rakic, 1989; Goldman & Galkin, 1978; Goldman-Rakic, 1987). Studies of normal children (e.g., Becker, Isaac,

& Hynd, 1987; Chelune & Baer, 1986; Levin et al., 1991; Welsh, Pennington, & Groisser, 1991) and of children with attention deficit disorder (Barkley, Grodzinsky, & DuPaul, 1992) and head injury (e.g., Dennis & Barnes, 1993; Fletcher, Levin, & Butler, 1995) have also been important for identifying potential behavioral correlates of frontal lobe development and, hence, the kinds of deficits that may accompany early frontal lobe damage. The study of children with focal frontal lobe damage, albeit rare, can provide instructive data about processing capabilities of the frontal lobes at various ages; organizational features of specialized regions; and compensatory patterns of functional reorganization, adaptation, and recovery that are possible. Understanding of these issues has been advanced by the handful of well-studied cases of childhood frontal lobe lesions (see Table 14.1 for summary description of these cases).

The findings from these studies address the following basic issues, which are briefly discussed:

- The importance of the prefrontal cortex for prosocial tendencies and social development
- Protracted postnatal development of prefrontal cortex operations responsible for higher level or executive abilities
- Interhemispheric effects between the prefrontal cortices during development
- Differentiation of rudimentary executive processes in early childhood
- Functional localization of supplementary motor area and associated pathways in the premotor cortex during middle childhood
- The fact that recovery from early prefrontal cortex lesion follows neither simple nor linear parameters
- Relative preservation of elementary cognitive abilities after early prefrontal cortex damage

Prefrontal Cortex and Social Development
Significant social and interpersonal impairments frequently develop and persist as a consequence of childhood prefrontal cortex damage. Such impairments may even appear to worsen over time as a widening discrepancy occurs between the expected and observed development of prefrontal lobe functions, especially in adolescence. Available data suggest that these difficulties contribute to disrupted adaptation throughout the life span more significantly than cognitive and sensorimotor impairments. For example, regardless of age of onset, none of the children with early prefrontal cortex damage summarized in Table 14.1 was able to develop and sustain meaningful friendships or family relationships over time.

Patient JP (Ackerly, 1964; Ackerly & Benton, 1947; Benton, 1991), with congenital bilateral prefrontal cortex damage, was one of the first cases to be identified with such a disproportionate impairment of social development and behavior. Although JP was described as having *social feeling*, this was of a shallow nature and limited to his immediate circumstances, with little generalization or elaboration once the other person was absent or the circumstances had changed. That is, JP could present himself as well mannered, opening doors for others, always standing when a woman entered the room, and addressing others in a polite manner, commensurate with community expectations. In fact, as a gas station attendant, he could be quite engaging and entice customers to purchase gas when they had stopped merely to ask for directions. Such manners and social conduct were the

Table 14.1. Summary of cases of childhood frontal lesion

Case	Reference	Chronological age of lesion onset	Age at time of study	Area of neuroanatomical involvement	IQ[a]	Primary deficits	Strengths
JP	Ackerly (1964); Benton (1991)	Congenital	12 yr	Extensive bilateral prefrontal	S-B IQ = 92; Army Alpha IQ = 100	Application of social knowledge; sustaining friendships; planning, impulse control; social self-regulation; learning from experience; abstraction beyond "materials in view"	Initiation, conversational language, elementary cognitive abilities, socially engaging at times
GK	Price, Daffner, Stowe, and Mesulam (1990)	Perinatal	28 yr	L>R frontal cortex and white matter to caudate nucleus	WAIS–R: VIQ = 102, PIQ = 90, FSIQ = 96	Serious behavior problems from 8 years of age; impulse control and social self-regulation; sustaining friendships; criminal behavior; learning from experience	Initiation, gregariousness, elementary cognitive abilities
PL	Marlowe (1992)	3 yr, 11 mo	6 yr, 1 mo	Right prefrontal cortex; Brodmann's areas 8, 9, 46, and 10 and subjacent white matter	WISC–R: VIQ = 119, PIQ = 132, FSIQ = 128	Self-regulation in complex social environments; novel problem solving in real world; visual-perceptual organization; learning from experience; impulse control, frustration tolerance	Utilization of verbal mediation and rehearsal, initiation, memory and language abilities, measured intellect
MH	Price et al. (1990)	4 yr	24 yr	Bilateral frontal lesions after head trauma	WAIS: VIQ = 78, PIQ = 83, FSIQ = 78	Impulse control with assaults; sustained friendships; sexual promiscuity; planning; academic achievement; judgment and learning from experience	Bravado, memory, language and visual-perceptual abilities

Reference			Lesion	IQ	Impaired functions	Spared functions
Eslinger, Grattan, Damasio, and Damasio (1992); Grattan and Eslinger (1991, 1992)	7 yr	33 yr	Left prefrontal cortex; Brodmann's areas 8, 46, and 32, white matter underlying areas 45 and 24; bilateral low cerebral blood flow in prefrontal regions (L>R)	WAIS–R; VIQ = 85, PIQ = 80, FSIQ = 83	Arrested social, emotional, and moral development; sustained attention and concentration; cognitive flexibility; organization of complex information for cognitive processing; using feedback to guide behavior; planning, judgment, and cognitive estimation	Initiation, elementary cognitive abilities, conversational language
Stelling, McKay, Carr, Walsh, and Baumann (1986)	10 yr, 8 mo	10 yr, 8 mo	Right mesial frontal lobe	None reported	Spontaneity and range of emotional expression; short-term contextual memory; difficulty using verbal instructions to regulate actions; confabulations	None reported
Hebb (1945); Hebb and Penfield (1940)	16 yr, 27 yr	27 yr	Resection at 27 years for bilateral frontal polar lesions sustained at 16 years	S-B IQ = 98	Impulse control, social self-regulation, and goal-directed behavior after injury at 16 years of age; lack of concern for distant future consequences after resection at 27 years	After resection at 27 years: could anticipate immediate behavioral consequences, initiation, inhibition of tactless and tasteless comments

[a]S-B, Stanford-Binet; WAIS–R, Wechsler Adult Intelligence Scale–Revised; VIQ, verbal IQ; PIQ, performance IQ; FSIQ = full-scale IQ; WISC–R, Wechsler Intelligence Scale for Children–Revised.

norm for the era and environment in which JP was raised. At other times, however, JP was short tempered and very critical, often regarding trivial matters such as a customer who had mud splashed on the side of a new car. He would also become upset when his routine was interrupted (e.g., when a customer would ask him to clean the windshield when he was checking the oil). Although JP achieved an acceptable level of social manners and conduct, at least for routine public or impersonal interactions, this did not facilitate the development of meaningful or productive social activities and relationships. Social relationships appeared to have little salience for JP at cognitive and emotional levels. Therefore, he remained socially and emotionally disconnected from those around him. Ackerly and Benton (1947) concluded that this pattern reflected a *primary social defect* that was life long and directly related to JP's bilateral prefrontal cortex lesion. Similar social impairments were described for GK and MH, who sustained early bilateral frontal lesions (Price, Daffner, Stowe, & Mesulam, 1990). In comparison with JP, however, both of these individuals were more aggressive in their behavioral violations.

Patient DT (Eslinger, Grattan, Damasio, & Damasio, 1992; Grattan & Eslinger, 1991, 1992) also had marked difficulties in social development and adaptation. When studied as an adult, 26 years after left prefrontal cortex damage, DT's social behavior was peppered with many expressions of strong emotions, ranging from total infatuation with unsavory characters to rage reactions, with minimal provocation. Moreover, she showed no insight into her behavior and no awareness of the inappropriateness of her unusual and ineffective social responses. As an adult, her social adaptation was immature, disorganized, and superficial, with unregulated emotional expression. Her personality structure can be described as simplistic and poorly integrated. She had a tendency to form dichotomous impressions of people and events and use basic rules of thumb to guide her behavior. In social situations, DT would jump to conclusions quickly and adhere to rigid beliefs even when confronting new and changing circumstances. Analysis of psychological test findings suggests that DT was also unable to develop a cognitive architecture that could support understanding, managing, and having insight into complex social experiences. Measurement of DT's level of moral reasoning indicated arrested development at the concrete level typically associated with middle childhood. Social perspective-taking and theory-of-mind abilities were minimal, precluding the capacity to be empathetic. In addition, DT was unable to develop a stable sense of identity, and her vocational planning capacities did not extend beyond early adolescent levels. Overall, her social development and adaptation were *arrested* at early adolescent levels, with increasing difficulties observed throughout adolescence and early adulthood.

Although DT's developmental impairments were inferred from retrospective analysis of records and extensive family interviews, recent data suggest that such deficits may be observed prospectively in childhood. At the time of last contact, patient PL (Marlowe, 1992) showed significant difficulties in establishing friendships and managing social situations at 6 years of age, approximately 2 years after onset of a right prefrontal cortex lesion. Although it has been observed that PL does not learn from positive and negative social experiences, the primary basis for his social and interpersonal difficulties is yet to be determined.

The study of case KM (Hebb, 1945; Hebb & Penfield, 1940) is marked by two types of social self-regulatory impairments: 1) the onset of socially inappropriate behavior with tactless and tasteless comments after traumatic frontal lobe injury at 16 years of age; and 2) the onset of a relatively pleasant, good-natured demeanor following bilateral prefrontal lobe resection at 27 years of age. His improvement may be attributed to resection of an irritative focus that was contributing to disinhibition and impulsivity and to postsurgical loss of motivation and drive, with a more passive social demeanor resulting from frontal resection.

Regardless of age of onset in childhood or specific location of lesion within the prefrontal cortex, all of these childhood cases had significant alterations in social development or behavior with generally preserved intellect, language, perception, memory, and daily instrumental skills. What varied among them was the particular forms of expression of emotional and social impairments and possibly some of the underpinnings of their deficits. Based on these cases, it can be concluded that the prefrontal cortex mediates a critical role in developing and establishing capacities for social self-regulation, attribution of social salience, perspective-taking ability, and social self-awareness.

Protracted Development of Prefrontal Cortex
The neurobiological events that mediate the extended course of development for executive and social processes continue to be investigated. These processes emerge throughout childhood, adolescence, and early adulthood and have been linked to prefrontal cortex maturation, yet their neurobiological basis remains unclear. The basic anatomical framework for the prefrontal cortex is evident in early infancy in humans and nonhuman primates and does not appear to lag behind other neocortical areas, at least in terms of projection and local circuitry neurons, synaptogenesis, and synaptic density (Bourgeois, Goldman-Rakic, & Rakic, 1994; Huttenlocher, 1979; Mrzljak, Uylings, van Eden, & Judáš, 1990; Rakic, Bourgeois, Eckenhoff, Zecevic, & Goldman-Rakic, 1986). Although there is a subsequent plateau and decline in neurons and synaptic density through adolescence, other neurobiological changes occur that may influence or reflect late-developing cognitive and social processes. These include increasing myelination of axons, elaboration of Layer III pyramidal neuron dendritic trees, a rise in local cerebral metabolic rate for glucose, and electrophysiological changes in coherence patterns between different neural regions (Chugani, Phelps, & Mazziotta, 1987; Mrzljak et al., 1990; Thatcher, 1991; Yakovlev & LeCours, 1967). The latter events may mediate the presumed pruning and sculpting of the basic anatomical framework of the prefrontal cortex that is stimulated by environmental demands, experience, and developmental neuroendocrine changes.

A prolonged, postnatal developmental course for the prefrontal cortex has also been suggested by neurobehavioral data showing that delayed onset of certain behavioral impairments can occur after early frontal lobe lesion (e.g., Ackerly & Benton, 1947; Eslinger et al., 1992; Goldman & Alexander, 1977; Price et al., 1990). This unusual pattern of recovery has been interpreted as a *failure of maturation* and is not readily demonstrated in adult-onset cases. The delayed onset of impairment was clearly evident in the retrospective study of patient DT (Eslinger et al., 1992; Grattan & Eslinger, 1992). With the exception of slower learning in school, behavioral difficulties in DT were not detected by family member and teacher reports until early adolescence, approximately 4 years after left prefrontal cortex lesion at 7 years of age. Thereafter a progressive deterioration in social, cognitive, and emotional domains was observed. We attributed this pattern of delayed progressive change to widening inability of a damaged neural system (i.e., the prefrontal cortex) to mediate the burgeoning cognitive, social, and emotional self-regulation tasks that escalate in adolescence and early adulthood. Animal model studies persuasively support this interpretation. For example, juvenile monkeys with dorsolateral frontal lesions showed immediate and significant impairment on tests of delayed responding. Similar lesions in infant monkeys did not have an immediate effect. However, as the infant monkeys matured, a deficit emerged in delayed responding that was attributed to functionally immature (i.e., damaged) dorsolateral frontal systems. In contrast, the effects of early and later orbital frontal lesions were the same—immediate impairment of delayed responding—regardless of age of injury. Postoperative training after an early orbital frontal lesion, however, resulted in some beneficial effect of such experience (Goldman, 1971; Goldman & Alexander, 1977; Goldman & Mendelson, 1977).

Interhemispheric Prefrontal Interactions in Childhood

There is preliminary evidence to suggest important interhemispheric influences between the prefrontal cortices in development. A potentially adaptive influence was identified from behavioral evidence in PL (Marlowe, 1992), who sustained a right dorsolateral prefrontal cortex lesion at about 4 years of age. During the ensuing 2 years, Marlowe observed that PL spontaneously used and benefited from verbally based strategies such as rules and guidelines to facilitate problem solving and guide social behavior. This process was mediated presumably by compensatory activity of the left frontal lobe when nonverbal perceptual and problem-solving situations were encountered. PL's verbal cognitive abilities in general remain within the high-average to superior range, suggesting no disruption of function or *crowding* in the language-dominant left prefrontal lobe.

In contrast, DT, who sustained a left prefrontal cortex lesion at 7 years of age, demonstrated the potential for untoward interhemispheric effects during development. Although her intraparenchymal hemorrhage was left-sided only, her cerebral blood flow study with xenon-144 as an adult indicated low flows in both *left* and *right* prefrontal regions. Brain magnetic resonance imaging (MRI) at that same time did not indicate detectable morphological lesions on the right. We hypothesized that the early left prefrontal cortex lesion may have had a disruptive effect on development of right prefrontal cortical function during development. Such an effect has not been reported, to our knowledge, with adult-onset cases. This bilateral physiological deficit may have contributed to the severe nature of DT's behavioral impairment, which became evident over the course of adolescence and has persisted into early adulthood. Whether early right prefrontal cortex damage, as in PL, will demonstrate a similar developmental effect over time is unclear, but we suspect that this will not be the case. The difference may be traced to a predominant role for the left prefrontal cortex in the verbal regulation of behavior, which can have a powerful influence on behavioral self-regulation in adolescence and early adulthood. Such asymmetry would not be unusual for the central nervous system, because a similar pattern of asymmetry has been observed with the anterior thalamus in adults, in whom left-sided lesions produce pervasive behavioral impairment in comparison with partial defects after right-sided lesions (Graff-Radford, Damasio, Yamada, Eslinger, & Damasio, 1985). There is also persuasive neurobiological data from an animal model indicating that a unilateral prefrontal cortex lesion at a very early age will result in anatomical abnormalities in the contralateral prefrontal region and hemisphere (Goldman & Galkin, 1978).

Early Differentiation of Executive Processes

There is increasing evidence from studies of normal and brain-injured children that development of executive processes begins at an early age. For example, spatial working memory, in the form of delayed responding and AB tasks, appears to develop within the first year of life and to be a sensitive marker of dorsolateral prefrontal cortex damage in developing nonhuman primates (Diamond & Doar, 1989; Diamond & Goldman-Rakic, 1989). Selective executive impairments can also be detected in children after congenital prefrontal cortex lesions as well as acquired lesions at 4 and 10 years of age. When formally tested, such children demonstrate problems in organizational capacities, shifting response set, self-regulation, and working memory (Ackerly & Benton, 1947; Marlowe, 1992; Stelling, McKay, Carr, Walsh, & Baumann, 1986). These impairments likely result from disruption of certain emerging abilities that are developing at the time of cerebral lesion and the subsequent lack of cognitive maturation over time.

Development of Supplementary Motor System

Available data provide evidence for functional development of the supplementary motor area and its projections by middle childhood. A superior mesial frontal lobe syndrome, similar to that observed in adults, was reported in Case 3 of Stelling and colleagues (1986). Specifically, this 10-year, 8-month-old child underwent a right frontal craniotomy for resection of a diencephalic craniopharyngioma (see Table 14.1 for summary). Her postoperative symptoms included loss of spontaneity (both verbal and behavioral) and significant reduction of emotional expression. Brain imaging studies were interpreted as showing abnormalities in the right dorsal frontal cortex and anterior horn of the lateral ventricle. It is plausible that the neural substrate for this syndrome is well established by 10 years of age, as suggested by the marked clinical defect. This is further supported by observation of a similar syndrome in a 7-year-old child that resulted from damage to the dentate nucleus of the cerebellum, which is interconnected with the dorsal frontal–supplementary motor area through the thalamus. In addition, we recently studied an adolescent female who sustained ischemic damage to the anterior thalamic relay for this circuit and demonstrated akinesia, reduction of emotional expression, and lethargy of cognitive processes during the early recovery phase, with mild residual impairment noted up to 2 years later (Herron, Grattan, Sloan, & Eslinger, in press). Although association areas of the prefrontal cortex do not complete myelination and functional development until late adolescence and early adulthood, the available clinical case data suggest that, by middle childhood, functional development of the superior mesial motor system may be established.

Recovery After Early Prefrontal Cortex Lesion

Data from the available childhood cases indicate that the earlier the onset of prefrontal cortex lesion, the less likely its immediate effects will reflect the specific impairments observed in adults. Benton (1985) noted that cerebral injuries acquired in adulthood involve dissolution of previously acquired abilities, whereas in childhood they involve impaired acquisition of developmental abilities. Contemporary data permit us to extend this line of reasoning and to hypothesize that altered development of new skills after early prefrontal cortex damage follows neither a simple nor a linear course. Assuming that brain damage early in life necessarily precludes normal ontogeny (Johnson & Almi, 1978), it is quite likely that early damage within any of the sectors of the prefrontal cortex will disrupt development and maturation of other regions with which it is interconnected. Depending on the age of onset and the particular location and size of the lesion, concepts of functional reorganization and crowding of function may help explain some of the altered developmental effects. Neurophysiological data regarding development of frontal lobe connections during childhood and adolescence further indicate a nonlinear pattern of differential left and right frontal lobe activity (Thatcher, 1991). Hence, early damage to such a dynamic system, with multiple connections to other brain areas, will produce neither simple nor linear neurobehavioral alterations.

Elementary Cognitive Abilities

Early prefrontal cortex damage does not appear to result in significant impairment of elementary cognitive abilities, that is, basic aspects of perception, speech and language, attention span, memory, motor skills, and spatial processing. With regard to measured intellect, IQ scores from the cases in Table 14.1 ranged from the higher end of the borderline range to superior. Because of the limited number of cases available, it remains unclear whether such measures remain stable over development or decline. For example, were DT's and MH's low average to borderline IQ scores higher in childhood, and will PL's superior IQ score in childhood decline in comparison with peers as he reaches adulthood? Furthermore, the effects of lateralized frontal lesions remain unclear. As Benton (1991) cautioned, it cannot be concluded that these data indicate entirely normal measured intellect among these childhood frontal lesion cases. In fact, there is a suggestion in several of the cases that, although the overall IQ level is within the broad normal range, it may be 10–20 points lower than that expected on the basis of family and academic history.

Summary

Review of childhood prefrontal cortex damage indicates a very small number of cases to draw upon but many interesting observations and descriptions. Although these are both informative and intriguing, they highlight the need for systematic and comprehensive research in this area to answer several important questions with modern experimental techniques. Toward this end, we suggest that the following may serve as some of the guiding questions for future research:

- What are the developmental cognitive alterations (beyond that measured by standard IQ tests) associated with childhood prefrontal cortex lesion?
- What are the developmental social-emotional alterations that occur and that can be empirically studied after childhood prefrontal cortex lesion?
- What consequences are evident in the early recovery phase, and what is the pattern of long-term recovery? What effects have a delayed onset?
- Does early prefrontal cortex damage influence long-term development of elementary cognitive and social competencies?
- Is the Kennard principle (i.e., that early brain damage leads to greater recovery than later damage) as accurate for executive functions and social behavior as for sensorimotor and language processes? How do effects of early prefrontal cortex damage compare with those of other cortical lesions and to damage in the thalamus and basal ganglia regions with which it is interconnected?

PROSPECTIVE EXPERIMENTAL AND CLINICAL STUDIES OF EARLY PREFRONTAL CORTEX DAMAGE

Bearing in mind the existing human cases and the aforementioned guiding questions, we recently initiated a research program to study children with early prefrontal cortex damage and their behavioral development in a prospective manner. This methodological approach has several advantages over retrospective study. First, it is possible to establish the early effects of prefrontal cortex lesions at different ages. With the increasing availability of age-appropriate neuropsychological measures and normative observations for developing cognitive processes in children, experimental and clinical studies in the early recovery phase are providing various indications of prefrontal cortex maturation, differentiation of cognitive and social-emotional processes, and emergence of integrative-regulatory mechanisms. However, very few data in humans are currently available (Grattan & Eslinger, 1991). These data are also critical for comparison with adult-onset cases and for formulating life-span models of how the prefrontal cortex and its related networks mediate cognitive and social-emotional development and regulation.

Second, the similarities and differences between early prefrontal cortex lesions and other disorders thought to be related to prefrontal cortex dysfunction can be directly compared empirically and clinically. Examples include attention-deficit/ hyperactivity disorder (ADHD), autism, mild phenylketonuria (PKU), closed head injury, fragile X syndrome in females, and conduct disorder. Although cognitive and behavioral impairments referable to prefrontal cortex dysfunction have been implicated in all of these disorders in various ways, there is very little understanding of why this should be the case and whether there is a single, unifying pathophysiology (e.g., dopamine deficiency) among these disorders or distinctive etiologies with some overlap to their behavioral and cognitive expression. A further possibility is that current methods of neuropsychological measurement are too gross to detect and characterize *component* differences in cognitive impairment among these disorders, creating a discriminant validity problem (Pennington, Bennetto, McAleer, & Roberts, 1996)

A third advantage to prospective study of early prefrontal cortex damage is that it permits examination of the course of recovery from initial deficits. The available data are very intriguing but limited in this regard. In nonhuman primate models, the studies of Kennard (see Finger, 1991, and Finger & Wolf, 1988, for reviews) have been widely interpreted as providing a guiding principle about greater plasticity after early cerebral injury. That is, early cerebral damage to motor and premotor cortices was found to lead to a much higher level of recovery of motor function in comparison with adult-onset cerebral damage. Kennard was quite cautious about the generalizability of these findings and, in fact, found this *not* to be the case with prefrontal cortex damage and other cortical lesions. The later studies of Teuber and Rudel (1962) in children and of Goldman in nonhuman primates (e.g., Goldman, 1971, 1978; Goldman & Alexander, 1977; Goldman & Galkin, 1978; Goldman & Mendelson, 1977; Miller, Goldman, & Rosvold, 1973) suggested a more complex picture and emphasized an important interaction between age of lesion onset and subsequent patterns of behavioral impairments. The results of early cerebral injury can range from immediate to delayed expression of behavioral impairments (depending on the age of the child and the behavioral processes under study) to recovery patterns that vary from complete to partial recovery with altered architectures. These variable effects and outcomes after early cerebral damage in humans have been confirmed and greatly extended scientifically by Aram and Ekelman (1986, 1988); Dennis (e.g., Dennis, 1991; Dennis & Barnes, 1993); Levin et al. (1988); Nass (e.g., Nass & Peterson, 1989; Nass, Sadler, & Sidtis, 1992); Stiles and Thal (see 1993 review); and studies in the rat model by Kolb (1987; Kolb & Gibb, 1990), among others. Obviously, the impact of cerebral damage to *developing* neural systems is different at different ages from damage to *mature* neural systems. However, the subject samples of Teuber and Rudel (Rudel & Teuber, 1971; Rudel, Teuber, & Twitchell, 1966, 1974; Teuber & Rudel, 1962) as well as more recent investigators (e.g., Aram & Ekelman, 1986, 1988; Ballantyne, Scarvie, & Trauner, 1994; Dennis, 1991; Nass & Peterson, 1989; Riva & Cazzaniga, 1986; Stiles & Thal, 1993) have not permitted much comparison of specific prefrontal cortex damage because of the very low base rate of such isolated lesions.

Finally, in prospectively examining the course of recovery from early prefrontal cortex damage, questions about *delayed effects* can be more clearly addressed on an empirical basis. This obtains not only for cognitive processes and especially development of executive functions but also for development of social cognition and behavior and what we have termed *social executors* (see Eslinger, Grattan, & Geder, 1995), which pertain to the complex regulation of social-emotional behavior. Both cognitive-executive and social-executive processes have a protracted course of postnatal development, as indicated by numerous neuropsychological studies (e.g., Chelune & Baer, 1986; Eslinger et al., 1992; Grattan & Eslinger, 1991; Miller et al., 1973; Passler, Isaac, & Hynd, 1985; Welsh & Pennington, 1988). Certain neurobiological data have also supported the concept of protracted development, particularly in prefrontal cortical systems (e.g., Mrzljak et al., 1990; St. James-Roberts, 1979; Thatcher, 1991; Yakovlev & LeCours, 1967), although the key neurobiological events that underlie continued emergence of executive functions in late childhood, adolescence, and early adulthood are not yet clear. Identifying such events within a developmental framework may help address the delayed effects issue and provide intervention possibilities.

An important advance in the study of prefrontal cortex systems has been the greater emphasis on the definition and operationalized measurement of the processes that it mediates, many of which are subsumed under the rubric of executive functions. Although there is no universally accepted definition of executive functions, these capacities have been conceptualized as involving mechanisms that provide control, organization, and direction to behavior. Eslinger (1996) defined *executive functions* as processes that have the purpose of

- controlling implementation of activation-inhibition response sequences . . .
- that is guided by diverse neural representations (verbal rules, biological needs, somatic states, emotions, goals, mental models) . . .
- for the purpose of meeting a balance of immediate situational, short-term, and long-term future goals . . .
- that span physical-environmental, cognitive, behavioral, emotional, and social spheres (p. 381)

Empirical measures of executive functions are more highly developed for cognitive and sensorimotor domains than for emotional and social domains. Executive function tests generally assess the following: 1) representation and maintenance of diverse information; 2) abilities to integrate and manipulate new representations (e.g., situational constraints or rules) with respect to knowledge and prior experiences; and 3) powerful access to control of the motor system and responding. Many empirical measures of executive functions involve processes of inhibition of behavior and working memory (Pennington et al., 1996), which we illustrate in case descriptions to follow.

Although prospective study of early frontal lobe damage in humans cannot command the experimental control possible in animal models, the rigor of such study has increased greatly since the 1960s. Brain imaging data are now much more available and more precise for establishing diverse neural alterations, lesion location, and size. The variety of neuropsychological instruments has increased, with more age-appropriate cognitive tasks and extensive normative observations. Standardized inventories for social and other behavioral domains have also been developed and typically cull observations and ratings from parents and teachers. Finally, the availability of specialists in developmental and pediatric neuropsychology in hospitals, schools, mental health facilities, and academic training programs has broadened the clinical services and research initiatives in this area and permitted a greater awareness of the need to evaluate and treat the untoward effects, both immediate and delayed, of pediatric brain injury.

NEW CASES OF CHILDHOOD PREFRONTAL CORTEX DAMAGE

In this section, we highlight findings from two new cases of childhood prefrontal cortex damage (cases JC and MJ) that are being studied prospectively. Both subjects sustained nontraumatic focal lesions to the right dorsolateral prefrontal cortex that required surgical treatment. Data gathered from anatomical, cognitive, and social-behavioral studies are summarized, together with behavioral observations offered by the parents of each child. The results from both cases strongly support the role of the prefrontal cortex in development of executive functions that influence learning, language, problem solving, and social behaviors. In the first case (JC), we emphasize the possible roles of the prefrontal cortex in regulation of cognitive-executive functions. Its role in regulation of social-executive functions is the focus of the second case (MJ).

Case JC

Illness and Developmental History   At 7 years, 9 months of age, this right-handed boy suddenly developed severe headache followed by vomiting, seizures, and then loss of consciousness. Brain CT scanning at a local hospital revealed a right frontal intraparenchymal hemorrhage, and JC was transferred to our medical center's neurosurgery service. On neurological exam, he was unresponsive to verbal stimuli but reacted to pain and moved all extremities. His pupils were 3 mm bilaterally and sluggishly reactive. His deep tendon reflexes were 2+ and symmetric. He immediately underwent a right frontal craniotomy with evacuation of hematoma and excision of an arteriovenous malformation (AVM) (anatomical details are summarized in the Lesion Localization section). Postoperatively, JC showed progressive improvement, answering questions and following commands within several days. He exhibited mild left facial palsy and mild left sixth nerve palsy, with motor strength 4+/5 on the left and 5/5 on the right. His sensory exam was intact. An angiogram revealed no evidence of residual AVM. He was noted to be emotionally labile and was transferred to a nearby rehabilitation center, where he continued to improve and was eventually discharged home with return to school. We first examined JC at 6 months and then again at 4 years after right frontal AVM resection.

Premorbidly, JC was the product of a full-term, uncomplicated pregnancy. He achieved all developmental milestones well within normal limits, walking at 9 months of age and speaking prolifically by 2 years of age. His parents are college-educated professionals, with no family history of learning disabilities, and JC achieved at above-average levels in school. For instance, on the Iowa Test of Basic Skills, completed just 2 months prior to his intraparenchymal hemorrhage, his scores all were above the 85th percentile, except for math computation, on which he scored at the 75th percentile. He completed the first grade with an A− in reading and math. Socially, he had many friends, was active in team sports such as hockey, and enjoyed skateboarding and other recreational activities. Therefore, no developmental cognitive or behavioral abnormalities could be identified.

Lesion Localization   Surgical approach to the hematoma was made through topectomy in the right middle frontal gyrus, following down to the head of the caudate, which was visualized but appeared to be normal and was not surgically invaded. The AVM was identified and resected, with coagulation and excision of feeding vessels laterally from the region of the insula and medially from above the head of the caudate. Analysis of a brain MRI scan taken 2 years after intraparenchymal hemorrhage indicated a focal area of hypodensity in the right dorsolateral frontal cortex (see Figures 14.1 and 14.2). T_1-weighted coronal slices of the frontal lobe are presented in Figure 14.1A, with localization of lesion on the best-fitting brain template according to the method of Damasio and Damasio (1989) shown in Figure 14.1B. Results indicated that the lesion compromised Brodmann's areas 9, 10, and 46 as well as areas 44, 45, and 47. A small dorsal portion of area 6, the anterior insula, and the deep white matter of the prefrontal cortex were also involved, extending to but not compromising the head of the caudate nucleus. As can be seen in the sagittal sections in Figure 14.2, there is sparing of the polar and orbital regions of the prefrontal cortex as well as most of the superior mesial structures of the anterior cingulate gyrus and supplementary motor area. Therefore, the lesion included a large portion of the right dorsolateral prefrontal cortex, with involvement of deep white matter.

Early Recovery Phase   After a brief stay in a rehabilitation center, JC was discharged home and returned to school after the summer break, 2.5 months after hemorrhage. He was noted to be more fidgety, distractible, and impulsive. He also was obsessed with smelling clothes, foods, and household items. He completed the second grade successfully, but several other changes in behavior were noted. JC talked excessively, often digressed from the topic, and had difficulty initiating as well as remaining on usual tasks. He required constant cuing to complete any multistep task, such as household chores and school assignments. His social behavior appeared to have regressed; he preferred to play with younger children and was unable to maintain solitary activities.

Neuropsychological exam at 6 months after AVM repair indicated a child who was distractible and impulsive but nonetheless cooperated with test procedures and appeared interested in doing well. Formal measures of intellect from the Wechsler Intelligence Scale for Children–Revised (WISC–R) (Wechsler, 1974) indicated a high-average level of intelligence with greater verbal than performance IQ score. (Scores are summarized in Table 14.2, where they are also compared with later testing.) Speech was fluent, nonparaphrasic, and well articulated, with above-average range of lexical access on the Boston Naming Test (Kaplan, Goodglass, & Weintraub, 1983). However, JC did not initiate much conversation or elaborate on his verbal responses. Measures of visual perception indicated normal object and word recognition, with a high-average score on discrimination of unfamiliar faces (Facial Recognition Test) but low-average spatial judgment (Judgment of Line Orientation) (Benton, Hamsher, Varney, & Spreen, 1983). Right–left discrimination was intact on himself and on confrontation testing. However, notable deficits were observed in constructional praxis and short-term visual memory for designs (Benton, 1974).

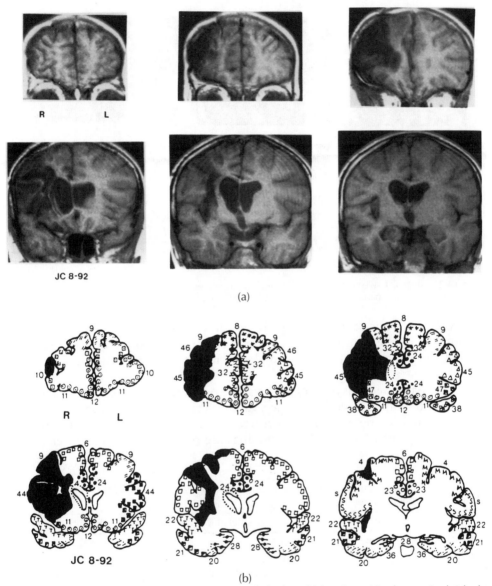

Figure 14.1.   (a) T$_1$-weighted coronal MRI cuts through the frontal lobe of case JC, who sustained right dorsolateral prefrontal cortex lesion from AVM resection at 7 years of age. (b) Best-fitting brain template for localization of the right frontal lesion, showing damage to Brodmann's areas 9, 10, 44, 45, 46, and 47; dorsal portions of 6; anterior insula; and deep white matter. The head of the caudate was not damaged.

Figure 14.3A presents examples of JC's immediate reproduction of a geometric shape (hexagon) after studying it for 10 seconds and then reproducing it from memory. He made two attempts at reproduction of the hexagon and showed spatial distortions in both cases. His clock drawing indicated marked left hemispatial neglect and spatial distortions, although all numbers and hands were included (Figure 14.3A). His spatial planning and construction of the complex figure of Rey-Osterrieth (Osterrieth, 1944; Rey, 1941) under standard administration conditions (see Figure 14.4A) indicated a drawing compressed along its horizontal axis, with spatial distortions and perseveration in line segments but an otherwise fair degree

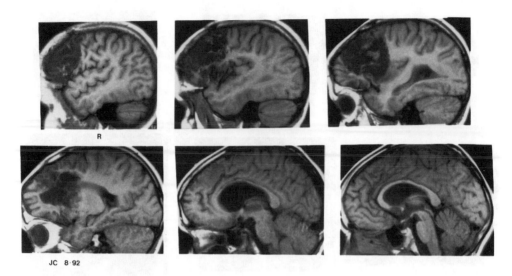

JC 8·92

Figure 14.2.   Sagittal T$_1$-weighted MRI cuts through the right hemisphere of case JC, showing dorsolateral frontal lobe lesion with sparing of the polar and orbital frontal cortices.

of internal detail. His score of 18.5 of 36 was in the markedly impaired range. JC's reproduction of the complex figure after a 20-minute delay was also markedly impaired, with spatial distortions and almost no features from the left side of the figure.

In summary, neuropsychological evaluation in the early recovery phase, approximately 6 months after AVM repair, gave several indications of specific dissociations in cognitive, memory, and executive abilities usually associated with right frontal lobe lesions in adults. These findings are remarkable for the extent of the

Table 14.2.   JC's performance on standard neuropsychological tests after AVM repair in the right dorsolateral prefrontal region

Test	Results at 4 years	Results at 6 months
Wechsler Intelligence Scale for Children III		
Verbal IQ score	125 (95th percentile, superior)	113
Performance IQ score	112 (79th percentile, high average)	106
Full-scale IQ score	121 (92nd percentile, superior)	111
Judgment of Line Orientation	26	14
Facial Recognition Test	43	40
Right–Left discrimination		
Self	12/12	12
Confrontation	7/8	8
Boston Naming Test	54	45
Benton Visual Retention Test		
Number Correct	6 (expect 7)	4
Number Errors	5 (expect 5)	12

Results on Wechsler Intelligence Scale for Children–Revised.

JC

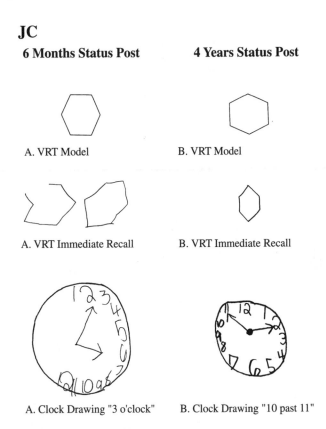

6 Months Status Post   **4 Years Status Post**

A. VRT Model   B. VRT Model

A. VRT Immediate Recall   B. VRT Immediate Recall

A. Clock Drawing "3 o'clock"   B. Clock Drawing "10 past 11"

Figure 14.3.   (A) Model of a geometric figure from the Benton Visual Retention Test (Benton, 1974) with JC's impaired attempts at immediate recall of that figure after its exposure for 10 seconds. His spontaneous clock drawing shows spatial distortion and left hemispatial neglect. These tasks were completed 6 months after right dorsolateral frontal lobe lesion at 7 years of age. (B) Performance on similar visual memory and constructional tasks at 4 years after lesion, showing marked improvement.

impairments 6 months after illness. His ability to handle daily living tasks and school assignments was now notably compromised by difficulty with spatial planning, sequencing, and keeping track of information in multistep tasks. JC also became more distractible, impulsive, disinhibited, and tangential in his speech and behavior. He did not initiate conversation or elaborate very much in verbal responses. A behavioral feature that may be somewhat unusual was his marked propensity to smell everything, even nonfood items such as clothing and furniture, to an obsessive degree. This may have resulted from a combination of disinhibition and utilization behavior. None of these difficulties was evident prior to his hemorrhage and AVM repair. In this recovery phase, his neurological exam remained remarkable only for mild left lower facial palsy and decreased left arm swing and left leg circumduction during gait. An electroencephalogram was normal, but he was continued on Dilantin on a prophylactic basis.

Chronic Recovery Phase   JC returned for comprehensive neuropsychological evaluation 4 years after AVM repair and right dorsolateral frontal cortex lesion. He had advanced into the sixth grade, with no medical complications or major changes

JC

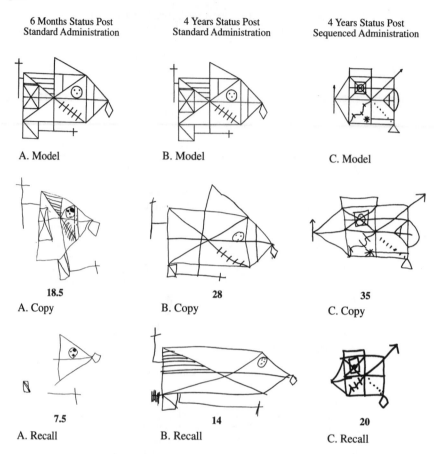

Figure 14.4.   (A) Copy of the complex figure of Rey-Osterrieth by JC at 6 months after lesion, with 20-minute delayed recall performance just below. (B) Performance on the same copy and recall task at 4 years after lesion, showing significant improvement. (C) Copy and delayed recall of the Taylor complex figure, which was presented by the examiner in a "sequenced administration" in which items of the figure were added to the central square in a series of 17 steps. This organizational strategy was beneficial to both copy and delayed recall of the stimulus figure.

in his psychosocial environment. We were able to complete more extensive cognitive and behavioral evaluations and also compare his recovery of function with the early-phase evaluation, with an eye toward identifying what impairments had resolved and what new difficulties may be emerging.

The first point of comparison involves JC's constructional praxis and visual memory performances, shown in Figures 14.3 and 14.4 for both the early and the chronic recovery phases. Specifically, in Figure 14.3B, it can be seen that his immediate reproduction of a comparable design from the Benton Visual Retention Test (Benton, 1974) indicated entirely normal construction and memory. His clock drawing was also remarkably improved, with very little evidence of spatial distortion and no evidence of left hemispatial neglect. In Figure 14.4B, his copy and recall of the Rey-Osterrieth complex figure showed marked improvement under standard administration conditions (score, 28 of 36). Despite this gain, difficulties were still observable in the spatial alignment of features and the omission of several details from the left side of the complex figure. A similar result was observed with his figure recall after a 20-minute delay interval (score, 14 of 36). To compare JC's self-generated constructional approach with an organizational strategy provided by the examiner, we presented the complex figure of Taylor (1959), under sequenced administration conditions (Eslinger et al., 1995). Specifically, the elements of the Taylor figure were presented one step at a time, beginning with the central square and continuing with an additional feature in each of 17 steps. Thus, the procedure required that JC construct the complex figure one step at a time as per the examiner's organizational strategy. His copy under this condition indicated entirely normal reproduction with very little evidence of spatial distortion (score, 35 of 36). His recall of the figure after a 20-minute delay also showed a beneficial effect of the organizational strategy on memory (score, 20 of 36). Therefore, although JC showed a significant improvement in his constructional and visual memory performance levels 4 years after the lesion, there was still residual evidence of spatial planning and spatial attentional defects that were remediable by providing an organizational strategy.

Comparison of results on several general cognitive measures with those of previous assessment (see Table 14.2) showed significant improvement on formal tests of intellect, spatial perception, facial pattern discrimination, naming ability, and short-term visual memory for designs. A discrepancy between verbal and performance IQ was still evident, although none of the subtest scores fell below the 50th percentile.

Executive Functions in Chronic Recovery Stage   One of the most intriguing areas to evaluate at this stage of recovery is the domain of executive functions. Concerns about confounding physiological effects of the lesion (e.g., edema, diaschisis, mass effects) have abated and impairments can be more reliably associated with the observed lesion site and neural networks. Table 14.3 provides a summary of the executive function measures that were presented to JC. As suggested from evolving definitions of executive functions (Denckla, 1996; Eslinger, 1996; Pennington et al., 1996), these necessarily span a number of processing domains, most importantly working memory, spatial planning, attention control and inhibition, processing speed, cognitive flexibility, learning, and language. The tasks were chosen to empirically measure registration, maintenance, manipulation, utilization, and organization of diverse information-processing features. Results indicated that impairments were evident in all of the domains.

Working Memory   Measures of verbal working memory were entirely normal. However, a marked defect was evident in spatial working memory, specifically delayed responding and to a lesser extent delayed alternation and delayed alternation responding (see Table 14.4). These tasks were presented in a computerized program (Carpenter, Randolph, & Gold, 1995). Delayed responding required the subject to retain the location of a colored square on either the left or the right side of the screen over several seconds' delay. JC achieved 55% accuracy of delayed responding, which was markedly impaired in comparison with 97.5% accuracy for 3 age- and sex-matched control subjects. The controls found this task easy, each performing it correctly on 39 of the 40 trials. JC's scores on the delayed alternation and delayed alternation responding tasks were also below controls, approximately 1.8 SD, placing him at less than the fifth percentile. Interestingly, JC has experienced persistent difficulties in keeping track of which end of the basketball court is offense

Table 14.3.   Executive function measures

Working memory
  Verbal
    Sentence span
    Counting span
  Visuospatial
    Delayed responding
    Delayed alternation
    Delayed alternation responding
Spatial planning
  Tower of Hanoi
  Rey-Osterrieth and Taylor complex figure constructions in standard and sequenced formats
Attentional control/inhibition
  Double simultaneous auditory stimulation (dichotic listening)
  Matching Familiar Figures Test
  Trail Making Test A & B
Processing speed
  Visual matching
  Visual search
  Rapid naming
Cognitive flexibility
  Reactive
    Wisconsin Card Sorting Test
    Woodcock-Johnson Tests of Cognitive Ability
    Concept Formation
  Spontaneous
    Verbal fluency—Letter stimulus, category stimulus, alternate uses
    Visual (nonverbal)—design fluency
Learning
  Serial position effects
  Subjective organization
Language
  Test of Language Competence–Expanded
  Analysis of narratives

and which is defense. Both spatial locations are the same and change within and between games, complicated by fast-moving action during the game. He is able to compensate, however, if a teammate or coach yells "offense" and "defense" as the team moves up and down the court.

Spatial Planning   The Tower of Hanoi task, as applied by Welsh et al. (1991) in their study of normal children, is a multistep task that requires spatial planning and problem-solving skills. Three- and four-ring problems are presented that require between 6 and 15 moves in order to match the goal configuration. The rings were of different sizes and colors and had to be moved one at a time, with the constraint that a larger ring could not be placed on top of a smaller ring. JC's performance, in terms of both total number of moves and latency, was comparable with controls. However, construction of the Rey-Osterrieth complex figure, as a multistep spatial planning task, was shown previously to be impaired.

Table 14.4.   Executive function impairments in Case JC

Task	Test results	
	JC	Controls ($\bar{x}$, SD)
Visuospatial working memory (percentage correct)		
Delayed responding	55.0	(97.5, 0)
Delayed alternation	47.5	(57.5, 5.4)
Delayed alternation responding	55.0	(66.0, 6.6)
Attention control/inhibition		
Dichotic Listening (percentage correct)		
Left ear	72	(101.5, 8.9)
Right ear	100	(105, 5.6)
Matching Familiar Figures Test		
Mean response time	11.12 sec	(35.5, 20)
Total errors	19	(4.2, 3.4)
Trail Making Test B		
Time to completion	121 sec	(95, 15.1)
Total errors	10	(1, 0.82)
Processing speed		
Visual matching	32	(5th percentile)
Visual search		
efficiency score	1.86	(1.40, 0.46)

Attention Control/Inhibition   Difficulties on three of these tasks are noteworthy. First, JC exhibited a relative left ear extinction in the dichotic listening task of word pairs (see Table 14.4). We have previously reported this pattern in adult-onset cases of right frontal lobe lesion and related it to impaired attentional control (Eslinger & Damasio, 1988). Second, JC's latency to respond on the Matching Familiar Figures Test (Kagan, Rosman, Day, Albert, & Phillips, 1964) was much quicker than controls, with a 4.5-fold increase in errors. These results indicated difficulty inhibiting responses to highly similar stimuli and poor control of attention to fine detail. Finally, although JC's performance on part A of the Trail Making Test (Reitan, 1979) was in fact quicker than that of the control subjects, his performance on Part B indicated increased latency and very frequent errors in completing the alternating number–letter sequence. This difficulty was unrelated to motor factors because finger tapping, grip strength, and pegboard scores of the right upper extremity were normal.

Processing Speed   JC's verbal processing speed was entirely normal in naming of objects, colors, numbers, and letters, as well as alternating stimuli (Denckla & Rudel, 1976; Wolf, 1986). In fact, his response latency was faster than that of controls. Measures of visuospatial processing speed varied from low-average to impaired (see Table 14.4). Specifically, speed of visual matching for numbers from the Woodcock-Johnson Psychoeducational Battery–Revised (Woodcock & Johnson, 1989) was at the fifth percentile, and efficiency of visual search for object drawings (Welsh et al., 1991) was 1 SD below controls.

Cognitive Flexibility   Two forms of cognitive flexibility were tested: reactive and spontaneous (Grattan & Eslinger, 1990). The reactive flexibility measures, the Wisconsin Card Sorting Test (WCST) (Heaton, Chelune, Talley, Kay, & Curtiss, 1993) and the Concept Formation task of the Woodcock-Johnson Tests of Cognitive Abil-

Table 14.5.   Executive function impairment: Fluency task results in Case JC

Test	Number of responses	Correct responses (%)		Perseverations (%)
Letter fluency	22	21	(95%)	0
	(21.3)[a]	(21.3)[a]	(100%)	(0)[a]
Category fluency	71	68	(96%)	0
	(51.3)	(49.7)	(97%)	(0)
Verbal ideational fluency	24	11	(46%)[b]	38%[b]
	(17.3)	(13.3)	(77%)	(9.6%)
Design fluency				
Free condition	11	5	(45%)[b]	29%[b]
	(15)	(13.7)	(91%)	(6.7%)
Fixed condition	11	6	(55%)[b]	0
	(15)	(13.7)	(91%)	(0)

[a]Numbers in parentheses are mean control values.
[b]Impaired relative to controls.

ity, require various aspects of establishing abstract relations among stimuli, utilizing examiner feedback and shifting response set. JC performed within the normal range for his age. His results on the spontaneous flexibility measures, which require generating a number of alternative responses to a simple question or rule, are summarized in Table 14.5. These involved measures of verbal associative fluency and design fluency (Benton & Hamsher, 1976; Jones-Gotman & Milner, 1977; McCarthy, 1972). JC was able to generate as many words according to a letter rule as normal controls, with no indication of perseverative tendencies. Generating words according to a semantic category rule (e.g., foods, animals, clothing, rides) revealed that JC in fact generated more correct responses than any of the controls, again with no perseverative tendencies. However, proficiency in verbal ideational fluency was difficult for JC. This task, adapted from Guilford's Alternate Uses Test (Guilford, Christensen, Merrifield, & Wilson, 1960), requires subjects to generate additional uses for common objects, such as other uses for a newspaper than reading and other uses for a pencil than writing. Although JC generated many more responses than controls, 54% of his responses were incorrect, and about a third of his responses were of a perseverative nature. The percentage of errors was twice that of controls, and the percentage of perseverative responses was four times greater than controls. Errors were a combination of unrealistic alternate uses for objects (e.g., wear a shoe as a hat, smash a key) or repeated, nonproductive uses such as throwing each of these items around. The alternate uses task differs from the letter and category fluency tasks in that it requires a higher degree of novel divergent production and possibly more spatially or visually based cognitive manipulation of the suggested stimulus items. This dissociation became much clearer in the design fluency task, on which JC's accuracy of spatial design productions was on average one-half that of controls. JC's percentage of perseverative responses under the free spatial design condition was four times greater than controls.

Organization to Verbal Learning   On the Children's Auditory Verbal Learning Test–2 (Talley, 1993), which is composed of a 16-word list drawn from four semantic categories, JC showed a flat learning curve (see Figure 14.5A). Although his standard score on Trial 1 was above average, his level of learning did not increase with subsequent repetitions of the same word list. His score drifts from the top toward the bottom of the normal range for his age over trials. This is also reflected in Figure 14.5B, where there is a notable drop from Trial 1 performance (Immediate

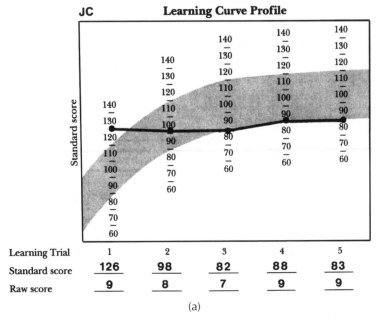

Learning Trial	1	2	3	4	5
Standard score	126	98	82	88	83
Raw score	9	8	7	9	9

(a)

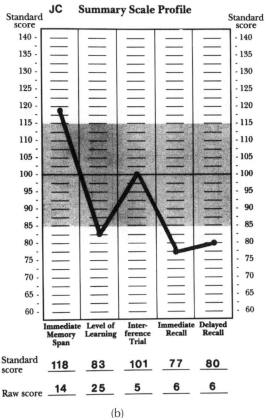

	Immediate Memory Span	Level of Learning	Inter-ference Trial	Immediate Recall	Delayed Recall
Standard score	118	83	101	77	80
Raw score	14	25	5	6	6

(b)

Figure 14.5. (a) Verbal learning curve of JC on the Children's Auditory Verbal Learning Test–2 (CAVLT–2), showing normal Trial 1 performance (normal range indicated by shaded area) but a flat learning curve with no improvement during subsequent learning trials. (b) Summary of several verbal learning and retention measures for JC on the CAVLT–2. Note particularly the poor recall performance in both immediate and delayed conditions.

Memory Span) to the Level of Learning composite score for subsequent trials. His single-trial learning performance again increases with the Interference Trial, but the Immediate and Delayed Recall of the original word list are quite poor (46% retention). This was unexpected, given the location of his cerebral lesion in the *right* dorsolateral prefrontal cortex and the highly verbal nature of the learning task, usually associated with left hemispheric function. Tulving, Kapur, Craik, Moscovitch, and Houle (1994), however, have indicated that the right prefrontal cortical region (including areas 10, 46, 9, and 6, which were damaged in JC) may play an important role in retrieval of explicit, episodic memory, based on positron emission tomography (PET) studies in normal subjects.

Because we know that JC processes verbal information quickly and is in the superior range of verbal intellectual ability, we examined indices of *organizational strategies* that JC may have used (or failed to use) in his verbal learning approach. The results were intriguing. First, we discovered that JC showed a delayed emergence of the typical serial position curve until the fifth learning trial. In contrast, adult-onset cases with right dorsolateral prefrontal cortex lesions quickly establish but are unable to maintain serial position effects (Eslinger & Grattan, 1994). When responses are plotted according to word list position, this generally results in a U-shaped curve with higher recall from the beginning (primacy effect) and end (recency effect) portions of the list and comparatively less recall from the middle stimulus items. This is a fundamental characteristic of serial learning that has been observed in human and nonhuman species, and JC's slowness to establish serial position effects may be related to altered temporospatial processing. A second indication of an organizational strategy can be garnered from Tulving's (1962) subjective organization index. This is a measure of how much of a sequential ordering strategy subjects apply in their verbal learning responses. In fact, JC's subjective organization index was quite high (.49), indicating that he recalled the same words in approximately the same order on each trial. However, this strategy accommodated only a few words, and he was unable to build upon the sequential ordering. Finally, we analyzed semantic clustering in his responses because the stimulus items were drawn from four semantic categories, and such clustering may provide an effective strategy for increasing learning across trials (e.g., Levin et al., 1991). The percentage of clustered responses was high but did not improve across trials, beginning at 56% of responses on Trial 1 and ending at 44% on Trial 5. Furthermore, most of these were couplets (two items from the same semantic category), with only one instance of a triplet on Trial 1. Therefore, we suggest that JC's verbal learning and memory deficit was very likely related to poor organizational strategies in handling the serial stimuli and possibly to a specific memory retrieval deficit. His most consistent strategy was to repeat back a small number of words in the same order from trial to trial, with only gradual emergence of a few additional items from the primacy portion of the curve across learning trials; obviously, this was not an effective verbal learning strategy in this task.

Discourse   In adults, lesions of the right frontal region can result in impairments in the pragmatic aspects of language that are necessary for understanding intention and context of meaning. We have shown that JC's basic language capacities, such as naming and vocabulary, are entirely normal and that his verbal intelligence is superior. For example, JC's word retrieval ability on the Boston Naming Test was above grade level, and his visual naming speed on rapid automatized naming (Denckla & Rudel, 1976) and rapid alternating stimulus naming (Wolf, 1986) was faster than controls. Similarly, he performed as well as or better than controls on measures of letter and category fluency. Therefore, we were interested in assessing his development of some discourse skills that are important to academic and social competence. Toward this end, we employed the Test of Language Competence–Expanded (TLC–E) (Wiig & Secord, 1988) and analyses of narratives.

The TLC–E is composed of four subtests that assess various aspects of children's communicative competence. JC performed within the average to above-average range on three of the subtests (see Table 14.6). On the fourth (Recreating Sentences), he performed in the low-average range. However, his behavior during the various tasks suggested cognitive inflexibility, impulsive responding, and a lack of planning. Results were as follows:

1. The Ambiguous Sentences subtest requires the subject to formulate two different meanings for one sentence that contains a lexical or syntactic ambiguity (e.g., "I saw the girl take his picture"). On this task, JC rapidly generated an initial response, but he had difficulty conceptualizing and shifting to a second possible meaning for 5 of the 13 items.
2. The Making Inferences subtest requires the child to listen to a stage-setting statement and an outcome statement and then infer two reasons for that outcome from among four choices. JC became confused and needed frequent redirection to complete this task. He often decided that the first inference ruled out the possibility of a second inferred meaning.
3. The Figurative Language subtest assesses the child's comprehension of metaphoric expressions. Although JC had no difficulty selecting a matching metaphor, his errors in all but one instance resulted from an inability to state the meaning of the metaphor in his own words.

Table 14.6.   Case JC: Results of language discourse assessment

Language measures	JC's score	Control mean or percentile
Test of Language Competence–Expanded		
Ambiguous Sentences	29	75th
Making Inferences	30	50th
Recreating Sentences	63	25th
Figurative Language	23	63rd
Narrative analysis		
Absolute measures		
Explicit propositions	18.0	21.33
Implicit propositions	3.0	1.67[b]
Repeated propositions	1.0	0.0[b]
Total dysfluencies	1.0	3.33
False starts	0.0	0.67
Fillers	1.0	2.33
Internal corrections	0.0	0.33
Level two propositions	15.0	9.67
Subordinate propositions	5.0	12.33[a]
Ratio scores		
Listener burden ratio	0.17	0.10
Redundancy ratio	0.05	0.0[b]
Dysfluency ratio	0.05	0.14
Density ratio	0.33	1.23[b]

[a]Score is 1.33 standard deviations below the control mean.

[b]Score is 1.66 standard deviations below the control mean.

4. The Recreating Sentences subtest requires the child to form a sentence using two or three key words, relating the sentence to the context shown in an illustration and also representing the intended meaning of the speaker in the picture. Although JC attempted to use the keywords, his sentences contained awkward phrasing (e.g., "Here nor the bakery down the street, these breads are more fresh"). He tended to make numerous revisions of his sentences, which indicated a lack of initial planning. It is notable that JC struggled with the Recreating Sentences subtest, given his superior verbal IQ, his intact naming and word retrieval ability, and the structured presentation of the task.

Overall, JC's performance on the TLC–E demonstrated relatively intact language abilities coexisting with impaired ability to formulate complex sentences. This comparative deficiency has also been noted by JC's teacher, who has identified difficulties with his formulation of essays and reports. Many children with traumatic brain injury have shown a similar pattern of results, with normal language and verbal intelligence scores but disrupted discourse (Chapman et al., 1992; Dennis, 1991; Dennis & Barnes, 1990; Dennis & Lovett, 1990; Mateer & Williams, 1991; Williams & Mateer, 1992; Ylvisaker, 1993). Nearly 80% of the children in the Dennis and Barnes (1990) study were impaired on at least one subtest of the TLC–E. This may be because the frontal lobe is often damaged from traumatic brain injury, and processes of planning, monitoring, and production of discourse can be compromised (Alexander, Benson, & Stuss, 1989).

A narrative generation task was also used to examine JC's ability to *spontaneously* organize discourse with minimal contextual support (see Liles, 1993). Six spontaneous personal narratives were elicited from JC using the conversational maps technique developed by Peterson and McCabe (1983). Dependency analysis (Deese, 1984; see Peterson & McCabe, 1983, for complete description and examples) provided a quantitative measure of narrative complexity, including syntax, dysfluencies, and repetitions. As part of the analysis, the narrative was divided into syntactic units called propositions. For example, the statement "I was stung by a bee last year" would be divided into three propositions: "I was stung" is the main proposition with "by a bee" and "last year" as modifying propositions. The results of the narrative analysis indicated that JC showed problems with planning and monitoring of discourse (see Table 14.6). On several measures, JC performed markedly worse than the controls. For example, he had significantly more implicit propositions (i.e., omitted information) in his narratives than did the controls. In addition, he made more repeated propositions. JC also generated fewer subordinate propositions than his peers, which indicated insufficient elaboration. On the remaining absolute measures of narrative ability, JC's performance was similar to that of controls. That is, he generated the same number of explicit (stated) propositions as his peers. He also had a similar number of level two propositions, which are the propositions at the level just below the superordinate organizing statement or theme for the narrative. In addition, JC had fewer dysfluencies than the controls. He made no false starts, used only one filler (e.g., "um"), and did not correct himself (internal correction) during his discourse.

The absolute measures were used to derive ratio scores. On two ratio measures, JC's performance was significantly worse than that of controls. The redundancy ratio, a measure of the speaker's repeated propositions relative to the total number of explicit propositions, indicated that JC was more repetitious than his peers. The lower density ratio, which compares the total number of subordinate propositions with the number of level two propositions, was indicative of JC's simpler narrative style than the controls. The listener burden ratio, which compares total implicit propositions with explicit propositions, was not statistically significant but conflicted with our clinical experience with JC. Although his generation of explicit (stated) propositions was comparable with that of normal controls, his narration style was actually much more restricted. He responded to the initial story prompt with only five propositions. In contrast, controls generated 13–33 propositions in response to the initial prompt, and 2 of the 3 controls required no additional prompting at all. The elaboration that JC could provide after neutral subprompts was simpler and less elaborate than that of his peers, as indicated by his use of fewer subordinate propositions. In comparison with controls, JC was more repetitive and omitted more information from his narrative. Although he made pronominal referencing errors, such as "I stung me," JC seemed unaware of these errors and did not correct himself. Like JC, children with traumatic brain injury have been reported to produce as much discourse as controls (Biddle, McCabe, & Bliss, in press). However, they did not adequately monitor their narratives and were less efficient and effective in their discourse delivery. The children with traumatic brain injury, 50% of whom had documented injuries to the frontal lobe, were more repetitive and omitted more information from their stories than controls, causing a significant listener burden.

Although the listener burden ratio (a measure of omitted information not statistically different in JC during this task) may capture certain aspects of the actual burden of the listener, JC's signficantly lower density ratio may create another form of listener burden. When he fails to elaborate during social discourse, it is quite possible that insufficient information is supplied to the listener. Consequently, the burden is placed upon the listener to ask questions or provide prompting in order to elicit a complete story from the speaker. In fact, JC's teacher has noted that she must provide additional prompting in order to elicit a complete written story from him. Although listener burden is not traditionally framed in this manner in dependency analysis (Deese, 1984), this hypothesis warrants further study.

In summary, despite entirely normal elementary language and verbal cognitive abilities, JC's performance indicated several pragmatic language difficulties, including impaired ability to formulate complex sentences; simpler and less elaborate narratives, even after several prompts; and impulsive responding at times. These difficulties are suggestive of impairments in the executive processes that manage discourse production, particularly the planning, organization, flexibility, and monitoring of discourse. This selective pattern was also evident on the verbal associative fluency measures. JC was able to generate responses when the demands were elementary and routine (e.g., animal names), but, as the task demands increased (e.g., alternative object uses), he was unable to elaborate a sufficient number of correct possibilities. We hypothesize that JC's discourse deficits are the result of impaired interaction between executive and linguistic systems following right dorsolateral prefrontal cortex injury. More generally, early injury to the prefrontal region may predispose the developing child to disturbances of discourse. This hypothesis warrants further investigation with a larger sample of children.

Social Behavior   The parent-, teacher-, and self-report forms of the Child Behavior Checklist (Achenbach & Edelbrock, 1983) were utilized to survey various aspects of JC's behavior and social interaction. Results indicated that JC did not identify any difficulties or concerns and described himself as "I'm nice. I'm a good friend, I'm nice to other people." Reports of his parents and teacher, however, indicated several areas of difficulty. Both identified attention problems, particularly difficulties concentrating, sitting still, and producing neat work. Parental responses also indicated elevation on the thought problems and anxiety-depression scales, related to occasional unusual behaviors and concerns about feeling different from others. The response pattern from his teacher indicated elevations on the social problems and aggressive behavior scales, related to being disturbing to others, showing off or clowning, teasing others a lot, and not managing the spatial coordination aspects of social interaction. Informal comments about JC's social behavior are also intriguing. For example, JC's parents report that "JC doesn't seem to understand a lot of the dynamics of his peer groups. He takes things very literally and very personally." However, JC is also described as a happy and loving child who can show a quick concern for others. He is still largely viewed by his family and by others as being sociable and outgoing, with a sense of humor.

Summary of Case JC   JC presents an intriguing array of information about the behavioral effects and pattern of recovery after AVM repair requiring tissue resection in the right dorsolateral prefrontal region at 7 years of age. In the early recovery phase, there were many similarities to adult-onset cases. Prominent deficits included left hemispatial neglect, constructional apraxia, poor visual memory for designs, and impaired attentional control, whereas speech and language as well as various measures of verbal and nonverbal intellectual ability were within the normal range. JC improved remarkably over the following 3.5 years, but results indicated much more clearly that certain impairments in executive functions were evident. These affected a number of domains, particularly those requiring visuospatial aspects of planning, fluency, and working memory. Executive function deficits were also observed in response inhibition and attentional control, application of organizational strategies to learning, and formulation and monitoring of discourse. On a daily basis, JC encounters his greatest difficulties in judging time, completing multistep tasks, and planning. In addition, he exhibits acquired characteristics of ADHD, combined type. Consequent to these difficulties, he has required a more structured approach to assignments and activities and often needs supervision in maintaining attention to task and completing multistep activities. Interestingly, JC's performance on a number of executive function measures often associated with the frontal lobe were entirely normal at this age, including the Wisconsin Card Sorting Test, the Tower of Hanoi, letter and category forms of verbal associative fluency, and verbal working memory. Unfortunately, these measures were not administered in the early recovery phase; hence, it is uncertain whether JC was entirely unaffected in these processes or recovered to age-appropriate levels. Study of new cases may answer this question. These findings indicate support for a model of selective differentiation of functions associated with the right dorsolateral prefrontal cortex and its associated networks by 7 years of age and persisting executive function deficits at least 4 years after cerebral lesion.

Although JC's postlesion development has not revealed major social or emotional abnormalities up to 11 years of age, there have been several behavior changes brought on by alterations in attentional, inhibitory, visuospatial, and working memory processes that affect his relationships. In addition, there appear to be emerging difficulties in his understanding group interactions, social discourse, and the social behavior of others. These have taken the forms of more literal or concrete social responses, disinhibited behavior, and limitations in following the flow of social interactions and changing circumstances. Despite this, JC has remained emotionally connected to family members and is largely perceived as an affectionate 11-year-old boy who is responsive to his family's emotional experiences.

Case MJ

For purposes of this chapter, we emphasized cognitive and linguistic aspects of behavior and executive functions with JC. We would like to contrast those results with elaboration of the social development of another case of right dorsolateral prefrontal cortex lesion in early childhood, case MJ. Being in middle adolescence at the time of evaluation, MJ has experienced a wider variety of social situations and has had to face several of the complex psychosocial challenges of adolescent development.

Developmental History and Illness   After an uncomplicated birth and normal developmental milestones up to 3 years of age, MJ developed symptoms of ear infection, progressing to meningitis that required hospitalization and treatment. After continued symptoms, brain CT scanning revealed an abscess in the right frontal lobe, which was surgically evacuated without complication at 3 years of age. MJ's recovery was considered excellent and has not been associated with any seizures or sensorimotor changes. MJ returned to his usual range of activities, although his mother observes that his personality has been different from the time of the right frontal lobe lesion. He began school at an appropriate age and has continued to advance, currently being in the middle high school years.

Lesion Localization   MJ had an MRI scan of the brain in 1992, 11 years after onset of the right frontal lobe lesion (see Figure 14.6). T_1-weighted slices through the coronal plane revealed a focal lesion in the right dorsolateral prefrontal cortex with minimal extension to the subjacent white matter. Lesion localization on the best-fitting template of Damasio and Damasio (1989) indicated that the lesion was limited to Brodmann's area 9 and partially to area 46, in the region of the middle frontal gyrus. There were no other indications of abnormality.

In comparison with JC, MJ's lesion in the right dorsolateral prefrontal cortex was more limited, involving the superior portions of this region and only minimal subjacent white matter. There was sparing of the inferolateral regions, as well as the polar, orbital, and superomesial frontal cortices.

Neuropsychological Results   MJ underwent neuropsychological evaluations at 8 and 14 years of age. More recently, at 16 years of age, he underwent a comprehensive cognitive examination similar to that described for JC. The earlier exams were prompted by difficulties "focusing" in school, tangential responses, disinhibited and acting-out behavior in school, and inability to establish friendships. In the elementary grades, MJ advanced in a grade-appropriate manner, even being somewhat above grade level in reading. His measured intelligence has consistently been in the average range, although difficulties with visual memory and mental control (e.g., freedom from distractibility) were found in the earlier evaluations. Mild perseverative tendencies, impulsive responding, and disinhibition were also observed during these evaluations. He has shown many characteristics of ADHD, inattentive type, and has required more supervision and cuing in completing daily activities and assignments than have his siblings.

An example of MJ's visual memory performance from our recent neuropsychological examination is presented in Figure 14.7, which shows immediate reproduc-

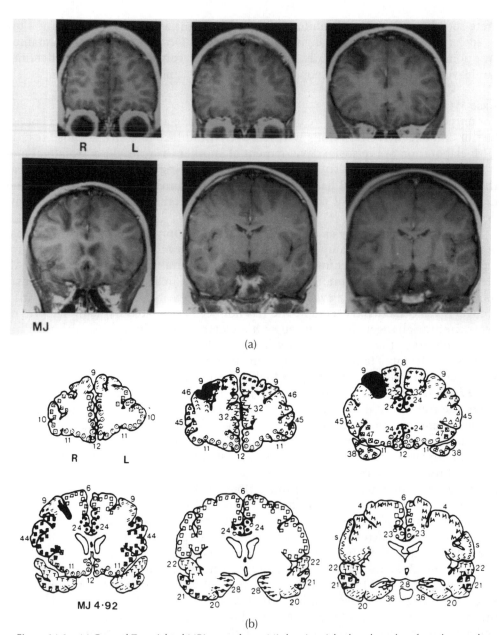

Figure 14.6.   (a) Coronal T$_1$-weighted MRI scan of case MJ showing right dorsolateral prefrontal cortex lesion. Scan was taken when MJ was 14 years of age, but lesion occurred from surgical evacuation of a hematoma at 3 years of age. (b) Best-fitting brain template showing localization of frontal lobe lesion to Brodmann's area 9 and a small extent of area 46.

tion of a simple and a complex design from the Benton Visual Retention Test (Benton, 1974). Unable to reproduce the hexagon in Figure 14.7A, MJ made two attempts and drew an octagon on each occasion. With the more complex model in Figure 14.7B, he reproduced the large triangle without difficulty (this was the first element reproduced) but erred with the internal detail of the right major figure and the shape and spatial placement of the peripheral figure. These errors, in fact, were perseverative from the prior set of figures in this task. At the bottom of Figure

MJ

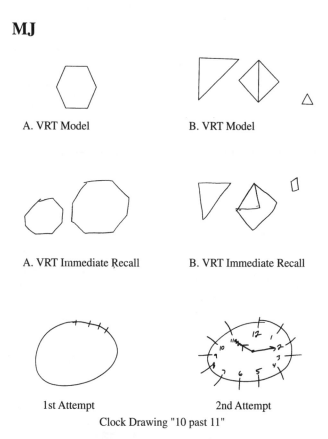

A. VRT Model   B. VRT Model

A. VRT Immediate Recall   B. VRT Immediate Recall

1st Attempt   2nd Attempt

Clock Drawing "10 past 11"

Figure 14.7.   (A) Immediate recall of a geometric figure from the Benton Visual Retention Test (Benton, 1974) in which MJ perseverated on an octagon rather than reproducing the hexagon model. (B) A second example of reproduction of a more complex geometric design from memory, showing distortion of internal detail and substitution of the peripheral figure. Below these examples are MJ's attempts to spontaneously draw a clock with hands set at "10 past 11."

14.7B are two attempts by MJ to spontaneously draw a clock with the hands placed at 10 past 11. His first attempt was quickly abandoned, presumably because of spatial compression of the hash marks along the rim of the circle. His final result was an adequate drawing, although with mild indications of spatial distortion in the placement of numbers and the need to use guiding hash marks placed around the circle. Figure 14.8 presents MJ's spatial planning and constructional performance in drawing the complex figures of Rey-Osterrieth and Taylor. The Rey-Osterrieth figure was copied in standard administration format, with a score in the low-average range. Mild spatial distortions can be observed with both internal detail and the overall gestalt of the figure. His retention of the figure after a 20-minute delay indicated an impaired level. In contrast, the examiner-presented sequential administration of the Taylor figure resulted in notable improvement in constructional performance. His score placed him at the 60th percentile. Retention of this design after a 20-minute delay was also significantly improved and was within the normal range. These data indicate impairments in visual memory and spatial planning–constructional performance 13 years after right dorsolateral pre-

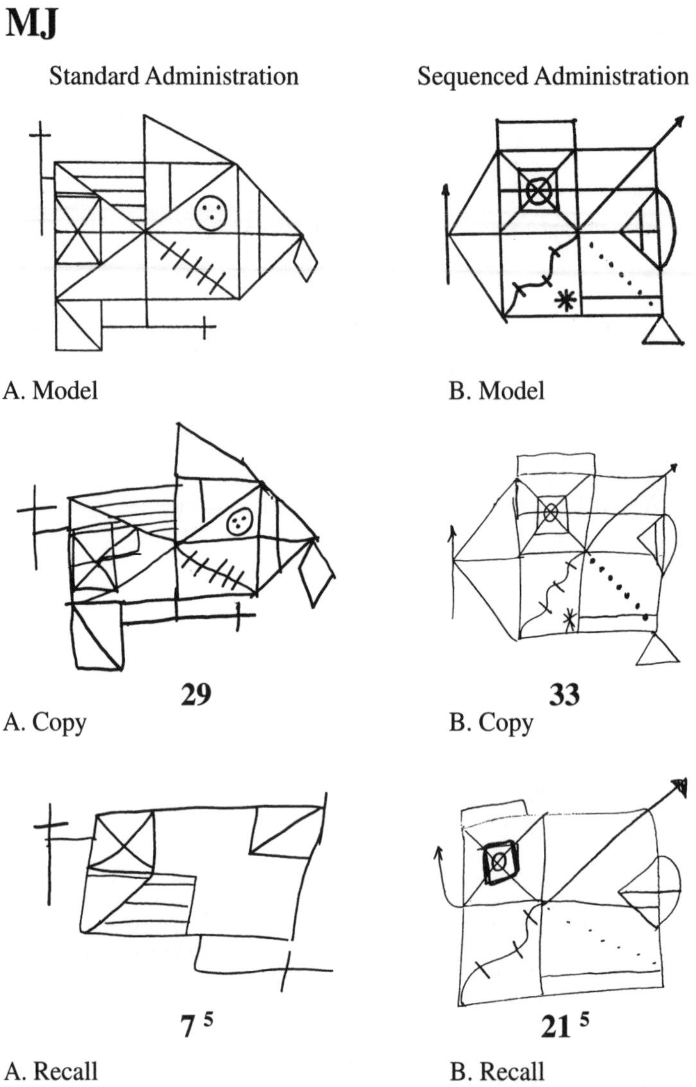

MJ

Standard Administration   Sequenced Administration

A. Model   B. Model

29   **33**

A. Copy   B. Copy

7 [5]   **21** [5]

A. Recall   B. Recall

Figure 14.8.   (A) Copy and 20-minute delayed recall of the complex figure of Rey-Osterrieth by patient MJ. His copy performance shows mild spatial distortion and disproportionate size of several features. Recall performance is in the impaired range. (B) Copy and 20-minute delayed recall of the Taylor complex figure, which was presented by the examiner in a sequenced administration. After the central square of the figure was presented by itself in Step 1, other features were added over a series of 17 steps. The effect of this organizational strategy was improved constructional performance and retention of the complex design.

frontal cortex lesion at 3 years of age. In addition, the data indicate the beneficial effect of providing an organizational strategy not only for reproductions but also for memory of the visuospatial material.

Although the remaining details of MJ's neuropsychological examination are not elaborated here because of space limitations, it is clear that his pattern of results was quite similar to that described for JC, showing disproportionate impairments in visuospatial aspects of executive processes and poor organizational strategies (e.g., in the verbal learning task, on which the pattern of results was similar to JC) but preservation of measured intellect, speech and language, visual perception, and routine problem-solving abilities. As with JC, MJ's results on several tests purported to measure frontal lobe function, including the Wisconsin Card Sorting Test and the Tower of Hanoi procedures, were again within the normal range.

Observations on Social Development   In this section, we briefly summarize several of the observations about MJ's social development, gathered from him, his family, and health care professionals. In the following section, we describe the results of several empirical measures of social behavior, including psychosocial development and empathy.

On the Achenbach Youth Self-Report form, MJ generally described himself as being average to above average in most domains. He denied any form of disability and any concerns about himself. He described himself as "athletic, nice." In contrast, parental report on the equivalent checklist form revealed concern about social appropriateness dating back to nursery school. Social behavior was rated as worse than average, with no friendships. In comparison with his preadolescent and adolescent siblings (all younger than him), MJ is in near-constant conflict with family members. His levels of empathy and reciprocity in relationships were rated as near zero, with little awareness of how his behavior affects others. MJ appears to have significant difficulty in reading the emotional facial expressions and emotional intonation of speech from family members. He reacts most frequently with indifference to the upset of others and will, for example, comfort another only if given specific verbal instructions on how to do so. However, he is kind to animals, including the dogs and cats about the house. He is described as an "animal person" and not a "people person," suggesting a preference for relationships that place simpler and more straightforward emotional and behavioral demands on him. With regard to moral development, his parents indicated that MJ knows what the legal bounds of acceptable behavior are. His understanding of what is fair and just behavior is strictly rule based. He has not had any inclination toward antisocial or criminal behavior. In fact, MJ is not considered a good liar and gets caught most of the time when he is trying to hide information. He has also not exhibited any abnormal sexual behavior and, if anything, becomes very embarrassed if a female classmate calls about a school assignment or the topic of sex is spoken about on television or among family members. His sense of humor is described as inappropriate, mostly from making jokes about others' misfortune and in a manner loud enough so others can hear. At this point in time, family members will warn him about inappropriate comments if they foresee such an instance. MJ has a preference for routine, nonambiguous settings. On a family vacation at a western ranch, where there was a fair degree of unstructured activity time, MJ ended up staying in his room but nonetheless reported that he had a good time.

In social settings, MJ exhibits a fair amount of discomfort, with awkward physical movements, variable eye contact, and limited facial expressions and modulation of voice. He frequently cuts into conversations and does not appear to get the gist of many intended meanings, with the exception of anger. It is hard to follow some of MJ's verbal responses because of the unusual juxtaposition of ideas and tangential remarks.

Empirical Measures of Social Functioning   Findings from empirical measures of empathy, psychosocial development, and self-awareness provided confirmatory data for MJ's observed interpersonal, social, and psychological difficulties and highlight specific domains of disturbance. On a self- and family member–report measure of cognitively based empathy (i.e., the Empathy Measure [Hogan, 1969]), responses from both MJ and his mother placed him at the lower end of the normal range for male adolescents. MJ has more difficulty than most of his peers in taking another person's perspective or in putting himself in their shoes. Componential analysis of responses on the Empathy Measure suggested relatively low self-confidence in social settings and an insensitivity to the thoughts or feelings of others, including what others think of him. In contrast, MJ demonstrated a relative strength in the ability to maintain even-temperedness with others (probably because he does not care what they think) and does not have antisocial or rebellious inclinations.

Responses on the affectively based empathy measure (Questionnaire Method of Emotional Empathy [QMEE]) (Mehrabian & Epstein, 1972) were consistently and significantly lower than that of the normal comparison group for both self- and family member–report. Results suggest that neither MJ nor his mother perceive him as someone who responds emotionally to others' emotional behaviors. This disturbance in affectively based empathy—or in the ability to be emotionally moved by or involved with the feelings of others—may contribute in part to his social insensitivity.

The pattern of responses on the Measures of Psychosocial Development (Hawley, 1988) indicated that both MJ and his mother view his autonomy as a relative strength. That is, he is fairly conscientious in his ability to initiate independent action, takes pride in being able to do things independently, and finds comfort in knowing that he is able to make his own decisions. Despite his personal sense of autonomy, both self-report and family member responses indicated that MJ is quite confused about how the outside world operates, where he fits within it, and how he can exert influence on its various activities and outcomes. MJ's mother perceived her son as living in an isolated and alienated world and, as a consequence, experiencing considerable distress. In contrast, MJ did not perceive himself as isolated and alienated from the outside world—he just found it confusing. As a result, MJ did not view himself as distressed.

Finally, when MJ's sense of behavioral competency was directly examined using the Patient Competency Rating Scale (Prigatano, Altman, & O'Brien, 1990), MJ consistently overestimated his capacities in social-emotional domains compared with the report of his mother. This raises the possibility that MJ may have a specific form of impairment in self-awareness, that is, social self-awareness (Eslinger et al., 1995). In all probability, it is the combination of MJ's social self-awareness deficiencies, social insensitivity, difficulty sharing the feeling states of others (i.e., empathy), and confusion regarding the complexities of the social world that contribute to many of his observed psychosocial difficulties. It is noteworthy, however, that his even-temperedness, lack of rebelliousness, and pride in independent accomplishment prevent him from demonstrating some of the more disruptive, antisocial behaviors observed in other childhood cases JP, KM, GK, MH, and DT—all of whom had *bilateral* prefrontal damage or physiological disruption.

CONCLUSIONS

The study of children with early lesions to the prefrontal cortex has historically provided a rich assortment of clinical observations and case histories that are fertile ground for generating testable hypotheses and models about cognitive and social development as well as cerebral plasticity. A major challenge at this time is advancement to stronger experimental and empirical scrutiny of such cases. The convergence of more precise anatomical imaging methods for lesion localization; new developmental neuropsychological measures of executive functions; and greater empirical analyses of social development, discourse, and emotional behavior potentially provide such techniques. There are also increasing linkages to the animal model literature, particularly anatomical and behavioral studies in nonhuman primates. We have begun to apply these advances to study of two new cases of early right prefrontal cortex damage. The findings from these and the other reviewed cases suggest several conclusions about development of the human prefrontal cortex.

First, the difficulties these children have shown in managing and completing school assignment, home, and social-recreational activities are not readily attributable to deficiencies in basic cognitive processing or other parameters of crystallized intelligence, which are within the normal range. Rather, the difficulties can be related to altered maturation of several executive processing domains after early prefrontal cortex damage. These domains are more accurately placed within the fluid aspects of intelligence. Their disruption by prefrontal lesion serves to limit how a person can register and maintain diverse information to guide subsequent behavior (i.e., working memory), shift and focus attentional resources, generate alternate possibilities to a problem, and plan as well as execute an effective approach to novel multistep assignments. Obviously, the correlation between standardized intelligence scores and executive function scores (as representative probes of crystallized and fluid intelligence, respectively) may be quite low in these cases. Examination by standardized intelligence testing alone, in fact, would be misleading with regard to the nature of the cognitive impairments after prefrontal cortex damage.

Second, the prefrontal cortex is intimately involved in development and regulation of personality and social-emotional processes from an early age. Damage to this region from birth at 3, 4, and 7 years of age has been associated with additional disruption to executive aspects of social-emotional processes, which we term *social executors*. These include disruption of social self-regulation, social self-awareness, social sensitivity (empathy), and social salience, which may represent some of the component impairments underlying a primary social defect. Marked personality alterations in childhood have been clearly reported only in cases of bilateral prefrontal damage. Unilateral lesions to the left and right prefrontal cortex have not been associated with bizarre, antisocial, or criminal behavior in childhood, although diminished social self-regulation, friendships, and social adaptation became progressively evident in adolescence; and clear personality alterations did become evident in adulthood.

Third, the comparison of effects from childhood versus adult-onset lesions to the prefrontal cortex remains largely anecdotal. Clear conclusions are not yet possible because of the small number of cases, differences in lesion size and location, and brevity of measures. Clinically, our impression has been that certain childhood-onset lesions can cause immediate deficits similar to those of adult-onset cases, but recovery is more complete. However, childhood-onset lesions can also cause long-term deficits that progressively emerge through adolescence and adulthood and are more problematic than observed in adult-onset cases. Therefore, notions of cerebral plasticity must be stated cautiously at this time. In one of our case studies, it was observed that JC showed a pattern of specific cognitive impairment similar to that of adults after right dorsolateral prefrontal AVM resection at 7 years of age. Whether this would also be the case at 3 and 5 years of age, for example, is unclear. His return to school, sports, and social activities, however, did appear more ambitious and successful up to 4 years later than would be expected in adults, but there are some indications of emerging social and achievement difficulties. Clearly, it can be concluded that the course of recovery is different in childhood- versus adult-onset prefrontal lesion cases and that further studies are needed to identify the parameters underlying recovery and delayed onset of impairments.

Fourth, disruption of the right dorsolateral prefrontal cortex may be linked in an important way to ADHD. Both cases reported showed behavioral and psychometric indications of impaired attentional control, with hyperactivity in one but not the other case. Comparison with left prefrontal and nonfrontal lesion cases is needed to establish the specificity of this finding. Similar comparison is needed with spatial aspects of executive functions, organization of learning, discourse, and social-emotional processing, which were also impaired developmentally after early right dorsolateral prefrontal cortex lesions.

There is clearly a need for study of larger subject samples over several epochs of development. Both longitudinal and cross-sectional approaches are informative. An important long-term goal is to construct much stronger models of normal and abnormal growth curves pertinent to cognitive, executive, and social-emotional domains. In cases of prefrontal cortex lesions, it is particularly important to identify which core deficits underlie the various expressions of executive impairments that limit development of self-regulated thought, action, and adaptation. Such models may prove beneficial to the study and management of a variety of other neurodevelopmental disorders that potentially affect the prefrontal cortex and its network systems, including traumatic brain injury; ADHD; autism with minimal supports; phenylketonuria; fragile X syndrome in females; and a variety of psychiatric categories such as conduct disorder, obsessive-compulsive disorder, and schizophrenia.

REFERENCES

Achenbach, T.M., & Edelbrock, C. (1983). *Manual for the Child Behavior Checklist and Revised Child Behavior Profile*. Burlington, VT: Queen City Printers.

Ackerly, S.S. (1964). A case of paranatal bilateral frontal lobe defect observed for thirty years. In J.M. Warren & K. Akert (Eds.), *The frontal granular cortex and behavior* (pp. 192–218). New York: McGraw-Hill.

Ackerly, S.S., & Benton, A.L. (1947). Report of a case of bilateral frontal lobe defect. *Proceedings of the Association for Research in Nervous and Mental Disease, 27*, 479–504.

Alexander, M.P., Benson, D.F., & Stuss, D.T. (1989). Frontal lobes and language. *Brain and Language, 37*, 656–691.

Aram, D.M., & Ekelman, B.L. (1986). Cognitive profiles of children with early onset of unilateral lesions. *Developmental Neuropsychology, 2*, 155–172.

Aram, D.M., & Ekelman, B.L. (1988). Scholastic aptitude and achievement among children with unilateral brain lesions. *Neuropsychologia, 26*, 903–916.

Ballantyne, A.O., Scarvie, K.M., & Trauner, D.A. (1994). Verbal and performance IQ patterns in children after perinatal stroke. *Developmental Neuropsychology, 10*, 39–50.

Barkley, R.A., Grodzinsky, G.M., & DuPaul, G.J. (1992). Frontal lobe functions in attention deficit disorder with and without hyperactivity: A review and research report. *Journal of Abnormal Child Psychology, 20,* 163–188.

Becker, M.G., Isaac, W.L., & Hynd, G.W. (1987). Neuropsychological development of nonverbal behaviors attributed to "frontal lobe" functioning. *Developmental Neuropsychology, 3,* 275–298.

Benton, A.L. (1974). *Revised Visual Retention Test.* New York: Psychological Corporation.

Benton, A.L. (1985). Child neuropsychology: Retrospect and prospect. In L. Costa & O. Spreen (Eds.), *Studies in neuropsychology: Selected papers of Arthur Benton* (pp. 274–294). New York: Oxford University Press.

Benton, A.L. (1991). Prefrontal injury and behavior in children. *Developmental Neuropsychology, 7,* 275–281.

Benton, A.L., & Hamsher, K. de S. (1976). *Multilingual aphasia examination.* Iowa City: University of Iowa Press.

Benton, A.L., Hamsher, K. de S., Varney, N., & Spreen, O. (1983). *Contributions to neuropsychological assessment.* New York: Oxford University Press.

Biddle, K.R., McCabe, A., & Bliss, L.S. (in press). Narrative skills following traumatic brain injury in children and adults. *Journal of Communication Disorders.*

Bourgeois, J.-P., Goldman-Rakic, P.S., & Rakic, P. (1994). Synaptogenesis in the prefrontal cortex of rhesus monkeys. *Cerebral Cortex, 4,* 78–96.

Carpenter, C.J., Randolph, C., & Gold, J.M. (1995). Prefrontal functioning in schizophrenia. *Journal of the International Neuropsychological Society, 1,* 173.

Chapman, S.B., Culhane, K.A., Levin, H.S., Harward, H., Mendelsohn, D., Ewing-Cobbs, L., Fletcher, J.M., & Bruce, D. (1992). Narrative discourse after closed head injury in children and adolescents. *Brain and Language, 43,* 42–65.

Chelune, G.J., & Baer, R.A. (1986). Developmental norms for the Wisconsin Card Sorting Test. *Journal of Clinical and Experimental Neuropsychology, 8,* 219–228.

Chugani, H.T., Phelps, M.E., & Mazziotta, J.C. (1987). Positron emission tomography study of human brain functional development. *Annals of Neurology, 22,* 487–497.

Damasio, H., & Damasio, A.R. (1989). *Lesion analysis in neuropsychology.* New York: Oxford University Press.

Deese, J. (1984). *Thought into speech: The psychology of language.* Englewood Cliffs, NJ: Prentice Hall.

Denckla, M.B. (1996). A theory and model of executive function from a neuropsychological perspective. In G.R. Lyon & N.A. Krasnegor (Eds.), *Attention, memory, and executive function* (pp. 263–278). Baltimore: Paul H. Brookes Publishing Co.

Denckla, M.B., & Rudel, R.G. (1976). Rapid automatized naming (R.A.N.): Dyslexia differentiated from other learning disabilities. *Neuropsychologia, 14,* 471–479.

Dennis, M. (1991). Frontal lobe function in childhood and adolescence: A heuristic for assessing attention regulation, executive control, and the intentional states important for social discourse. *Developmental Neuropsychology, 7,* 327–358.

Dennis, M., & Barnes, M.A. (1990). Knowing the meaning, getting the point, bridging the gap, and carrying the message: Aspects of discourse following closed head injury in childhood and adolescence. *Brain and Language, 39,* 428–446.

Dennis, M., & Barnes, M. (1993). Developmental aspects of neuropsychology: Childhood. In D. Zaidel (Ed.), *Handbook of perception and cognition: Vol. 15. Neuropsychology* (pp. 219–246). New York: Academic Press.

Dennis, M., & Lovett, M. (1990). Discourse ability in children after brain damage. In Y. Joanette & H.H. Brownell (Eds.), *Discourse ability and brain damage: Theoretical and empirical perspectives* (pp. 199–223). New York: Springer-Verlag.

Diamond, A., & Doar, B. (1989). The performance of human infants on a measure of frontal cortex function: The delayed response task. *Developmental Psychology, 22,* 271–294.

Diamond, A., & Goldman-Rakic, P.S. (1989). Comparison of human infants and rhesus monkeys on Piaget's A$\bar{\text{B}}$ task: Evidence for dependence on dorsolateral prefrontal cortex. *Experimental Brain Research, 74,* 24–40.

Eslinger, P.J. (1996). Conceptualizing, describing and measuring components of executive function: A summary. In G.R. Lyon & N.A. Krasnegor (Eds.), *Attention, memory, and executive function* (pp. 367–395). Baltimore: Paul H. Brookes Publishing Co.

Eslinger, P.J., & Damasio, H. (1988). Anatomical correlates of paradoxic ear extinction. In K. Hugdahl (Ed.), *Handbook of dichotic listening: Theory, methods and research* (pp. 139–160). Chichester, England: John Wiley & Sons.

Eslinger, P.J., & Grattan, L.M. (1994). Altered serial position learning after frontal lobe lesion. *Neuropsychologia, 32,* 729–739.

Eslinger, P.J., Grattan, L.M., Damasio, H., & Damasio, A.R. (1992). Developmental consequences of childhood frontal lobe damage. *Archives of Neurology, 49,* 764–769.

Eslinger, P.J., Grattan, L.M., & Geder, L. (1995). Impact of frontal lobe lesions on rehabilitation and recovery from acute brain injury. *NeuroRehabilitation, 5,* 161–182.

Finger, S. (1991). Brain damage, development and behavior: Early findings. *Developmental Neuropsychology, 7,* 261–274.

Finger, S., & Wolf, C. (1988). The "Kennard Effect" before Kennard: The early history of age and brain lesions. *Archives of Neurology, 45,* 1136–1142.

Fletcher, J.M., Levin, H.S., & Butler, I.J. (1995). Neurobehavioral effects of brain injury on children: Hydrocephalus, traumatic brain injury, and cerebral palsy. In M.C. Roberts (Ed.), *Handbook of pediatric psychology* (2nd ed., pp. 362–383). New York: Guilford Press.

Goldman, P.S. (1971). Functional development of the prefrontal cortex in early life and the problem of neuronal plasticity. *Experimental Neurology, 32,* 366–387.

Goldman, P.S. (1978). Neuronal plasticity in primate telencephalon: Anomalous projections induced by prenatal removal of frontal cortex. *Science, 202,* 768–770.

Goldman, P.S., & Alexander, G.E. (1977). Maturation of prefrontal cortex in the monkey revealed by local reversible cryogenic depression. *Nature, 267,* 613–615.

Goldman, P.S. & Galkin, T.W. (1978). Prenatal removal of frontal association cortex in the fetal rhesus monkey: Anatomical and functional consequences in postnatal life. *Brain Research, 12,* 451–485.

Goldman, P.S., & Mendelson, M.J. (1977). Salutary effects of early experience on deficits caused by lesions of frontal association cortex in developing rhesus monkeys. *Experimental Neurology, 57,* 588–602.

Goldman-Rakic, P.S. (1987). Development of cortical circuitry and cognitive function. *Child Development, 58,* 601–622.

Graff-Radford, N.R., Damasio, H., Yamada, T., Eslinger, P.J., & Damasio, A.R. (1985). Nonhaemorrhagic thalamic infarction: Clinical, neuropsychological, and electrophysiological findings in four anatomical groups defined by computerized tomography. *Brain, 108,* 485–516.

Grattan, L.M., & Eslinger, P.J. (1990). Higher cognition and social behavior: Cognitive flexibility and empathy after brain injury. *Neuropsychology, 3,* 175–185.

Grattan, L.M., & Eslinger, P.J. (1991). Frontal lobe damage in children and adults: A comparative review. *Developmental Neuropsychology, 7,* 283–326.

Grattan, L.M., & Eslinger, P.J. (1992). Long-term psychological consequences of childhood frontal lobe lesion in patient DT. *Brain and Cognition, 20,* 185–195.

Guilford, J.P., Christensen, P.R., Merrifield, P.R., & Wilson, R.C. (1960). *Alternate uses manual of instructions and interpretations.* Orange, CA: Sheridan Psychological Services.

Hawley, G.A. (1988). *Measures of psychosocial development: Professional manual.* Odessa, FL: Psychological Assessment Resources.

Heaton, R.K., Chelune, G.J., Talley, J.L., Kay, G.G., & Curtiss, G. (1993). *Wisconsin Card Sorting Test manual.* Odessa, FL: Psychological Assessment Ressources.

Hebb, D.O. (1945). Man's frontal lobes: A critical review. *Archives of Neurology and Psychiatry, 54,* 10–24.

Hebb, D.O., & Penfield, W. (1940). Human behavior after extensive bilateral removal from the frontal lobes. *Archives of Neurology and Psychiatry, 44,* 421–438.

Herron, J.E., Grattan, L.M., Sloan, M.A., & Eslinger, P.J. (in press). Recovery from left anterior thalamic infarction in an adolescent: Neuropsychological and neuroanatomic findings. *Developmental Neuropsychology.*

Hogan, R. (1969). Development of an empathy scale. *Journal of Consulting and Clinical Psychology, 33,* 307–316.

Huttenlocher, P.R. (1979). Synaptic density in human frontal cortex: Developmental changes and effects of aging. *Brain Research, 163,* 195–205.

Johnson, D., & Almi, C.R. (1978). Age, brain damage, and performance. In S. Finger (Ed.), *Recovery from brain damage* (pp. 115–134). New York: Plenum.

Jones-Gotman, M., & Milner, B. (1977). Design fluency: The inventions of nonsense drawings after focal cortical lesions. *Neuropsychologia, 15,* 653–674.

Kagan, J., Rosman, B.L., Day, L., Albert, J., & Phillips, W. (1964). Information processing in the child: Significance of analytic and reflective attitudes. *Psychological Monographs, 78*(1, Whole No. 578).

Kaplan, E., Goodglass, H., & Weintraub, S. (1983). *Boston Naming Test.* Philadelphia: Lea & Febiger.

Kolb, B. (1987). Recovery from early cortical damage in rats. I. Differential behavioral and anatomical effects of frontal lesions at different ages of neural maturation. *Behavioral Brain Research, 25,* 205–220.

Kolb, B., & Gibb, R. (1990). Anatomical correlates of behavioral change after neonatal prefrontal lesions in rats. *Progress in Brain Research, 85,* 241–255.

Levin, H.S., Culhane, K.A., Hartmann, J., Evankovich, K., Mattson, A.J., Harward, H., Ringholz, G., Ewing-Cobbs, L., & Fletcher, J.M. (1991). Developmental changes in performance on tests of purported frontal lobe functioning. *Developmental Neuropsychology, 7,* 377–395.

Levin, H.S., High, W.M., Ewing-Cobbs, L., Fletcher, J.M., Eisenberg, H.M., Miner, H.E., & Goldstein, F.C. (1988). Memory functioning during the first year after closed head injury in children and adolescents. *Neurosurgery, 42,* 1043–1052.

Liles, B.Z. (1993). Narrative discourse in children with language disorders and children with normal language: A critical review of the literature. *Journal of Speech and Hearing Research, 36,* 868–882.

Marlowe, W. (1992). The impact of right prefrontal lesion on the developing brain. *Brain and Cognition, 20,* 205–213.

Mateer, C.A., & Williams, D. (1991). Effects of frontal lobe injury in childhood. *Developmental Neuropsychology, 7,* 359–376.

McCarthy, D. (1972). *Manual for the McCarthy Scales of Children's Abilities.* New York: Psychological Corporation.

Mehrabian, A., & Epstein, N. (1972). A measure of emotional empathy. *Journal of Personality, 40,* 525–553.

Miller, E.A., Goldman, P.S., & Rosvold, H.E. (1973). Delayed recovery of function following orbital prefrontal lesions in infant monkeys. *Science, 182,* 304–306.

Mrzljak, L., Uylings, H.B.M., van Eden, C.G., & Judáš, M. (1990). Neuronal development in human prefrontal cortex in prenatal and postnatal stages. *Progress in Brain Research, 85,* 185–222.

Nass, R., & Peterson, H. de C. (1989). Differential effects of congenital left and right brain injury on intelligence. *Brain and Cognition, 9,* 258–266.

Nass, R., Sadler, A.E., & Sidtis, J.J. (1992). Differential effects of congenital vs. acquired unilateral brain injury on dichotic listening performance: Evidence for sparing and asymmetric crowding. *Neurology, 42,* 1960–1965.

Osterrieth, P.A. (1944). Le test de copie d'une figure complexe. *Archives de Psychologie, 30,* 206–356.

Passler, M.A., Isaac, W., & Hynd, G.W. (1985). Neuropsychological development of behavior attributed to frontal lobe functioning in children. *Developmental Neuropsychology, 1,* 349–370.

Pennington, B.F., Bennetto, L., McAleer, O.K., & Roberts, R.J. (1996). Executive functions and working memory: Theoretical and measurement issues. In G.R. Lyon & N.A. Krasnegor (Eds.), *Attention, memory, and executive function* (pp. 327–348). Baltimore: Paul H. Brookes Publishing Co.

Peterson, C., & McCabe, A. (1983). *Developmental psycholinguistics: Three ways of looking at a child's narrative.* New York: Plenum.

Price, B.H., Daffner, K.R., Stowe, R.M., & Mesulam, M.-M. (1990). The comportmental learning disabilities of early frontal lobe damage. *Brain, 113,* 1383–1393.

Prigatano, G.P., Altman, I.M., & O'Brien, T. (1990). Behavioral limitations that traumatic brain-injured patients tend to underestimate. *Clinical Neuropsychologist, 4,* 163–176.

Rakic, P., Bourgeois, J.-P., Eckenhoff, M.F., Zecevic, M., & Goldman-Rakic, P.S. (1986). Concurrent overproduction of synapses in diverse regions of primate cerebral cortex. *Science, 232,* 232–234.

Reitan, R.M. (1979). *Manual for administration of neuropsychological test batteries for adults and children.* Tucson, AZ: Reitan Neuropsychological Laboratories.

Rey, A. (1941). L'examen psychologique dans les cas d'encéphalopathie traumatique [Psychological examination of cases of traumatic encephalopathy]. *Archives de Psychologie, 28,* 286–340.

Riva, D., & Cazzaniga, L. (1986). Late effects of unilateral brain lesion sustained before and after age one. *Neuropsychologia, 24,* 423–428.

Rudel, R.G., & Teuber, H.-L. (1971). Spatial orientation in normal children and in children with early brain injury. *Neuropsychologia, 9,* 401–407.

Rudel, R.G., Teuber, H.-L., & Twitchell, T.E. (1966). A note on hyperesthesia in children with early brain damage. *Neuropsychologia, 4,* 351–356.

Rudel, R.G., Teuber, H.-L., & Twitchell, T.E. (1974). Levels of impairment of sensori-motor functions in children with early brain damage. *Neuropsychologia, 12,* 95–108.

St. James-Roberts, I. (1979). Neurological plasticity, recovery from brain insult, and child development. *Advances in Child Development and Behavior, 14,* 253–319.

Stelling, M.W., McKay, S.E., Carr, A., Walsh, J.W., & Baumann, R.J. (1986). Frontal lobe lesions and cognitive function in craniopharyngioma survivors. *American Journal of Diseases of Children, 140,* 710–714.

Stiles, J., & Thal, D. (1993). Linguistic and spatial cognitive development following early focal brain injury: Patterns of deficit and recovery. In M.H. Johnson (Ed.), *Brain development and cognition* (pp. 643–664). Oxford, England: Blackwell Scientific.

Talley, J.L. (1993). *Children's Auditory Verbal Learning Test–2: Professional manual.* Odessa, FL: Psychological Assessment Resources.

Taylor, E.M. (1959). *The appraisal of children with cerebral deficits.* Cambridge, MA: Harvard University Press.

Teuber, H.-L., & Rudel, R.G. (1962). Behavior after cerebral lesions in children and adults. *Developmental Medicine and Child Neurology, 4,* 3–20.

Thatcher, R. (1991). Maturation of the human frontal lobes: Physiological evidence for staging. *Developmental Neuropsychology, 7,* 397–419.

Tulving, E. (1962). Subjective organization in free recall of unrelated words. *Psychological Review, 69,* 344–354.

Tulving, E., Kapur, S., Craik, F.I.M., Moscovitch, M., & Houle, S. (1994). Hemisphere encoding/retrieval asymmetry in episodic memory: Positron emmission tomography findings. *Proceedings of the National Academy of Sciences of the United States of America, 91,* 2016–2020.

Wechsler, D. (1974). *Wechsler Intelligence Scale for Children–Revised.* New York: Psychological Corporation.

Wechsler, D. (1991). *Wechsler Intelligence Scale for Children* (3rd ed.). New York: Psychological Corporation.

Welsh, M.C., & Pennington, B.F. (1988). Assessing frontal lobe functioning in children: Views from developmental psychology. *Developmental Neuropsychology, 4,* 199–230.

Welsh, M.C., Pennington, B.F., & Groisser, D.B. (1991). A normative-developmental study of executive function: A window on prefrontal function in children. *Developmental Neuropsychology, 7,* 131–149.

Wiig, E.H., & Secord, W. (1988). *Test of Language Competence: Expanded edition.* San Antonio, TX: Psychological Corporation.

Williams, D., & Mateer, C.A. (1992). Developmental impact of frontal lobe injury in middle childhood. *Brain and Cognition, 20,* 196–204.

Wolf, M. (1986). Rapid alternating stimulus naming in the developmental dyslexias. *Brain and Language, 27,* 360–379.

Woodcock, R.W., & Johnson, M.B. (1989). *Woodcock-Johnson Psychoeducational Battery–Revised.* Allen, TX: DLM.

Yakovlev, P.I., & LeCours, A.R. (1967). The myelogenetic cycles of regional maturation of the brain. In A. Minkowsky (Ed.), *Regional development of the brain in early life* (pp. 3–70). Oxford, England: Blackwell Scientific.

Ylvisaker, H. (1993). Communication outcome in children and adolescents with traumatic brain injury. *Neuropsychological Rehabilitation, 3,* 367–387.

15

Sexually Dimorphic Brain–Behavior Development
A Comparative Perspective

William H. Overman, Jocelyne Bachevalier,
Elena Schuhmann, and Patricia McDonough-Ryan _____

Although a complete review of human gender differences is beyond the scope of this chapter, it is important to note that there are several categories of cognitive behavior that show reliable gender differences. These gender differences appear to be related to the levels of gonadal hormones during development and to the development of particular brain structures. A partial list of these behaviors includes patterns of childhood play behavior, tendencies for physical aggression, sexual orientation, and behaviors related to language and visuospatial abilities.

During play behavior, boys and girls generally prefer different types of toys (Connor & Serbin, 1977; Liss, 1991), and these differences in toy preference appear to be both learned through social modeling (Bussey & Bandura, 1984) and influenced by hormones. In the latter case, young girls with congenital adrenal hyperplasia (CAH) prefer boys' toys (Berenbaum & Hines, 1992). (CAH is an enzymatic defect resulting in high levels of adrenal androgens beginning in utero.)

With regard to sexual orientation and aggression, women exposed prenatally to excess testosterone or estrogen show increases in homosexual fantasy and experience (Erhardt, Meyer-Bahlburg, & Rosen, 1985; Money, Schwartz, & Lewis, 1984), and women exposed to androgens show increased aggression (Reinisch, 1981; Resnick, Berenbaum, Gottesman, & Bouchard, 1986). In contrast, boys whose mothers have been treated during pregnancy with estrogens display less aggressive behavior than normal, and they have poorer athletic skills and spatial ability than their normal untreated siblings or matched controls (Yalom, Green, & Fisk, 1973). In men, testosterone enhances overall sexual activity (Davidson, Carmargo, & Smith, 1979); the frequency of sexual thoughts; and the level of subjective arousal by erotic stimuli (Alexander & Sherwin, 1991; O'Carrol, Shapiro, & Bancroft, 1985).

_____

This chapter was supported by National Institute of Mental Health Grant R01 MH50724-02 to William H. Overman.

Regarding gender differences in cognition, men excel on certain tasks of visuo-spatial abilities, particularly on tasks requiring mental rotation of objects and on tasks requiring imagining what an object would look like from a different vantage point (Linn & Petersen, 1985; Maccoby & Jacklin, 1974). In contrast, women excel on certain tasks of verbal abilities, especially those of expressional fluency, word fluency, and associational fluency (Hines, 1990; Linn & Petersen, 1985). The gender difference in verbal abilities appears to be related to language lateralization in the brain. Although most men and women have a left hemispheric dominance for language, the degree of this dominance is greater in men than in women (Hines, 1990). Furthermore, some of these patterns can be reversed by abnormal exposure to go-nadal hormones: Women with CAH show enhanced performance on visuospatial tasks, and men with lower-than-normal levels of androgen show reduced visuospa-tial abilities (Resnick et al., 1986). Women who were exposed to high prenatal lev-els of estrogen because their mothers were prescribed synthetic estrogen (diethyl-stilbestrol) during pregnancy show increased language lateralization (Hines & Shipley, 1984).

In addition to correlation with levels of hormones, some human behaviors ap-pear to be related to the size-specific brain structures. Two studies (Allen, Hines, Shryne, & Gorski, 1989; Swaab & Fliers, 1985) have reported sex differences in the human preoptic area–anterior hypothalamus, an area of the brain known to be in-volved in sexual behavior in primates and rodents. LeVay (1991) has reported that one of the anterior interstitial hypothalamic nuclei in homosexual men was smaller than that in heterosexual men and about the same size as that of women. In addition, there have been several reports of gender differences in the anatomy of the corpus callosum (e.g., Hines, 1990; Witelson, 1989).

The data strongly indicate that underlying biological factors account for some of the sexually dimorphic cognitive behaviors in adult humans. However, with most of the behaviors listed previously, one could also argue that gender differences are due, to some extent, to differential postnatal environmental or social factors or both. Therefore, the major problem in the study of sex-specific mental abilities is how to separate biological factors from social-learning factors.

For any given mental ability, the weighting of social factors would be reduced if gender differences were found to exist in very young, normal children by using tests that were originally used to demonstrate cognitive gender differences in monkeys. The argument for biological influences would be even stronger if the gen-der direction of the cognitive differences were reversible in monkeys by experi-mental manipulations of steroidal gonadal hormones, perinatal lesions of the brain, or both.

There are, in fact, two such cognitive tests that show significant and hormon-ally controlled gender differences in infant monkeys: object reversal, on which young males are superior, and concurrent object discrimination, on which young females are superior. We have evaluated young children on these two tests of cogni-tion and found that the same pattern of gender-specific cognitive behavior also ex-ists in humans early in ontogeny. These results are consistent with the idea that bi-ologically based cognitive gender differences exist in children, as is the case for infant monkeys, and that gender differences in frontal and temporal lobe function appear in infancy.

BIOLOGICALLY BASED COGNITIVE
GENDER DIFFERENCES IN INFANT MONKEYS

Male Superiority on the Object Reversal Task

On the object reversal task, a subject is first taught to discriminate between and consistently respond to one of two stimuli; then the reinforcement contingencies are reversed without warning so that the previously positive stimulus becomes nonrewarded and the previously negative stimulus becomes rewarded. Once the subject learns the new contingencies, they are reversed to the original format, and the subject must return to the original response patterns. Typically, the subject is taught five such reversals, and reversal learning is reported as the number of errors made on each reversal and the total number of errors across all reversals.

On this task, it has been shown that 75-day-old male rhesus macaques perform significantly better than age-matched females (Clark & Goldman-Rakic, 1989). This gender difference is absent in juvenile monkeys (Goldman, Crawford, Stokes, Galkin, & Rosvold, 1974) and therefore appears to be ontogenetically transient. Neonatal manipulations of androgen levels reverse this gender difference, as evidenced by the finding that androgenized infant females perform as well as normal males and better than normal females (Clark & Goldman-Rakic, 1989). Furthermore, neonatal ablations of the orbital prefrontal cortex (a region known to be crucial for normal performance on this task [Mishkin, 1964]) impair object reversal performance of both normal infant males and androgenized infant females, but these lesions do not impair the performance of normal infant females (Clark & Goldman-Rakic, 1989; Goldman et al., 1974). These findings suggest that functional maturation of the orbital prefrontal cortex occurs earlier in life for males than for females and is influenced by steroid gonadal hormones (Goldman et al., 1974).

Female Superiority on the Concurrent Discrimination Task

On the concurrent discrimination task, the subject is consecutively shown several pairs of objects. One member of each pair conceals a reward (positive pair member) and one does not (negative pair member). Each day the subject sees the same object pairs, in the same order, with left and right positions of the positive and negative pair members randomized. Over the course of training, the subject learns to respond consistently to the positive pair member; that is, the subject learns a list of simultaneous object discriminations.

On this task, it has been shown that 90-day-old female monkeys perform significantly better than age-matched males, but the gender difference is not found in 6-month-old monkeys (Bachevalier, Hagger, & Bercu, 1989). In addition, castrated males perform as well as normal females and significantly better than normal males (Hagger, Bachevalier, & Bercu, 1987), whereas neonatal ablations of area TE in the inferior temporal cortex (a temporal cortical area crucial for normal performance on this task) (Phillips, Malamut, Bachevalier, & Mishkin, 1988) impair concurrent discrimination performance in normal females, but not in infant males (Bachevalier, Brickson, Hagger, & Mishkin, 1990). Infant females who are ovariectomized and androgenized at birth are inferior to normal females and perform poorly like normal males (Hagger et al., 1987). Finally, high levels of circulating testosterone in males are positively correlated with poor performance (Bachevalier et al., 1989). Therefore, it appears that, at 3 months of age, area TE is more fully developed in females than in males and that the maturation of this area is influenced by steroid gonadal hormones.

Summary of Animal Testing

As summarized in Figure 15.1, these results provide strong evidence that, at an early age, some cognitive gender differences are due to differential maturation rates of neural systems that are under the influence of circulating hormones. Because the animals in these studies were reared in controlled conditions and without socialization from adult conspecifics, this double dissociation in infant monkeys is the strongest evidence to date that, in primates, gender differences in mental abilities can have a biological basis that is independent of social factors.

COGNITIVE GENDER DIFFERENCES IN INFANT HUMANS

In order to determine whether a similar behavior pattern exists in humans, we tested normal children and adults on these two tests using animal procedures—that is, using nonverbal, operant procedures in a Wisconsin General Test Apparatus (WGTA). First we describe the general testing procedures, then the specific procedures for the object reversal and concurrent discrimination tasks, and finally the results of testing children.

General Testing Procedures

Since 1990, the general testing methods have been standardized in our laboratory for adults and for children between the ages of 12 and 60 months to ensure that subjects will work reliably and consistently on the tasks (Overman, 1990; Overman, Bachevalier, Miller, & Moore, 1996; Overman, Bachevalier, Sewell, & Drew, 1993; Overman, Bachevalier, Turner, & Peuster, 1992). Experimenters are given extensive training in testing procedures before working with subjects. In all testing situations, there are two experimenters, one who sits behind the WGTA and manipulates the stimuli and rewards and another who either holds the subject (young child) or sits beside the subject (older child or adult) on the other side of the WGTA. A guillotine-type door separates the two experimenters, and, on each trial, it is raised about 3 inches, just enough to slide out a stimulus tray that contains three shallow food wells in a horizontal display. With the door raised, the experimenter cannot see the subject's body or the face of the other experimenter. Each experimenter serves on alternate days as the tester or the person with the subject. Experimenters are blind to any hypotheses guiding this research. Although the majority (80%) of the experimenters are female, data collected in our laboratory have failed to reveal significant differences in children's or adults' performance with these nonverbal, operant procedures when using female versus male experimenters. Behavior testing for children was conducted with parental consent at local preschools, and adults were tested in our laboratory at the university.

For all tasks, the subjects undergo brief preliminary training in which, by nonverbal successive approximations, they learn to displace objects covering the food wells and to retrieve a concealed food reward (Cheerios or Froot Loops for children and M&M's for adults). Throughout testing, reinforcement for correct responses consisted of food reward and social reinforcers ("Good boy" or "Good girl" for children and "Good" for adults). Obviously, one procedural difference between monkeys and humans concerns food restrictions. Because food restriction could not be used with human subjects, we attempted to increase their motivation level by us-

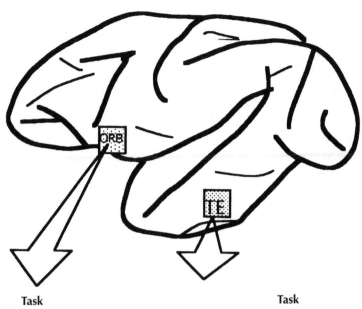

Task

Object reversal

1. 75-day-old males perform better than 75-day-old females.[a]
2. Androgenized females perform as well as males and better than normal females.[a]
3. Early lesions in males, but not in females, impair performance when tested at 75 days.[b]
4. Early lesions do not impair normal females until they are 15–18 months of age.[b]
5. Early lesions in androgenized females impair performance when tested at 75 days, as is the case for early-lesioned males.[a]

Conclusion: The orbital prefrontal cortex develops earlier in males than in females, under the influence of testosterone.

Task

Concurrent discrimination

1. 90-day-old females perform better than 90-day-old males.[c]
2. Castrated males perform as females and better than normal males.[d]
3. Ovariectomized/androgenized females are inferior to normal females.[d]
4. Neonatal lesions in females, but not in males, impair performance.[c]
5. In males, high levels of testosterone are correlated with poor performance.[c]

Conclusion: Area TE develops earlier in females than in males.

Figure 15.1.   Summary of research showing biological bases of cognitive gender differences in monkeys. Left column indicates that the orbital prefrontal cortex (ORB) subserves object reversal learning and that younger males are superior to younger females. Right column indicates that area TE in the inferior temporal cortex subserves concurrent discrimination learning and that younger females are superior to younger males. ([a]Clark & Goldman-Rakic [1989]; [b]Goldman et al. [1974]; [c]Bachevalier et al. [1989]; [d]Hagger et al. [1987].)

ing social reinforcement. This has proved to be successful because, with these procedures, even 12-month-old children rapidly master object discriminations in about 50 trials (Overman et al., 1992). Other than the social reinforcer, no verbalizations were made about the task, the apparatus, or the nature of the experiment. Stimulus objects were plastic, three-dimensional, abstract-shaped objects varying in color, size, and texture that were glued to plastic bases large enough to cover the food wells (see Overman et al., 1992, for examples of stimulus objects). The objects used for these studies were screened to ensure that there was no gender preference, and, in the case of pairs of objects (concurrent discriminations), the stimuli had been screened to ensure equal preference for each member of a pair (Overman et al., 1992).

Object Reversal

In this task, without verbal instructions and over the course of several days, the subject learned, at 15 trials per day, to discriminate between two objects (Problem 1), one of which always concealed a food reward (positive) and one of which did not (negative). After the subject reached criterion (two successive 15-trial sessions with 13 of 15 correct), the subject learned, to criterion, a second discrimination between two new objects (Problem 2). These first two discrimination problems provided the subject an opportunity to learn the general testing procedure and served as control tasks for general learning ability. On the test day after reaching criterion on the second discrimination problem, the reward contingencies were reversed without warning; that is, the previously negative object became positive. The subject learned this reversed discrimination to criterion, whereupon the reward contingencies were reversed again, and so forth for five reversals. The subject's score for this task was the number of errors on each reversal as well as the total number of errors made over five consecutive reversals. This object reversal procedure was identical to that used previously with monkeys (Clark & Goldman-Rakic, 1989; Goldman et al., 1974), except that monkeys were taken through six reversals.

Concurrent Discrimination

For this task, monkeys learned a list of 20 object pairs; that is, they learned which member of 20 pairs of objects was consistently reinforced (Bachevalier et al., 1990). In the study with children, we used a list of only eight pairs of objects because previous research showed that 12- to 18-month-old children required up to 56 days to learn lists of 20 pairs (Overman et al., 1992), and, during this prolonged training, many of the younger children became difficult to test. The eight pairs of stimulus objects were similar in shape, color, and size to those used for object reversal. As for the previous task, no verbal instructions were given. For each pair, one member was arbitrarily designated as positive (always concealed a food reward), and the other was negative. On each of the eight daily trials, one pair of objects was presented over two food wells, and the subject was allowed to displace one of them. Displacement of the positive stimulus was rewarded with food and a social reinforcer. After a 15-second intertrial interval, a second pair was presented for choice, and so forth, until all eight pairs had been presented once each. The same series was then shown once every 24 hours on weekdays. As was the case in studies with monkeys (Bachevalier et al., 1990), the baited and unbaited object within each pair as well as the serial order of the pairs remained constant across daily sessions, but the left–right positions of the pair members were randomized each day. The subject's score for this task consisted of the total number of errors to criterion (90% correct for 2 consecutive days).

Determination of the Age Range of Subjects

Comparative studies on the development of the visual system (Atkinson, 1977; Boothe, Williams, Kiorpes, & Teller, 1980; Teller, Morse, Borton, & Regal, 1974) and the development of several learning abilities (Gunderson, Grant-Webster, & Fagan, 1987; Overman et al., 1992; Williams, 1979) have indicated a developmental ratio of approximately 4:1 between humans and macaques. In other words, 4 months for humans correspond, roughly, to 1 month for monkeys in the maturation of visual learning behavior. This 4:1 developmental ratio, along with the ages at which gender differences occurred in monkeys (75 days and 90 days of age for object reversal and concurrent discrimination, respectively) led to the prediction that, if cognitive gender differences were to be found in human infants, then they should be evident as early as 300–360 days of age (10–12 months). The age at which these gender differences should no longer be present, however, was more difficult to predict from the existing literature on monkeys. This is because none of the studies with monkeys attempted to precisely determine the age at which gender differences disappear. In one case (Goldman et al., 1974), the older monkeys were 1.5 to 2 years of age, and, in the other case (Bachevalier et al., 1989), the older monkeys were 6 months of age. These two older groups correspond to approximately 6–8 years and 24 months, respectively, in humans. Based on these data, we began our study by testing children as young as 13 months of age, an age at which gender differences should clearly be detectable, and by testing children up to 3 years of age in order to assess the period at which the gender differences were no longer measurable.

Gender Differences in Object Reversal Abilities in Humans

The subjects were 62 experimentally naïve children and 10 adults. The children, 34 boys and 28 girls, ranged in age from 15 to 54 months. The adults, 4 men and 6 women, were college students between 17 and 36 years of age (mean, 25.3 years).

Object Reversal Scores   The results for this task are presented as a function of age for each male and female child (Figure 15.2 top). Best-fit regression curves showed that both boys' and girls' scores had different but statistically significant negative error–age slopes. As shown on the scatterplots, girls younger than approximately 30 months of age appeared to make more errors than age-matched boys, but boys and girls older than 30 months of age appeared to make approximately equal numbers of errors. An age-bin statistical analysis (Overman, Bachevalier, Schuhmann, & Ryan, 1996) resulted in a separation of the children into a Younger group (15–30 months of age; $n = 34$, 17 boys and 17 girls) and an Older group (31–54 months of age; $n = 28$, 17 boys and 11 girls).

The error scores for all age groups are presented in Table 15.1 for each of the two discriminations and five reversal problems. The results for adult subjects showed no gender differences on either discrimination or any reversal (p values $> .05$), because all subjects learned each problem with zero errors to criterion. (*Note:* A score of 13 of 15 correct responses for two sessions met the definition of *criterion*, and, because we measured errors *to* criterion, not including errors made on criterion days, a subject could learn with "zero" errors.) Because there was no variance in the adults' scores, this group could not be included in the analysis of variance for the children's learning scores; however, nonparametric comparisons (Mann-Whitney U tests) showed that the adults were superior to both groups of children on all discriminations and reversals (p values $< .05$). For either age group of children, there were no gender differences on the first two object discriminations (Mann-Whitney U tests, p values $> .05$), showing that general learning and performance abilities were equal in boys and girls. However, for the reversal learning, an analysis of variance showed significant effects of age and gender as well as a significant age–gender interaction (all p values $< .05$). These results are depicted in Figure 15.3, together with the results of reversal learning in infant monkeys reported above (Clark & Goldman-Rakic, 1989).

As shown in Figure 15.3, Older children performed better than Younger children, and Younger boys learned the first three reversals with significantly fewer errors than did Younger girls (p values $< .05$), who caught up with boys (p values

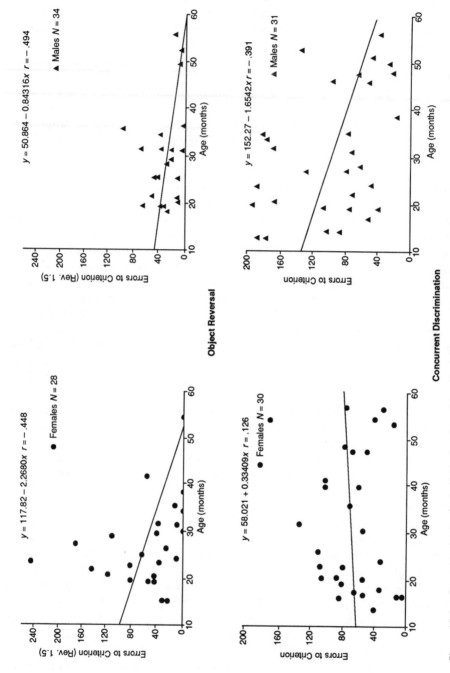

Figure 15.2. Errors to criterion for individual male and female children on the object reversal task (top) and the concurrent discrimination task (bottom). Best-fit regression lines, regression equations, and Pearson's correlations show that, on the object reversal task, errors declined as a function of age for both boys and girls; however, the slopes of the regression lines were different for boys and girls. For the concurrent discrimination task (bottom), errors declined as a function of age for the boys but not for the girls (nonsignificant Pearson's r).

Table 15.1.   Mean group errors preceding criterion on each phase of the object reversal task and on the concurrent discrimination task[a]

| Group | Object reversal task[b] | | | | | | | Concurrent discrimination task |
	D1	D2	R1	R2	R3	R4	R5	
Younger boys	19.2	2.8	10.2	6.1	5.2	5.5	2.5	118.4
			*	*	*			*
Younger girls	21.3	3.3	23.1	17.9	21.6	7.9	6.8	66.3
Older boys	12.7	0.5	7.1	2.9	2.8	2.2	2.0	62.8
Older girls	2.3	1.3	7.5	0.0	1.3	1.1	0.5	72.5
Adult men	0.5	0.0	0.0	0.0	0.0	0.0	0.0	13.1
Adult women	0.5	0.0	0.0	0.0	0.0	0.0	0.0	12.7

[a]Most adults learned the first two discrimination problems with zero errors; consequently, their scores could not be included with the children's scores in a parametric analysis of variance. Nonparametric paired comparisons showed that adult subjects of either sex were equally proficient in solving the two discrimination problems as well as all subsequent reversals (Mann-Whitney U tests, p values $> .05$). Boys and girls did not differ in the rate of learning on the first two discrimination problems (Fisher's protected t tests, p values $> .05$), although the difference between Older boys and Older girls approached significance. For the first three reversal problems, Younger boys were superior to Younger girls ($p < .05$); for the concurrent discrimination task, Younger girls were superior to Younger boys ($p < .05$).

[b]D, object discrimination task; R, reversal task. Asterisks indicate significant differences between the scores above and below the asterisks.

$> .05$) by the fourth reversal. These results are almost identical to those reported for infant monkeys (Figure 15.3 inset), with the exception that the female monkeys did not catch up with the males until the fifth reversal (Clark & Goldman-Rakic, 1989). In both species, the gender difference appeared only in the initial reversals and, therefore, appeared to be ontogenetically transient. For Older children, there were no gender differences on any reversal problem (p values $> .05$), and, by 30 months of age, both male and female children made very few errors subsequent to the first reversal problem, as was the case for juvenile monkeys (Clark & Goldman-Rakic, 1989).

Types of Errors on Object Reversal for Boys and Girls   Jones and Mishkin (1972) divided errors made on the object reversal task by monkeys into three types: Stage I errors, in which a subject has a high level of responding to the previously positive stimulus (i.e., the subject is "stuck in set" and fails to change the previous response pattern); Stage II errors, in which the subject shows equal levels of responding to both stimuli (i.e., the subject responds to the new positive stimulus on some trials but to the previously positive stimulus on other trials); and Stage III errors, in which the subject responds to the newly positive stimulus above chance levels, but not yet at criterion levels.

Because this type of analysis provides more details about behavior during object reversal, we analyzed the error types in boys and girls of the Younger group; the results are shown in Figure 15.4. This analysis revealed that, although there were no gender differences between Older boys and girls, the Younger girls made significantly more Stage I and Stage II errors than did the Younger boys. Thus, at the beginning of a reversal, the Younger girls failed to shift their responding to the newly positive stimulus as readily as did boys. Furthermore, in subsequent test sessions, after the shift to the new stimulus had occurred, they continued to occasionally

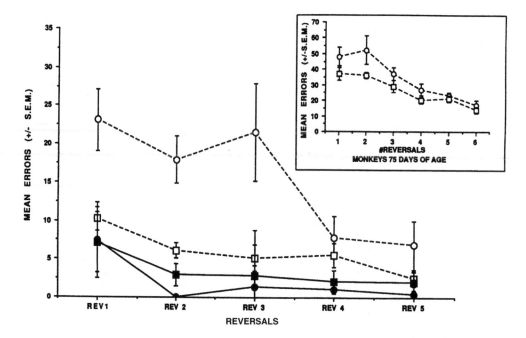

Figure 15.3.   Mean errors to criterion for five reversals of an object discrimination for male and female children 15–30 months of age (Younger group) and 31–54 months of age (Older group). Inset shows previously collected data with monkeys: mean errors to criterion for each of six reversal problems for normal male (---□---) and female (---○---) monkeys tested at 75 days of age. Vertical bars indicate standard error of the mean for all graphs. (---○--- = younger females, ---□--- = younger males, —●— = older females, —■— = older males.) (Inset adapted from Clark & Goldman-Rakic [1989].)

and erroneously respond to the previously positive stimulus, as if they were not sure of the reversed contingencies. This checking behavior transpired for a full week or more after the start of a reversal and prevented the Younger girls from attaining learning criterion as rapidly as their male counterparts.

In addition, there was another behavioral difference between Younger girls and Younger boys on the object reversal task. Approximately 15% of the girls demonstrated extreme emotional behavior upon the start of the first reversal problem. This emotional reaction was so severe in six of the girls that they were dropped from the study (their data are not part of this data set) because they became untestable when the reversal portion of the study began. Reactions of this severity were not observed in a single boy, younger or older. It is not stated in previous studies with monkeys whether young females demonstrated emotional reactions upon reversal demands (Clark & Goldman-Rakic, 1989; Goldman et al., 1974). The exact meaning of this gender-specific reaction is unclear; however, it may be related to the neural input to the orbital frontal cortices from the limbic system, a neural circuit implicated in the regulation of emotions.

Gender Differences in Concurrent Discrimination Abilities in Humans

For the concurrent object discrimination test, new groups of 61 experimentally naïve children (31 boys and 30 girls, ranging in age from 13 to 54 months) and 22 adults (11 men and 11 women, ranging in age from 17 to 24 years) were studied. The general training procedures for this task were described earlier.

The results obtained on this task are presented in terms of errors to criterion as a function of age for each child subject (Figure 15.2 bottom). Best-fit regression lines showed that boys' scores declined with age (significant slope) but that girls' scores were constant across all ages (nonsignificant slope). Inspections of these regression lines suggested that, under the age of about 35 months, boys made more errors than did girls but that above this age boys and girls performed equally.

Based on a statistical age-bin analysis of the regression data (Overman et al., 1996), the children were divided into two groups, a Younger group (15–35 months of age; $n = 40$, 21 boys and 19 girls) and an Older group (36–54 months of age; $n = 21$, 10 boys and 11 girls). A two-way analysis of variance (three age groups and two gender groups) showed a significant effect of age and a significant age–gender interaction (p values $< .05$). The results (Figure 15.5) show that adults learned significantly faster than either group of children (p values $< .05$), and there were no gender differences among adults. Younger girls learned with significantly fewer errors than did younger boys ($p < .05$); however, by the age of 35 months, there were no differences between the boys and the girls ($p > .05$). These results are almost identical to those with monkeys discussed earlier (Figure 15.5 inset) (Bachevalier et al., 1989).

The learning curves for Younger and Older children on the concurrent discrimination task (Figure 15.6) indicate that all children, regardless of age, began learning at chance levels. Older boys and girls learned at equivalent rates, attaining criterion in about 50 sessions. In contrast, although Younger boys and girls began training at chance levels, Younger girls showed a steeper and more positively accelerated learning curve than age-matched boys. In fact, 29% of the Younger boys failed to reach criterion in 50 sessions, at which time training stopped.

COGNITIVE GENDER DIFFERENCES IN PRIMATES

Taken together, the data from the two tasks reveal a double dissociation in early learning by male and female children. This is shown in Figure 15.7, which plots the data as population scores grouped by gender: Each bar represents the score of a single child. Figure 15.7A shows the error scores of young children (15–29 months of age) on Reversals I–III, and Figure 15.7B shows errors to criterion of individual young children (15–35 months of age) on concurrent discrimination learning. It is clear that, on object reversal learning, Younger boys are superior to Younger girls and, on concurrent discrimination, Younger girls are superior to Younger boys. In both infant humans and infant monkeys, the gender scores of particular age groups overlap but are statistically different on both tasks.

Given the close parallel in learning behavior in infant humans and infant monkeys, it is reasonable to propose that the gender differences are mediated by similar biological mechanisms in both species. Therefore, in children, as in infant monkeys, there may be a more rapid maturation of orbital prefrontal circuits in boys and a more rapid maturation of inferior temporal circuits in girls. There are strong arguments in favor of this biological hypothesis, and some alternative arguments for differential socialization can be eliminated. These topics are discussed next.

Development of Orbital Prefrontal Cortex in Humans and Monkeys

Our data with children and previous data with monkeys lead us to hypothesize that the orbital prefrontal cortex develops earlier in infant male children than in infant female children. We reach this hypothesis because the Younger girls were slower than Younger boys to master the object reversal task and because normal infant female monkeys as well as infant male monkeys with orbital prefrontal damage were slower to learn the same task relative to normal infant male monkeys (Clark

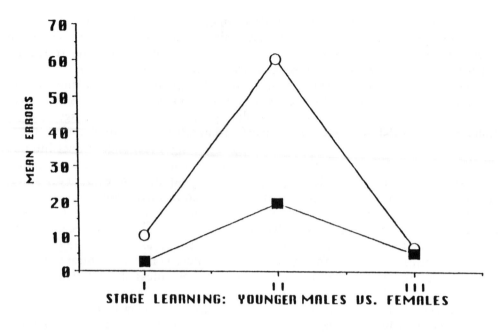

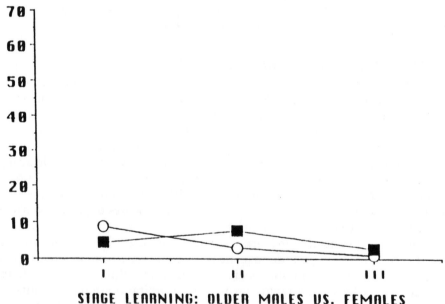

Figure 15.4.   Mean errors made by younger boys and younger girls (15–30 months of age) and by older boys and older girls (31–54 months of age) on each of three stages of learning across all five object reversals. (—O— = females [N = 16], —■— = males [N = 17]; Stage I, responding to old stimulus above chance; Stage II, responding to new stimulus at chance; Stage III, responding to new stimulus above chance.)

& Goldman-Rakic, 1989; Goldman et al., 1974). This conclusion was strengthened by the fact that both the learning performance and the emotional behavior of the Younger girls were highly similar to that of adult monkeys with damage to the orbital prefrontal cortices. Regarding learning performance, it is known that damage to this region impairs object reversal learning in adult rhesus monkeys by increasing the number of perseverative Stage I errors and, to a lesser extent, Stage II errors (Jones & Mishkin, 1972). This was the case for the Younger female children on object reversal. Regarding emotional behavior, it is known that lesions of the orbital prefrontal cortex in rhesus monkeys result in emotional changes such as decreased aggression, increased aversion, and hyperreactive responses to arousing stimuli (Butter & Snyder, 1972). In the human study, only the Younger girls exhibited increased emotionality during reversal learning. Finally, it is interesting to note that neuroanatomical data show significant gender differences in the cross-sectional size of that portion of the corpus callosum that contains axons emanating from the orbital frontal cortex (Cowell, Allen, Zalatimo, & Denenberg, 1992). In that study, female human subjects did not attain a maximum callosal size in this region until middle adulthood (41–50 years of age), whereas males attained peak values at 20 years of age and declined thereafter. These findings provide further evidence that gender differences in the orbital prefrontal cortex not only exist but occur, perhaps, across the life span.

Development of Inferior Temporal Cortex in Humans and Monkeys
The data with children lead us to hypothesize that the inferior temporal cortex in humans develops earlier in girls than in boys. We reach this hypothesis because the Younger boys were slower than girls to learn the concurrent discrimination task and because normal infant male monkeys and infant female monkeys with lesion of Area TE in the inferior temporal cortex were slower than normal females to learn the same task (Bachevalier et al., 1989, 1990). Furthermore, in adult monkeys, performance on this task depends upon the integrity of area TE (Phillips et al., 1988) as well as on the level of circulating hormones in young males (the higher the level of testosterone, the poorer the performance) (Bachevalier et al., 1989). Our hypothesis is further corroborated by evidence from other lines of research showing that the inferior temporal cortex matures earlier in life in females than in males. For example, individual visual neurons in the inferior temporal cortex have been found to be less responsive and more variable in infant male monkeys than in females (Rodman, 1994). Taylor (1969, 1971) has reported that the onset of temporal lobe seizure activity begins to decline markedly during the second year of life in girls but not until the fourth year of life in boys, indicating an earlier maturation of temporal lobe circuits in girls. Finally, there are reports of gender differences in the maturation of occipitotemporal systems for object perception: Girls demonstrate earlier abilities in visual habituation (Tighe & Powlison, 1978), visual resolution (Held, Bauer, & Gwiazda, 1988), and binocularity (Bauer, Shimojo, Gwiazda, & Held, 1986). Collectively, these findings suggest earlier development of portions of the inferior temporal cortex in females than in males.

Similar Hormonal Development in Humans and Monkeys
Another argument in favor of similar biological foundations for cognitive gender differences in children and infant monkeys lies in the similarity of their perinatal hormonal development. In both species, there is a significant prenatal blood testosterone elevation in males and a lesser prenatal testosterone surge in females, followed by a postnatal decline to a plateau at about 9 months of age in humans and age 3 months in monkeys, after which the level remains constant until puberty (Bachevalier et al., 1989; Corbier, Edwards, & Roffi, 1992; Stahl, Gotz, Poppe, Amendt, & Dorner, 1978). Thus, at the time of testing, both infant humans and

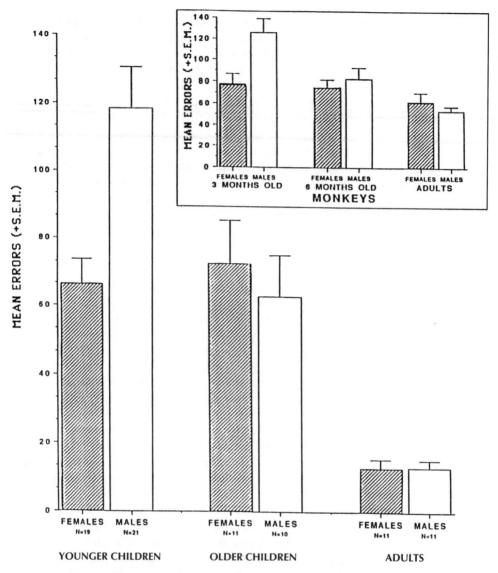

Figure 15.5.   Mean errors to criterion on eight-pair concurrent discrimination task for male and female children 13–35 months of age (Younger) and 36–54 months of age (Older), and adults. Vertical bars show standard error of the mean. Inset shows mean errors to criterion on a 20-pair concurrent discrimination task for young, juvenile, and adult monkeys. (Inset adapted from Bachevalier, Hagger, & Bercu [1989].)

monkeys had recently experienced the perinatal hormone surge and were in the initial stages of their prepubertal hormonal plateau. Because it has been experimentally demonstrated that, in monkeys, perinatal testosterone contributes significantly to the cognitive gender dimorphism, it is reasonable to suppose that similar hormonal process might also contribute to the gender dimorphism on the two cognitive tasks in human infants.

Developmental Time Course of Cognitive Gender Differences

The present data clearly show that, early in life, boys and girls perform differently on two cognitive tasks. However, the data do not allow firm conclusions about the

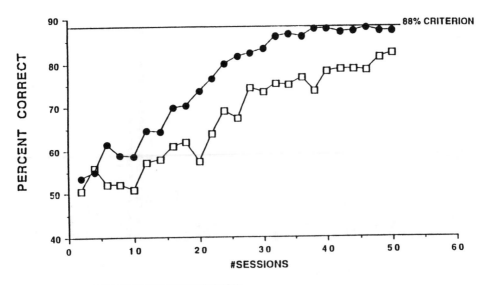

CONCURRENT DISCRIMINATION:
YOUNGER MALES VS. FEMALES LEARNING TO CRITERION

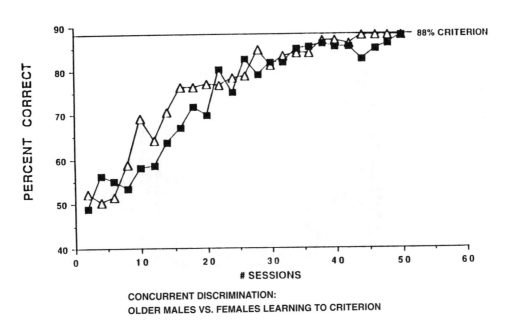

CONCURRENT DISCRIMINATION:
OLDER MALES VS. FEMALES LEARNING TO CRITERION

Figure 15.6.   Learning curves on concurrent discrimination task for male and female children 13–54 months of age (top) (—□— = young males [N = 21], —●— = young females [N = 19]) and 36–54 months of age (bottom) (—△— = older males [N = 10], —■— = older females [N = 11]).

ontogenetic duration of the cognitive gender dimorphisms. We do know that there were no significant gender differences on the object reversal task in children older than 30 months of age or on the concurrent discrimination task in children older than 35 months of age. There are at least three possible explanations for these findings.

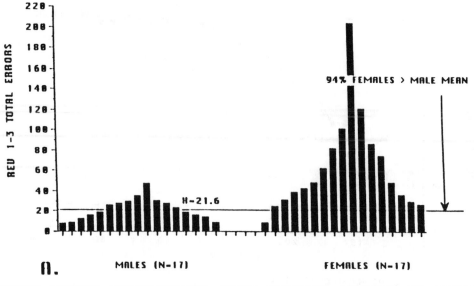

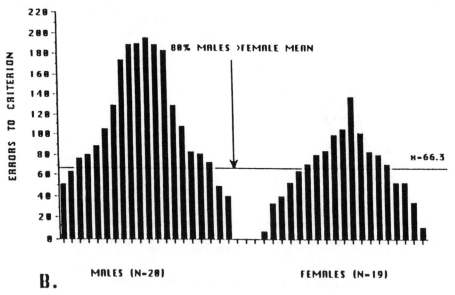

Figure 15.7.   Scores of individual children plotted as "population" scores on two tasks: Each bar represents the score of a single child. (A) Total errors to criterion on reversals one through three for individual male and female children 15–29 months of age. (B) Total errors to criterion on concurrent discrimination task for individual male and female children 13–35 months of age.

First, it is possible that, by 30–35 months of age, the males' and females' orbital prefrontal and inferior temporal brain regions had become functionally equivalent.

Although little is known about postnatal development of specific regions or early gender differences of the human brain, there is information about widespread development after birth (see Kolb & Fantie, 1989). During the postnatal period relevant to the present study (i.e., about 1–3 years of age), neuronal division, migration, and lamination should have been complete, and most changes would involve decreasing synaptic density resulting in an increase in functional neuronal interconnections (Goldman-Rakic, 1987; Huttenlocher, 1979; Kolb & Fantie, 1989; Marin-Padilla, 1970). Therefore, it is possible that, in the present study, by 3 years of age, the interconnections within the orbital frontal and inferior temporal cortices had become functionally equivalent, and earlier cognitive gender differences disappeared. Future studies of neuroanatomical development will provide more information about this possibility.

The second explanation for the absence of gender differences in older children and adults is that there may have been a floor effect for older subjects on the two relatively simple tasks. This was certainly the case for the object reversal task, on which subjects over 30 months of age made virtually no errors. Therefore, the present findings may indicate that cognitive gender differences were masked by the simplicity of the tasks. If this interpretation is correct, then gender difference may be discovered in older children when tested on more cognitively challenging tasks.

The third possibility regarding the absence of cognitive gender differences in older children is that the gender differences may exist only when there are gender differences in circulating hormones. At about 3 years of age, children have entered their prepuberty hormonal plateau, during which both boys and girls have very low levels of circulating hormones. Therefore, the earlier cognitive gender differences that occurred during the high-hormonal perinatal period may have subsided. Support for this circulating hormone hypothesis comes from studies with young monkeys showing a significant correlation between levels of circulating testosterone and performance on the concurrent discrimination task. Bachevalier et al. (1989) found an inverse correlation so that, in male monkeys, the higher their testosterone level, the poorer their performance on concurrent discrimination tasks. If, in fact, performance were dependent upon levels of circulating hormones, then one would expect that cognitive gender differences would reappear at postpuberty ages. Although in the present study the relative simplicity of the particular tasks may have masked cognitive gender differences in older children and adults, there is strong evidence from other lines of research for adult gender differences in brain anatomy and function.

In adult subjects, brain imaging studies indicate gender differences in the functions of orbital frontal and inferior temporal systems. Positron emission tomography studies have revealed a higher metabolic rate of glucose utilization for men in temporal–limbic regions (Gur et al., 1995), for women in orbital prefrontal areas (Andreason, Zametkin, Guo, Baldwin, & Cohen, 1993), and for women in the middle and posterior cingulate gyrus (Gur et al., 1995). In addition, data from magnetic resonance imaging studies show that gender differences in the frontal lobe and, to a lesser extent, in the temporal lobes continue into advanced age (Cowell et al., in press). It is possible that the data with children presented here reflect the earliest manifestations of lifelong gender differences in regional brain function.

Cognitive Gender Differences and Socialization

The joint findings of monkey and human infant cognitive gender differences in the form of a double dissociation strongly suggest that socialization has little or no impact on the appearance of the differences. Both cognitive tasks in the present study required the same perceptual skills (i.e., discriminating between two simultaneously presented objects) as well as the same motor skills (i.e., displacing objects for reward). Thus, gender differences in performance cannot be attributed to factors such as motivation, perception, or motor performance. Although the two tasks differ in the number of daily trials and the number of discriminants, they differ most importantly in their cognitive demands, which are known to be mediated by different brain systems (Bachevalier et al., 1989; Goldman et al., 1974). Considering these facts, it is difficult to imagine that differential socialization of males and females can explain the gender differences on these two tasks in either humans or monkeys. This is particularly true in the case of the monkeys, who were reared without physical contact with adult conspecifics in controlled laboratory conditions (Bachevalier et al., 1989; Goldman et al., 1974). Considering the similarity of the two tasks and the similarity of the perinatal hormonal environments in humans and monkeys, the most parsimonious explanation of the behavioral data is that, very early in life, sex-linked, hormonally induced differences in functional maturation of specific brain systems result in cognitive gender differences in both species. The male superiority on object reversal, the female emotionality on this task, and the data from ablation and hormone studies in monkeys all suggest that, in primates, the orbital prefrontal cortex develops earlier in life in males under the accelerating influence of testosterone. The female superiority on the concurrent discrimination task, together with the data from ablation and hormone studies in monkeys, suggests that Area TE in the inferior temporal lobe develops earlier in life in females and that its development is retarded in males by some yet unknown function of testosterone.

REFERENCES

Alexander, G.M., & Sherwin, B.B. (1991). The association between testosterone, sexual arousal and selective attention for erotic stimuli in men. *Hormones and Behavior, 25,* 367–381.

Allen, L.S., Hines, M., Shryne, J.E., & Gorski, R. (1989). Two sexually dimorphic cell groups in the human brain. *Journal of Neuroscience, 9,* 497–506.

Andreason, P.J., Zametkin, A.J., Guo, A.C., Baldwin, P., & Cohen, R.M. (1993). Gender-related differences in regional cerebral glucose metabolism in normal volunteers. *Psychiatry Research, 51,* 175–183

Atkinson, J. (1977). The development of optokinetic nystagmus in the human infant and monkey infant: An analog to development in kittens. *Developmental Neurobiology of Vision, 27,* 277–287.

Bachevalier, J., Brickson, M., Hagger, C., & Mishkin, M. (1990). Age and sex differences in the effects of selective temporal lobe lesions on the formation of visual discrimination habits in rhesus monkeys (*Macaca mulatta*). *Behavioral Neuroscience, 104,* 885–889.

Bachevalier, J., Hagger, C., & Bercu, B. (1989). Gender differences in visual habit formation in 3-month-old rhesus monkeys. *Developmental Psychobiology, 22,* 585–599.

Bauer, J.A., Shimojo, S., Gwiazda, J., & Held, R. (1986). Sex differences in the development of human infants. *Investigative Ophthalmology and Visual Sciences, 27*(Suppl.), 265–273.

Berenbaum, S.A., & Hines, M. (1992). Early androgens are related to childhood sex-typed toy preferences. *Psychological Science, 3,* 203–209.

Boothe, R.G., Williams, R.A., Kiorpes, L., & Teller, D.Y. (1980). Development of contrast sensitivity in infant Macaca nemistrina monkeys. *Science, 208,* 1290–1292.

Bussey, K., & Bandura, A. (1984). Influence of gender constancy and social power on sex-linked modeling. *Journal of Personality and Social Psychology, 47,* 1292–1303.

Butter, C.M., & Snyder, D.R. (1972). Alterations in aggressive and aversive behaviors following orbital frontal lesions in rhesus monkeys. *Acta Neurobiologiae Experimentalis, 32,* 525–565.

Clark, A.S., & Goldman-Rakic, P. (1989). Gonadal hormones influence the emergence of cortical function in non-human primates. *Behavioral Neuroscience, 103,* 1287–1295.

Connor, J.M., & Serbin, L.A. (1977). Behaviorally based masculine- and feminine-activity-preference scales for preschoolers: Correlates with other classroom behaviors and cognitive tests. *Child Development, 48,* 1411–1416.

Corbier, P., Edwards, D.A., & Roffi, J. (1992). The neonatal testosterone surge: A comparative study. *Archives Internationales de Physiologie, de Biochimie et de Biophysique, 100,* 127–131.

Cowell, P.E., Allen, L.S., Zalatimo, N.S., & Denenberg, V.H. (1992). A developmental study of sex and age interaction in the human corpus. *Developmental Brain Research, 66,* 187–192.

Cowell, P.E., Turetsky, B.I., Gur, R.C., Shtassel, D.L., & Gur, R.E. (in press). Sex differences in aging of the human frontal and temporal lobes. *Journal of Neuroscience.*

Davidson, J.M., Carmargo, C.A., & Smith, E.R. (1979). Effects of androgens on sexual behavior of hypogonadal men. *Journal of Clinical Endocrinology and Metabolism, 48,* 955–958.

Ehrhardt, A.A., Meyer-Bahlburg, H.F.L., & Rosen, L.R. (1985). Sexual orientation after prenatal exposure to exogenous estrogen. *Archives of Sexual Behavior, 14,* 57–77.

Goldman, P.S., Crawford, H.T., Stokes, L.P., Galkin, T., & Rosvold, H.E. (1974). Sex-dependent behavioral effect of cerebral cortical lesions in the developing rhesus monkey. *Science, 186,* 540–542.

Goldman-Rakic, P. (1987). Development of cortical circuitry and cognitive function. *Child Development, 58,* 601–622.

Gunderson, V.M., Grant-Webster, K.S., & Fagan, J.F., III. (1987). Visual recognition memory in high- and low-risk infant pigtailed macaques (*Macaca nemistrina*). *Developmental Psychology, 23,* 671–675.

Gur, R.C., Mozley, L., Mozley, P.D., Resnick, S., Karp, J., Alavi, A., Arnold, S., & Gur, R.E. (1995). Sex differences in regional cerebral glucose metabolism during a resting state. *Science, 267,* 528–531.

Hagger, C., Bachevalier, J., & Bercu, B.B. (1987). Sexual dimorphism in the development of habit formation: Effects of perinatal steroidal gonadal hormones. *Neuroscience, 22*(Suppl.), S520.

Held, R., Bauer, J., & Gwiazda, J. (1988). Age of onset of binocularity correlates with level of plasma testosterone in male infants. *Investigative Ophthalmology and Visual Sciences, 29*(Suppl.), 60.

Hines, M. (1990). Gonadal hormones and cognitive development. In Balthazart (Ed.), *Hormones, brain, and behavior in vertebrates: 1. Comparative physiology* (pp. 51–63). Basel, Switzerland: Karger.

Hines, M., & Shipley, C. (1984). Prenatal exposure to diethylstilbestrol and development of sexually dimorphic cognitive abilities and cerebral lateralization. *Developmental Psychology, 20,* 81–94.

Huttenlocher, P.R. (1979). Synaptic density in human prefrontal cortex: Developmental changes and effects of aging. *Brain Research, 163,* 195–205.

Jones, B., & Mishkin, M. (1972). Limbic lesions and the problem of stimulus–reinforcement association. *Experimental Neurology, 36,* 362–377.

Kolb, B., & Fantie, B. (1989). Development of the child's brain and behavior. In C.R. Reynolds & E. Fletcher-Janzen (Eds.), *Handbook of clinical child neuropsychology* (pp. 17–39). New York: Plenum.

LeVay, S. (1991). A difference in hypothalamic structure between heterosexual and homosexual men. *Science, 253,* 1034–1037.

Linn, M.C., & Petersen, A.C. (1985). Emergence and characterization of sex differences in spatial ability: A meta-analysis. *Child Development, 56,* 1479–1498.

Liss, M.B. (1991). Patterns of toy play: An analysis of sex differences. *Sex Roles, 7,* 1143–1150.

Maccoby, E.E., & Jacklin, C.N. (1974). *The psychology of sex differences.* Stanford, CA: Stanford University Press.

Marin-Padilla, M. (1970). Prenatal and early-postnatal ontogenesis of motor cortex: A Golgi study. *Neuropsychologia, 13,* 489–497.

Mishkin, M. (1964). Perseveration of central sets after frontal lesions in monkeys. In J.M. Warren & K. Akert (Eds.), *The frontal granular cortex and behavior* (pp. 219–241). New York: McGraw-Hill.

Money, J., Schwartz, M., & Lewis, V.G. (1984). Adult erotosexual status and fetal hormonal masculinization and demasculinization: 46, XX congenital virilizing adrenal hyperplasia and 46, XY androgen-insensitivity syndrome compared. *Psychoneuroendocrinology, 9,* 405–414.

O'Carrol, R., Shapiro, C., & Bancroft, J. (1985). Androgens, behaviour, and nocturnal erection in hypogonadal men: The effects of varying the replacement dose. *Clinical Endocrinology, 23,* 527–538.

Overman, W.H. (1990). Performance on traditional match-to-sample, non-match to sample, and object discrimination tasks by 12–32-month-old children: A developmental progression. In A. Diamond (Ed.), *The development and neural basis of higher cognitive function* (Vol. 608, pp. 365–383). New York: New York Academy of Science Press.

Overman, W.H., Bachevalier, J., Miller, M., & Moore, K. (1996). Children's performance on "animal tests" of oddity: Implications for cognitive processes required for tests of oddity and delayed nonmatch-to-sample. *Journal of Experimental Child Psychology, 62,* 223–242.

Overman, W.H., Bachevalier, J., Schuhmann, E., & Ryan, P. (1996). Cognitive gender differences in very young children parallel biologically based cognitive gender differences in monkeys. *Behavioral Neuroscience, 110*(4), 673–684.

Overman, W.H., Bachevalier, J., Sewell, F., & Drew, J. (1993). A comparison of children's performance on two recognition memory tasks: Delayed nonmatch-to-sample vs visual paired comparison. *Developmental Psychobiology, 26,* 345–357.

Overman, W.H., Bachevalier, J., Turner, M., & Peuster, A. (1992). Object recognition versus object discrimination: Comparison between human infants and infant monkeys. *Behavioral Neuroscience, 106,* 15–29.

Phillips, R.R., Malamut, B.L., Bachevalier, J., & Mishkin, M. (1988). Dissociation of the effects of inferior temporal and limbic lesions on object discrimination learning with 24-h intervals. *Behavioral Brain Research, 27,* 99–107.

Reinisch, J.M. (1981). Prenatal exposure to synthetic progestens increases potential for aggression in humans. *Science, 211,* 1171–1173.

Resnick, S.M., Berenbaum, S.A., Gottesman, I.I., & Bouchard, T.J. (1986). Early hormonal influences in cognitive functioning in congenital adrenal hyperplasia. *Developmental Psychology, 22,* 191–198.

Rodman, H.R. (1994). Development of inferior temporal cortex in the monkey. *Cerebral Cortex, 5,* 484–498.

Stahl, F., Gotz, F., Poppe, I., Amendt, P., & Dorner, G. (1978). Pre- and early postnatal testosterone levels in rat and human. In G. Dorner & M. Kawakami (Eds.), *Hormones and brain development* (pp. 99–109). New York: Elsevier/North Holland.

Swaab, D.F., & Fliers, E. (1985). A sexually dimorphic nucleus in the human brain. *Science, 228,* 1112–1114.

Taylor, D.C. (1969). Differential rates of cerebral maturation between sexes and between hemispheres: Evidence from epilepsy. *Lancet, ii,* 140–142.

Taylor, D.C. (1971). Ontogenesis of chronic epileptic psychoses: A reanalysis. *Physiological Medicine, 1,* 247–253.

Teller, D.Y., Morse, R., Borton, R., & Regal, D. (1974). Visual acuity for vertical and diagonal gratings in human infants. *Vision Research, 14,* 1433–1439.

Tighe, T.J., & Powlison, L.B. (1978). Sex differences in infant habituation search: A survey and some hypotheses. *Bulletin of the Psychonomic Society, 12,* 337–340.

Williams, A.E. (1979). A longitudinal study of object concept development in pigtail macaques (*Macaca nemestrina*). *Dissertation Abstracts International, 40,* 2868B. (University Microfilms No. 79-27, 889)

Witelson, S. (1989). Hand and sex differences in the isthmus and genu of the human corpus callosum. *Brain, 112,* 799–835.

Yalom, I., Green, R., & Fisk, N. (1973). Prenatal exposure to female hormones: Effects on psychosexual development in boys. *Archives of General Psychiatry, 28,* 554–556.

16

The Work in Working Memory
Implications for Development

Karl H. Pribram

> The frontal "association areas," sometimes referred to as "the organ of civilization," are intimately connected with the limbic systems to form the internal core of the forebrain. This most forward portion of the primate frontal lobe appears to us to serve as a "working memory" where Plans can be retained temporarily when they are being formed, or transformed, or executed.
>
> Miller, Galanter, and Pribram (1960, p. 207)

Much evidence has accrued since 1960 to bear out this proposal regarding frontal lobe function encapsulated in the term *working memory*. The paragraph from which the quotation is taken goes on to state that "this speculation appears to be consistent with the fact that animals with lesions in the frontal lobes have difficulty with the delayed reaction and the delayed alternation tests." It is also consonant with the warning issued by Jacobsen (1928, 1931, 1935, 1936) when he first demonstrated the relation between the performance of these tasks and the integrity of the far frontal cortex: The notion of an immediate or short-term memory interpretation is too simple, and some more sophisticated conception is needed. Nissen (1951) pointed out that these tasks form a category that he called *one trial learning tasks*, and Mishkin (1966) has called them *trial unique*. Further work by Jacobsen and his colleagues Wolfe (Jacobsen, Wolfe, & Jackson, 1935); Finan (1939); Nissen (Jacobsen & Nissen, 1937); and Malmo (1942) demonstrated the importance of attention to the performance of these tasks both during the predelay period and in sustaining performance in the face of distraction during the delay itself.

In this chapter, I recount the path of frontal lobe research that has been taken from the early demonstrations and recent confirmations of the importance of attention to the concept of work—that is, allocation of resources—in a working memory. Even the concept *attention* has proved to be insufficiently precise. Frontal lobe lesions lead to a susceptibility to be distracted, an appetite for novelty—in short, the failure of the ability to disattend distraction. A similar deficit can be shown to impair the carrying out of a behavior sequence. It is as if the frontally lesioned primate becomes bored and thus distractible in tasks that control subjects pursue. Such lack of persistence can be due to a lack of motivation or to an inability to maintain concentration, disparate descriptions that may apply to the same basic phenomenon. Alternatively, the disability may be due to a deficiency in a process that flexibly organizes and reorganizes our attention (control of sensory input), intention (control of behavioral output), and even thought (memory processing). The experiments reviewed here indicate that it is this organizing function that is disturbed by frontal lesions. A computational model is presented that shows how such an organizing process might operate. Finally, data are presented that relate developmental stages in brain electrical activity to the maturation of frontal lobe function—maturation that remains incomplete as late as the ages of 17–21 years.

PARCELLATION

What, then, is working memory? How does it become implemented? A short answer given by Deeke, Kornhuber, Long, and Schreiber (1985) was that human subjects with frontal cortex damage were deficient in their ability to know what to do, when to do, and how to do. These three factors composing working memory are linked to separate subsystems of the far frontal lobe.

As was Caesar's Gaul, the far frontal cortex can be divided anatomically into three parts, and each part has been shown to have somewhat different relations to behavior consonant with the connectivity of the parts. An orbitofrontal sector can be identified with heavy connections to the amygdala, anterior insula, and temporal pole through the uncinate fasciculus. This sector has been shown to be especially involved in processing novelty and in establishing a familiar context within which subsequent processing occurs. It is this sector that is related to the functions of the visceroautonomic system through connections with the amygdala and hypothalamus. Visceroautonomic responses to novel cues (as part of the orienting reaction) were shown to be necessary to the development of familiarity. On the basis of clinical data (Konow & Pribram, 1970; Luria, Pribram, & Homskaya, 1964; Poppen, Pribram, & Robinson, 1965), the orbitofrontal sector has been shown to utilize familiarity in the service of propriety—that is, to determine what is and what is not appropriate behavior in any particular situation.

A second sector encompassing the dorsal part of the far frontal cortex is related to the hippocampal system through connections with the cingulate cortex. The hippocampal system was shown to be involved in the processing of spatial and temporal cues into a context that organizes maximally efficient action (see reviews by Pribram, 1986, 1991). It is this sector, therefore, that deals with assessing priorities. The dorsal frontal cortex modifies this organization when the situation demands flexibility to act effectively.

The third sector takes up the middle of the far frontal cortex. This sector connects to the remainder of the cortex and can be further subdivided according to the locus of connections to the various sensory modalities (Pribram, 1987). It is this middle sector of the far frontal cortex that integrates the functions of the other two sectors with those of the rest of the brain, thus ensuring practicality in the execution of actions.

The processing of propriety, priority, and practicality entails the processing of "what, when, and how" when these are not completely specified by the situation in which an action is to be undertaken (Deeke et al., 1985). The "what" must primarily be based on familiarity, a particular kind of memory. The "when" is primarily based on sustaining attention and noticing when efficient, automatic processing becomes ineffective. The "how" is primarily based on assessing what works (what is appropriate) and when it is working and when it is not. Therefore, when we state that lesions of the far frontal cortex result in defects in *working* memory, we mean that under certain conditions attentional and intentional processes necessary to the processing of "one trial learning" tasks are disrupted.

What makes a task "trial unique," and what are the conditions that must be present to make one-trial learning necessary? The short answer to these questions is flexibility in the face of spatial or temporal ambiguity, or both.

Why are spatial and temporal ambiguity so critical to bringing out the frontal lobe deficit? When I have an intention, I certainly know how to go about implementing it—if I make a mistake, I rectify my behavior; if all goes well, I proceed. Thus, it is clear that I can evaluate mistakes and successes. When we examine patients with frontal lobe pathology, they are found to be deficient in carrying out their intentions; therefore, we infer that they have difficulty in evaluating their errors and successes (Luria et al., 1964). However, when examining such patients, I noted that they were cursing whenever they made a mistake—it was obvious that they recognized the incorrect outcome of their behavior. Nonetheless, their next attempt did not profit from that recognition. I therefore concluded that such patients could not *utilize* their errors (Konow & Pribram, 1970).

In economics, a utility function is composed of the desirability of a transaction and the momentary estimation of the probability that the transaction can be executed. Could this formulation be effectively applied to all intentional behavior? If so, the experiment showing that far frontal resections disrupt the probability distribution of responses in a fixed internal experiment (see Figure 16.5 on page 368) can be taken as an indication that it is the execution of the probability distribution of a behavior, not its desirability, that suffers in the frontal lesion patient.

This interpretation is congruent with Milner's (1974) finding of intralist order disturbances in recall. It is serial position, the ability to monitor probability distributions, that becomes muddled; patients fail in their ability to temporally tag events. It is therefore the ability to monitor serially, whether in relation to attention or to intended behavior, that constitutes the work in working memory. The following experiments made with monkeys support and extend this conclusion.

ATTENTION

With regard to attention, Bolster and Pribram (1993), in a series of experiments, showed that recordings of brain electrical activity could be used to differentiate the brain systems involved in automatic, para-attentional parallel processing of visual stimuli from those involved in controlled, consciously attended procedures demanding an effective sampling of the feature array. A modification of Treisman's (1969) tasks was used: a distinct-feature array tested for automatic processing and a shared-feature array tested for controlled scan (Figure 16.1). Figure 16.2 shows the effect the number of shared features has on the response latency (reaction time) of

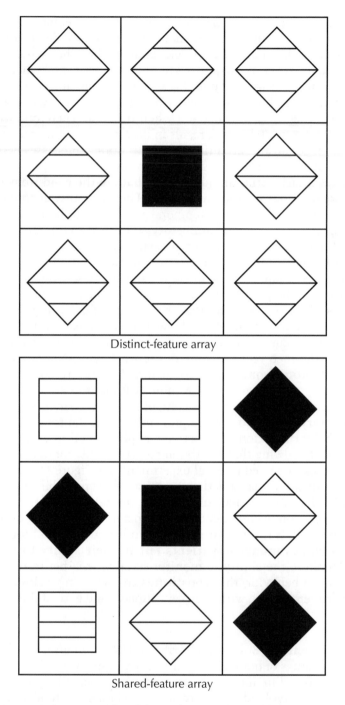

Distinct-feature array

Shared-feature array

Figure 16.1.   Examples of distinct-feature and shared-feature arrays with the target (solid square) shown in the central position. (From Bolster, B., & Pribram, K.H. [1993]. Cortical involvement in visual scan in the monkey. *Perception and Psychophysics, 53,* 507; reprinted by permission.)

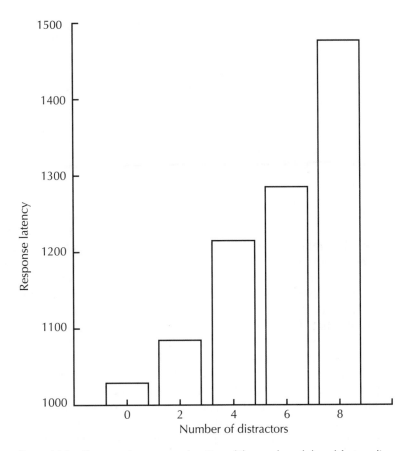

Figure 16.2.   Response latency as a function of the number of shared-feature distractors present in the stimulus array. (From Bolster, B., & Pribram, K.H. [1993]. Cortical involvement in visual scan in the monkey. *Perception and Psychophysics, 53,* 507; reprinted by permission.)

the monkeys tested, confirming the assumption that shared features increase search of the array.

Recordings were made of event-related local field potentials placed over the primary visual projection cortex (V1) of monkeys and over parietal, frontal, and inferior temporal "association" areas. Changes in field potentials recorded from the primary visual projection cortex changed as a function of the total number of features, never as a function of shared features; by contrast, changes in the number of shared features produced changes recorded from all three "association" areas. With regard to the changes in local field potentials recorded from the frontal cortex, we concluded that the difficulty in search over the cues with the shared features was a function of the fact that these shared features composed a *distractor* set. In earlier experiments, we had found that performance of monkeys with far frontal cortex resections suffers when the location of distractors is randomized over nine positions, as in the Discrimination Apparatus for Discrete Trial Analysis (Drake & Pribram, 1976; Pribram, 1969; Pribram, Gardner, Pressman, & Bagshaw, 1962) used in those and the current experiments. The deficiency becomes especially apparent when compared with performance on the Wisconsin General Test Apparatus, where randomization is limited to two locations (Brody & Pribram, 1978; Brody, Ungerleider, & Pribram, 1977; Pribram, Konrad, & Gainsburg, 1966). The nine-location randomization was instituted to deter monkeys (especially those with far frontal cortex resections) from falling into position habits. In this the technique was successful, but the changes in location of a cue pose an especially potent distractor for monkeys (Douglas & Pribram, 1969), especially for those with far frontal cortex damage (Grueninger & Pribram, 1969). Therefore, in the current experiments, one source of difficulty is the fact that manipulations were made of the number of shared features that constituted a *distractor* set.

A distractor set provides the context, the contingencies, within which the rewarded target must be chosen. Fuster (1988) conceptualized this context–reward relationship in terms of cross-temporal contingencies. However, experiments in our laboratory in which spatial context is manipulated, as in variants of delayed response tasks that related them to Piaget's findings on object constancy (Anderson, Hunt, Vander Stoep, & Pribram, 1976), showed that the relationship can be spatiotemporal as well as temporotemporal. In these tasks, the monkeys had to remember *where* an object had been hidden on a previous occasion. In fact, in other experiments (Brody & Pribram, 1978; Pribram, Plotkin, Anderson, & Leong, 1977), we presented data that showed far frontal cortex involvement whenever behavior is influenced by two or more distinct sets of covarying contingencies, even when both are spatial. In these experiments, the monkeys had to remember in which location they had received a reward and to avoid that location on the subsequent trial(s).

More generally, therefore, the far frontal cortex becomes implicated whenever perception entails relating current contingencies to a context computed from prior relevant contingencies. The computation of this covariation demands that cross-temporal, spatiotemporal, and cross-spatial contingencies be perceived. In classic and operant conditioning, the consequences of behavior are contiguous in time and place with the stimulus conditions that initiate the behavior. When contiguity is loosened, stimulation that intervenes between initiation and consequence has the potential to distract and thus to prevent the processing of covariation. Perception is perturbed and processing is destabilized. Perturbation is controlled only if a stable state, an established set of contingencies—that is, a stable context—instructs and directs the process (Pribram, 1987).

It is from the effects of interference on the establishment of such a stable state that one is able to discern the powerful role of context in controlling trial-unique processing. When the interfering effect of distractors is removed (e.g., by darkening the testing chamber) during trial-unique tasks such as delayed response, monkeys with far frontal cortex resections perform the task as well as their controls (Malmo, 1942; Pribram, 1961). The effects of interference occur primarily during stimulus presentation or shortly thereafter, not during the delay period (Pribram, 1961; Stamm, 1969). Interference therefore is with the organization of a perceptual context within which subsequent performance occurs.

The impairment is also shown by patients with damage to the frontal cortex. These patients fail to remember the place in a sequence in which an item occurs. They lose the ability to "temporally tag" events, that is, to *monitor* and place them within the episode. With such patients, Milner (1974; see also Petrides & Milner, 1982) performed a series of experiments demonstrating how the processing impairment affects the middle portions of an episode. In her studies, it is *relative recency*, the *serial position* of the sequence, that becomes muddled. Other patients with frontolimbic damage, described by Kinsbourne and Wood (1975), also show that the impairment in processing serial position is due to a derangement in monitoring and therefore in organizing contextual structure of an episode.

To summarize, the involvement of the far frontal cortex in visual scans of shared feature arrays entails a stable state within which search for the rewarded target can be performed. This state is characterized as establishing and mapping (Schneider & Shiffrin, 1977), a serial search within a context of contingencies that show covariation over successive trials. In Efron's (1989) terms, this context forms a flexible yet stable "scanplan" within which shared features can be searched. Efron showed that such a scanplan does not depend on actual receptor scanning; rather, the scan is an internal process attributable to the mind's eye or ear.

INTENTION

The results of these experiments suggest that the relationship of the far frontal cortex to attention involves some deeper function. This function, a scan *plan* in the previously noted experimental results, is the intentional aspect of attention.

In an earlier series of experiments, Pribram (1960, 1961), having confirmed the earlier conclusion regarding the importance of attention, added as a result of his experiments that "frontal lesions apparently interfere with the organizational process that must take place in normal subjects when events that serve as guides to subsequent actions occur in relatively unreliable situations" (Pribram, 1961, p. 462). Some of the critical experiments that show that the far frontal cortex is involved in the organization of intention (i.e., "guides to subsequent actions") are described here.

Performance on Nonspatial Object Alternation Tasks

Twelve animals were given 50 trials a day for a total of 1,200 trials on a nonspatial object alternation. For the first 500 trials, two objects, a tobacco tin and an ashtray, were presented on a board that contained two holes 1.5 inches in diameter and 3 feet apart. For the remaining 700 trials, these objects were presented on a board that contained six holes, each with a diameter of 1.5 inches, arranged in a circle with a diameter of 2 feet. Each object could cover one hole completely, and a peanut could therefore be concealed by the object. The holes were given numbers, and on each trial the objects were placed over the holes according to a random number table. On successive trials, a peanut was placed alternately under one and then the other object irrespective of the placement of the object on the board. Trials were separated by the interposition of an opaque screen between the monkey and the test object. The animals were not allowed to correct if they made an error; that is, on any one trial, a monkey was allowed to manipulate only one object and to uncover one hole to see if a peanut was there. On the next trial, the alternative object was baited and so on throughout the 50 alternations. Trials were spaced approximately 5 seconds apart. As can be seen from Figure 16.3, monkeys with resections of the frontal cortex are impaired to a considerable extent (although not completely) in their ability to maintain their "set" to respond on each trial, a deficit that can be interpreted to be due to a change in motivation or in memory.

Performance on a Multiple-Choice Task

To further explore this relationship between memory and motivation, a multiple-choice task reward reversal was devised. Reversal was instituted after five trials as

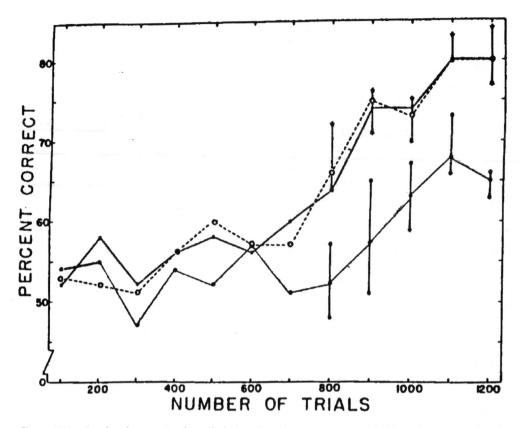

Figure 16.3.   Results of comparing frontally lesioned monkeys on a nonspatial object alternation task with unoperated and temporal cortex resected controls. Monkeys with frontal resections reach only a 65%–70% performance level, indicating that the spatial parameter is not the only one responsible for the frontal lobe deficit in alternation performance. (■——■, normals; ○——○, temporals; ●——●, frontals; ⏄, range.)

in the previous experiment, but now a sequence of 12! (twelve factorial) tasks was given in which, after each set of reversals among a given number of cues was completed, a novel cue was added until a total of 12 cues were presented to the monkey on each trial. The locations of the cues were randomized from trial to trial among 12 possible positions. The results showed that the monkeys with far frontal cortex resections responded immediately to the novel cue when it was introduced, whereas the control subjects tended to respond more to the previously rewarded (familiar) cues (see Figure 16.4). Furthermore, the monkeys with frontal lesions failed to sustain their intention to respond to the rewarded cue for the five consecutive trials necessary to reach criterion before reward reversal was instituted (see Figure 16.5), despite the fact that they have shown (statistically) that they "know" which one shelters the reward. These results show that the reinforcing consequences of the monkeys' behavior had less impact on their future behavior than these consequences had on that of the control subjects. Alteration in intention (organizing behavior on the basis of consequences, i.e., reinforcement) was thus shown to affect "memory."

The results of these experiments also tell once more the twice-told tale. After the completion of search (see Figure 16.7 on page 370), frontal lesions produced perseveration of the set of responses that had proved useful to the subject in the imme-

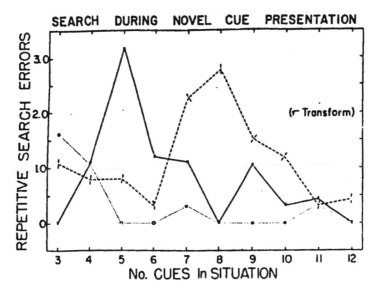

Figure 16.4.   Graph of the average of the number of repetitive errors made in the multiple-choice experiment during the search trials when the novel cue is presented. (——— = normals, - - - - = temporals, ... = frontals.) Note that, although records of the control groups show peaks that indicate confusion between novel and familiar cues, the monkeys with frontal lesions are not confused.

diately preceding circumstance. During search, in contrast, the frontally lesioned monkeys tended to shift their responses.

What features distinguish search and postsearch situations? After search, the reward contingencies are held constant for the duration of a problem, then changed. During search, the reward situation varies. Specifically, the cue–reinforcement contingencies had remained consistent during a period sufficient for the subject to develop an identifiable (adaptive) response pattern; perseveration (response to the novel cue) occurs in frontally lesioned primates when the cue–reinforcement contingencies are then changed to another but equally consistent cue–reinforcement configuration. During the postsearch period, characterized by varying cue–reinforcement contingencies trial by trial, frontally lesioned monkeys react with an increased (compared with controls) variability in response pattern. In general, therefore, these results can be summarized by stating that perseveration occurred with *inter*problem change and an increased tendency to shift occurred with *intra*problem change of the cue–reinforcement configuration.

In this experiment, paradoxically, perseveration consisted of responding to a novel cue. This suggests that frontally lesioned primates are especially susceptible to distraction (see also results obtained by Grueninger & Grueninger, 1973; Grueninger & Pribram, 1969), which accounts for both the increased variability and the perseveration obtained in these and other experiments. Distractibility interferes with working memory—but the question remains as to whether this is due to lowered motivation or to a more rapid decay in a memory trace. Or both? Or neither?

Performance on a Fixed Interval Task
The results of these experiments were inconclusive regarding the relationship of the anterior frontal cortex to motivation and of motivation to memory. To resolve

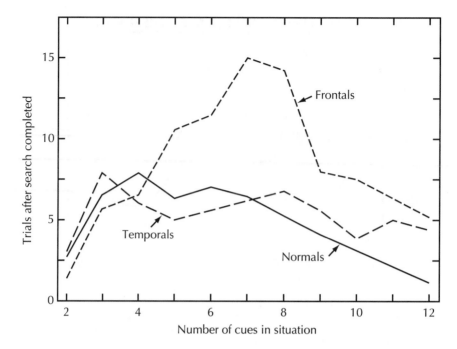

Figure 16.5. Graph of the average of the number of trials to criterion taken in the multiple-object experiment by each of the groups in each of the situations after search was completed (i.e., after the first correct response). The difference between the curves for the controls and for the frontally operated group is significant at the .05 level by an analysis of variance ($F_{2,6} =$ 8.19) according to McNemar's procedure performed on normalized (by square-root transformation) raw scores.

these issues, a set of experiments was undertaken in which the effects of starvation were compared with the effects of frontal cortex resection. Twelve rhesus monkeys were trained to press a lever in an experiment where a reward was delivered on a "fixed-interval" schedule. The monkeys were fed a sufficient amount of laboratory chow immediately after each training session to maintain them at approximately 80% of the weight they had attained after a 3-week period of *ad libitum* feeding.

In addition to the usual cumulative record obtained, counters were so arranged as to sum the number of responses an animal made during six equal periods into which the total 2-minute interval was divided. From the numbers recorded on the counters, performance graphs were constructed. These graphs show the distribution of responses across as many of the 2-minute intervals as desired. Therefore, the total performance of any monkey could be measured—an advantage not given by inspection of the ordinary representative cumulative curve. Also, in this way, averages of the responses of groups of animals could be taken and the variations between individual animals statistically analyzed.

The actual experiment consisted of the following procedure. Ten 2-hour sessions were given. Then each animal was subjected to a 72-hour fast and retested for one session, after which the usual feeding schedule was immediately resumed and testing continued as in the prefast period for 10 sessions. The entire procedure was repeated another time with the interposition of 118 hours of fasting before the critical test session.

The results are shown in Figure 16.6. As can be clearly seen, the effect of food deprivation (i.e., of starvation) is upon the rate and not upon the distribution of monkeys' responses during an interval. The percentage of total responses made during any particular portion of the interval appears to remain remarkably constant despite marked changes in the total number of responses an animal makes. Also, there is remarkable consistency of results and little variation between animals. When monkeys are starved for 3–5 days, their total rate of response increases—but the way in which they distribute these responses during an interval does not change. (Similar changes are observed when monkeys are sated. Fixed-interval performance when the animals are kept in an *ad libitum* feeding situation shows a lower overall rate.)

The same group of animals were used to assay the effect of selective brain resections on performance in the fixed-interval operant task. Three of them were given ablations of the frontal eugranular isocortex, and three others were given control lesions that consisted of resection of the inferior portion of the temporal isocortex. Four of the remaining animals served as unoperated controls.

Figure 16.7 graphs the results obtained following these procedures. When rate of response of the operated and control groups is compared, no differences are apparent. However, for the frontally operated group, the *distribution of responses* across the interval is markedly different, whereas that of the control monkeys remains unchanged. This effect of the frontal lesion is in direct contrast to the effect of starvation. Here, instead of a deficit in monitoring, in constructing a scanplan that relates to searching the environment, the deficiency in planning entails instrumental behavior. Neither motivation per se nor the ability to remember per se is affected by the frontal resection. The frontally lesioned monkeys respond *precisely* to the timing of the reward. Therefore, neither timing nor general memory is affected (see also Stamm, 1963). Rather, it is monitoring the distribution and therefore *the allocation of effort* that constitutes the work in working memory.

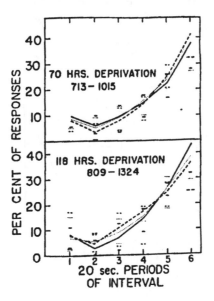

Figure 16.6.   Graph showing the effect of food deprivation on monkeys' rates of lever-pressing response to food (a small pellet of laboratory chow), which became available every 2 minutes. (——— = prehunger, ... = hunger, - - - - = posthunger.) The change in total rate is indicated by numbers under the deprivation label. The lack of change in the distribution responses is shown by the curves. Each curve represents the average of the responses of 10 monkeys; each point represents the average rate during a period of the interval over 10 hours of testing. Variance is indicated by the short horizontal bars.

COMPUTER SIMULATION

In order to determine how such a process might operate, I turned to computer simulations, which, much as in vitro experiments in biochemistry, can often help to clarify processes that are difficult to examine in vivo. The following is an excerpt from a paper presented during a conference on frontal lobe function in 1964:

Because simulation can be made precise with the use of computers, erroneous or vague models can be readily rejected. The experimentalist is therefore given a limited number of models, i.e., hypotheses about mechanism, that are found to fit the data. These he can then test against the real nervous system. By the use of this intervening step of model building, the neurological scientist can test notions about neural mechanism instead of notions directly derived from behavioral observation such as "perseveration of set," "tendency to shift," or even "immediate memory."

A model worth serious consideration derives from the work of Newell et al. (1958). These investigators have simulated the human cognitive, i.e., problem-solving, process by devising a hierarchically organized computer program composed of lists of items, each item capable of referring to another list. The structure of such programs can be variously represented as an English teacher's outline, a mathematician's branching set theoretical tree, or a systems engineer's flow diagram. Once such a computer program has been engaged it runs its problem-solving course relentlessly. Erroneous or nonsense solutions indicate errors in programs, errors that must be painstakingly sought out and corrected.

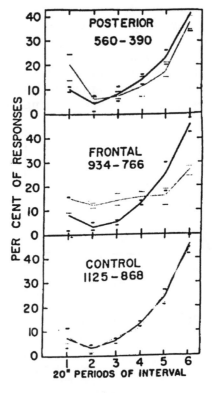

Figure 16.7.   Graph showing the change in distribution on monkeys' response rates following frontal ablation (three monkeys). (—— = preoperation, ... = postoperation.) Note that the distribution of rate over the interval is not affected in the controls (four monkeys) and after inferotemporal (posterior) ablations (three monkeys). Also note that the total rate of response did not increase; rather, the rate was somewhat decreased in all groups, probably as a result of the *ad libitum* feeding period that all groups were given prior to operation—approximately 2 weeks before postoperative testing.

Instruction Programs

One of the most recent of these continually evolving problem-solving programs is EPAM II (Feigenbaum, 1959, 1961; Feigenbaum & Simon, 1961a, 1961b, 1961c; Newell, 1961). In this program, as in most others, a recurrent difficulty had to be met. Once the stored lists that compose a complex program reach a certain number, access to the list structure needs itself to be programmed to "get the show on the road," as it were. Three types of such instruction programs have to date been found useful.

The first type (type I) of instruction is contained in the problem itself; for instance, in its simplest form it will be an instruction that reads "find item X." This instruction both sets the problem and indicates that the computer's stored list structure is to be systematically searched until an item that matches X is found.

The second type (type II) of instruction program is closely related to the first, but is more complicated. This instruction reads that the first step in problem solving is to run the problem program through the computer's *permanently stored* list structure and to report the items on the problem list that match the items in the stored program. The residue, the items that fail to match, are also reported as such and stored in new locations in the permanently stored list structure.

The third, and for our purposes the most interesting, type of instruction program (type III) has an "iffy" nature. This type is a somewhat complex and hierarchically organized list structure independent of both the problem programs and the computer's stored list structure. The lists that comprise this program contain items such as "(1) take the problem program and search part A of the stored list structure for its match; (2) if no match is found, search part B; (3) and so on until a match is obtained." However, this routine is not fixed. Another set of items states: "Shuffle the *order* in which these items of instruction are to be tried in such a way that the instruction that has proved repeatedly successful is tried first, i.e., is placed first on the list." This is accomplished by temporarily storing the information about the outcome of prior searches (through A or B or . . .). This temporary storage must take place not in the computer's permanent memory where it would do little good, but in the instruction program itself. Needless to say, there is a limit to the complexity which such a flexible set of temporary instructions can attain if they are to remain an efficient tool for problem solving.

These temporary instruction programs are called noticing orders; those that shift the order of the items on their lists on the basis of the outcomes of searches through their memories are known as flexible noticing orders. Noticing orders and the current problem program are kept separate from the computer's main storage facility in a "working" or temporary memory that is at all times immediately accessible to the programmer and computer.

To pursue the analogy: the primate brain must solve the same tasks that the computer has been programmed to solve. Since the computer processes were composed in order to simulate "primate" problem-solving processes, the processes are likely to be similar if not yet identical. However, this does not mean that the brain mechanism need mirror the computer mechanism that is set up to accomplish a particular process.

Noticing Order in a Working Memory

Noticing order is a process used by EPAM II and other problem-solving programs based on list structures. If noticing order is a process used by the primate brain when the subject is solving problems, several statements can be made about noticing order and the performance of frontally lesioned monkeys.

First, on problems where noticing order is unimportant, or where it is determined by the situation, frontally lesioned monkeys have no difficulty. This is especially apparent when the situation is novel.

Second, on problems where noticing order is determined by running the problem through the subject's fixed store of representations of past experiences, the frontally lesioned monkeys also have no difficulty. Discrimination performances and discrimination learning have repeatedly been shown [to be] unaffected by frontal lesions. Matching from sample remains unimpaired. And, in the multiple-choice problem analysis, sampling and search, though different from controls because of irrelevant interproblem changes, are also essentially unimpaired.

When, however, problem solution demands a noticing order that is not contained in the problem itself nor in the permanently fixed store of representations of past experience of the subject, frontally lesioned primates have difficulty. Such problems have in common the factor of change, not in the stimuli per se, but in the way in which the already-experienced stimuli (e.g., cues and reinforcements) covary to form the context for the new problem. The organism must react to these changes much as does the computer program: it must reshuffle the order in which the stimuli are processed. When change is occasional, i.e., when the change occurs between problems, the frontal defect is minimal and shows up as perseveration of set since noticing order within each problem proceeds, once the frontally lesioned subject catches on that a change has taken place, according to the type I or type II process of noticing order. When, however, the change occurs within a problem; i.e., when the appropriate behavior sequence depends solely on the outcome of the immediately preceding application of the noticing order, the frontal defect shows up full-blown.

As a rule, the monkey returns to random behavior since his apparatus for shifting noticing order is broken down with the result that the various behaviors tried all result in the same number of reinforcements. But perseveration may also be shown; when frontally lesioned monkeys are tested in the delayed-response or delayed-alternation situation, they frequently—more frequently than their controls—develop a position habit, since this behavior mode obtains as many reinforcements as random behavior does. The results of the experiment show that frontally lesioned monkeys are no more prone to position habits than unoperated monkeys are. My view is that frontally lesioned monkeys, just as unoperated monkeys, take position habits whenever they need not or cannot cope with a task, i.e., whenever the number of reinforcements they gain remains constant irrespective of their responses. Since frontal lesions impair delayed response and alternation learning, the operated subjects tend to take position habits—but no more so than their controls would if they could not cope with the problem. Support for this view comes from the observation that inferotemporally lesioned monkeys, when they have difficulty with visual discrimination problems, also slip easily into position stereotypes. At present, however, there is as yet no quantitative comparison of the relative proneness to stereotypy by frontally and inferotemporally lesioned monkeys in an insoluble problem.

In a sense, this explanation of the frontal defect in terms of impairment of a flexible noticing order is in partial agreement with the explanation made by Brush et al. (1961). They hypothesize that regression to a more primitive innate performance set occurs whenever the frontally lesioned primate cannot change this innate response tendency through learning. When, however, a task has already been learned, this performance is perseverated. As already noted, we could say the same, even for our results with respect to tendency to shift, were we to interpret the data in the multiple choice experiments as perseveration of some initial "set to explore" or set to behave randomly, which is overcome by the controls as a result of reinforcing contingencies which do not affect the frontally lesioned group. As Wilson points out, however (1962), the notion of perseveration of set so conceived can be stretched over any data set since all that need be done is to specify after the fact which response tendencies are resistant to change. Does not the stretching go too far when it is made to cover random responses and response to novelty? The explanation in terms of impairment of a flexible noticing order is considerably more predictive, yet captures the spirit of the intent of the perseveration of set hypothesis.

The suggestion is, therefore, that the frontally lesioned primate is defective in problem solving whenever a process that corresponds to a flexible noticing order is demanded. From the analysis made above, it follows that a disruption of the mechanism that allows monitoring of stimuli that temporarily covary would impair this process. It follows also that this temporary flexible monitoring of stimulus-covariation is separable from the process that allows more permanent storage of invariant representations of experiences, (e.g., in a discrimination tree).

Stimulus Covariation and Dominant Foci
Neurologically, the search is shifted. Earlier notions of the short or immediate memory process led to hypotheses about memory trace formation and decay, and to experiments aimed at uncovering reverberatory circuits in the brain. The concept of a flexible noticing order within a working memory leads instead to tracking down the mechanism of tempo-

rary, flexible stimulus covariation, perhaps through the formation of readily shifted dominant neural foci (see review by E.R. John, 1961; Pribram 1971). Such dominant foci can be
manipulated in a classical Pavlovian situation, for instance, by training a dog to raise his
right hind leg to a signal. When the response had been well established, the dog's right motor cortex was exposed and a patty of strychnine sulfate–soaked filter paper was placed
over the area that controls the left foreleg. While the strychnine was effective, the dog was
placed in a conditioning situation. Now he raised his left foreleg instead of his right hind
leg whenever the signal was given.
      The production and shift of dominant foci have recently been repeatedly studied (Mor-
rell, 1961; Rusinov, 1956; Ukhtomski, 1927). Could frontal lesions be shown to alter the
time course of the establishment or of the shift of such dominant foci? If for no other reason than that the direction of experimentation has been altered, the experiments and
analyses reported here may thus be shown by future events to have been worthwhile.
(Pribram, Ahumada, Hartog, & Roos, 1964, pp. 47–52)

      With currently available tools, noticeably 128-electrode geodesic scalp record-
ing arrays with which to assay brain electrical activity, a first step toward demonstrating a frontal influence on an evoked visual response in the occipital cortex has
been taken. Tucker, Liotti, Potts, Russell, and Posner (1994) have shown a "reinforcement" of an occipitally evoked response by a "reprise" that issues from that
response to the frontal cortex and then back again to the occipital cortex. The relationship of the reprise to working memory must now be shown.

IMPLICATIONS FOR DEVELOPMENT

Thatcher (1994a, 1994b; see also Chapter 5) has analyzed the process of maturation
of brain electrical activity and correlated it with a variety of anatomical and other
physiological indicators. In his analysis, Thatcher has mapped coherence among
recordings from different brain sites. The maturation process was shown to proceed
in cycles, each cycle consisting of rapid change (spurts) followed by a plateau. Three
"stages" were identified: one occurring in early childhood, a second during what is
sometimes called the latency period, and another following puberty.
      Specifically, the physiological processes observed in the study are 2-year
growth spurt cycles in the strength of intrahemispheric couplings, which are nested
within 4-year interhemispheric rotations. Figure 16.8 is a diagrammatic representation of the structure of cycles and subcycles as observed in the electroencephalographic coherence data. In summary, there are three main cycles separated by at
least two bifurcations or phase transitions (see also a bifurcation between ages
4 and 5 in the right frontal regions; Thatcher, 1994b). Phase transition 1 occurs in
the left hemisphere between ages 5 and 7, and phase transition 2 occurs in the right
hemisphere between ages 9 and 11. Cycle I is from approximately age 1.5 years to
age 5.0, cycle II is from approximately ages 5 to 10, and cycle III is from approximately ages 10 to 14. For continuity, the Fischer (Fischer, 1980; Fischer & Ferrar,
1987) and Case (1985, 1987) descriptions of cognitive development are used.
      Hudspeth and Pribram (1992) performed a somewhat different analysis using
the increase in desynchronization of brain electrical activity as our indicator. We
found three stages spanning much the same age ranges as those found by Thatcher.
The first stage of maturation, which spans the period between 1 and 6 years of age,
is characterized by rapid maturation in all brain regions. The frontal executive (FT),
visuospatial (PO), somatic (CC), and visuoauditory (TT) functions reach their
respective peaks almost simultaneously (i.e., within 6-month intervals of each

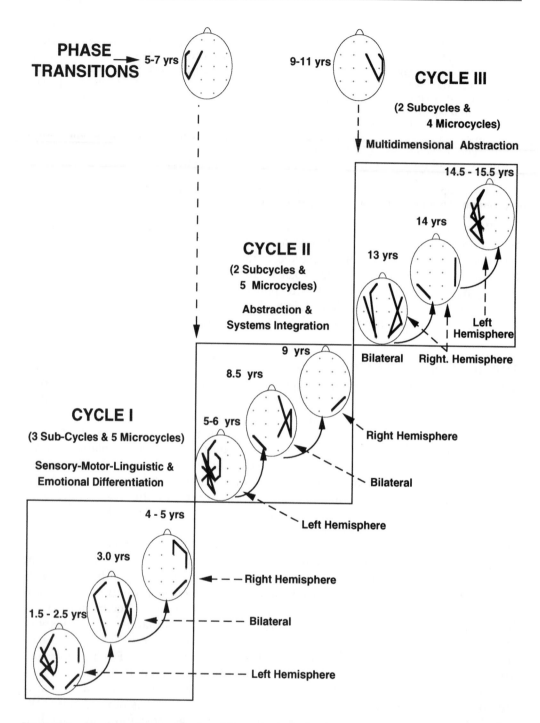

Figure 16.8.   Diagrammatic representation of the predominant developmental cycles and subcycles of neocortical reorganization. A designation of "Left hemisphere," "Bilateral," or "Right Hemisphere" emphasizes the predominant growth spurts during a given age range. This figure illustrates the combination of punctuated equilibria and the presence of a "spiral staircase" process of cyclical reorganization during postnatal cerebral development. (Adapted from Thatcher [1994b].)

other). This suggests that the executive control exercised by the far frontal cortex is primarily directed toward regulating body functions (e.g., going to the toilet at appropriate times and places).

In a second stage of maturation that spans the period between 6 and 10.5 years of age, rates are synchronized across the sensory and motor systems (PO, TT, CC), with all reaching a peak at 7.5–8 years of age. A mild acceleration in development in the frontal executive region (FT) starts only then (7.5 years) but terminates synchronously with that of the rest of the brain at 10.5 years. The early part of this period is therefore a continuation of the maturation of sensorimotor functions, whereas the latter part, beginning at age 7.5, heralds some enhancement of executive control, perhaps over sensory input (attention).

The third stage of maturation spans the period between 10.5 and 17 years of age. The third stage appears to be initially devoted to the elaboration of visuospatial (PO) functions. At the same time, however, maturation of the visuoauditory (TT) function starts and slowly accelerates, to be followed by successive maturation of another phase of visuospatial (PO) and somatic (CC) functions, with each region reaching its maturational peak with 1-year intervals (i.e., at 14, 15, and 16 years, respectively). The frontal executive region remains unchanged at this time.

However, our data permitted us to extend our analysis to age 21. Much to our surprise, a sizable acceleration of maturation of the electrical activity recorded from the frontal cortex occurred during the ages of 17–21 years. These changes can be attributed to the development of monitoring the controls over behavior, that is, the development of intentions. This is the age range of students in college, a period of intense cognitive and social activity. It is at the college level that many students become exposed to the variety of viewpoints, the variety of subcultures with which they must cope during life. It has been said that the far frontal cortex is the organ of civilization. Should our findings hold up, they emphasize the importance to our civilization of college and university education—the period when the plasticity of the frontal cortex can be challenged to provide a responsible, rich, and productive life in an environment replete with ambiguities and change.

These stages are in close correspondence with those delineated by Piaget and Inhelder (1966) (see also Kramer, 1983; Riegel 1973, 1975). Other stage-based theories for the maturation of emotion (Freud, 1932; Sullivan, 1953), moral judgment (Kohlberg, 1969), and psychosocial adaptation (Erikson, 1963) delineate roughly the same age boundaries as those described in this chapter (however, see also critique by McGuinness, Pribram, & Pirnazar, 1988). The theories are based on a wide range of observed behaviors. Therefore, a considerable amount of variation is to be expected when attempts are made to delineate maturational stages with behavioral criteria alone. The fact that stages could be gleaned from such evidence at all strongly suggests that biological factors are entailed in the processes denoted by these behavioral indices. Further refinements in these biobehavioral relationships would be expected when maturation in specific brain subsystems can be linked to maturation in specific behavioral subsystems.

REFERENCES

Anderson, R.M., Hunt, S.C., Vander Stoep, A., & Pribram, K.H. (1976). Object permanency and delayed response as spatial context in monkeys with frontal lesions. *Neuropsychologia, 14,* 481–490.

Bolster, B., & Pribram, K.H. (1993). Cortical involvement in visual scan in the monkey. *Perception and Psychophysics, 53*, 505–518.

Brody, B.A., & Pribram, K.H. (1978). The role of frontal and parietal cortex in cognitive processing: Tests of spatial and sequence functions. *Brain, 101*, 607–633.

Brody, B.A., Ungerleider, L.G., & Pribram, K.H. (1977). The effects of instability of the visual display on pattern discrimination learning by monkeys: Dissociation produced after resections of frontal and inferotemporal cortex. *Neuropsychologia, 15*, 439–448.

Brush, E.S., Mishkin, M., & Rosvold, H.E. (1961). Effects of object preferences and aversions on discrimination learning in monkeys with frontal lesions. *Journal of Comparative Physiological Psychology, 54*, 319–325.

Case, R. (1985). *Intellectual development: Birth to adulthood*. New York: Academic Press.

Case, R. (1987). The structure and process of intellectual development. *International Journal of Psychology, 22*, 571–607.

Deeke, L., Kornhuber, H.H., Long, M., & Schreiber, H. (1985). Timing function of the frontal cortex in sequential motor and learning tasks. *Human Neurobiology, 4*, 143–154.

Douglas, R.J., & Pribram, K.H. (1969). Distraction and habituation in monkeys with limbic lesions. *Journal of Comparative and Physiological Psychology, 69*, 473–480.

Drake, K.U., & Pribram, K.H. (1976). DADTA IV: A computer based video display and recording system for behavioral testing. In P.B. Brown (Ed.), *Computer terminology in neuroscience* (pp. 509–528). New York: John Wiley & Sons.

Efron, R. (1989). *The decline and fall of hemispheric specialization (MacEachran lectures)*. Hillsdale, NJ: Lawrence Erlbaum Associates.

Erikson, E.H. (1963). *Childhood and society* (2nd ed.). New York: Norton.

Feigenbaum, E.A. (1959). *An information processing theory of verbal learning*. Paper P-1817, Rand Corp.

Feigenbaum, E.A. (1961). The simulation of verbal learning behavior. *Proceedings of the Western Joint Computer Conference, 19*, 121–132.

Feigenbaum, E.A., & Simon, H.A. (1961a). Forgetting in an association memory. *Proceedings of the 1961 National Conference of the Association for Computing Machinery, 16*, 202–205.

Feigenbaum, E.A., & Simon, H.A. (1961b). *Performance of a reading task by an elementary perceiving and memorizing program*. Paper P-2358, Rand Corp.

Feigenbaum, E.A., & Simon, H.A. (1961c). A theory of the serial position effect. Paper P-2375, Rand Corp.

Finan, J.L. (1939). Effects of frontal lobe lesions on temporally organized behavior in monkeys. *Journal of Neurophysiology, 2*, 208–226.

Fischer, K.W. (1980). A theory of cognitive development: The control and construction of hierarchies of skills. *Psychological Review, 87*, 477–531.

Fischer, K.W., & Ferrar, M.J. (1987). Generalizations about generalization: How a theory of skill development explains both generality and specificity. *International Journal of Psychology, 22*, 643–677.

Freud, S. (1932). *New introductory lectures in psychoanalysis*. London: Hogarth Press.

Fuster, J.M. (1988). *The prefrontal cortex: Anatomy, physiology and neuropsychology of the frontal lobe* (2nd ed.). New York: Raven Press.

Grueninger, W.E., & Grueninger, J. (1973). The primate frontal cortex and allassostasis. In K.H. Pribram & A.R. Luria (Eds.), *Psychophysiology of the frontal lobes* (pp. 253–290). New York: Academic Press.

Grueninger, W., & Pribram, K.H. (1969). The effects of spatial and nonspatial distractors on performance latency of monkeys with frontal lesions. *Journal of Comparative and Physiological Psychology, 68*, 203–204.

Hudspeth, W.J., & Pribram, K.H. (1992). Psychophysiological indices of cognitive maturation. *International Journal of Psychophysiology, 12*, 19–29.

Jacobsen, C.F. (1928). Recent experiments on the function of the frontal lobes. *Psychological Bulletin, 25*, 1–11.

Jacobsen, C.F. (1931). A study of cerebral function in learning: The frontal lobes. *Journal of Comparative Neurology, 52*, 271–340.

Jacobsen, C.F. (1935). Functions of frontal association area in primates. *Archives of Neurology and Psychiatry, 33*, 558–569.

Jacobsen, C.F. (1936). The functions of the frontal association areas in monkeys. *Comparative Psychology Monographs, 13,* 3–60.

Jacobsen, C.F., & Nissen, H.W. (1937). Studies of cerebral function in primates: IV. The effects of frontal lobe lesions on the delayed alternation habit in monkeys. *Journal of Comparative Psychology, 23,* 101–112.

Jacobsen, C.F., Wolfe, J.B., & Jackson, J.A. (1935). An experimental analysis of the functions of the frontal association areas in primates. *Journal of Nervous and Mental Disorders, 82,* 1–14.

John, E.R. (1961). High nervous functions: Brain function and learning. *Annual Review of Physiology,* 451–484.

Kinsbourne, M., & Wood, F. (1975). Short term memory processing and the amnesic syndrome. In J.A. Deutsch (Ed.), *Short term memory* (pp. 257–291). New York: Academic Press.

Kohlberg, L. (1969). Stage and sequence: The cognitive developmental approach to socialization. In D. Gosline (Ed.), *Handbook of socialization theory and research* (pp. 347–480). Chicago: Rand McNally.

Konow, A., & Pribram, K.H. (1970). Error recognition and utilization produced by injury to the frontal cortex in man. *Neuropsychologia, 8,* 489–491.

Kramer, D.A. (1983). Post-formal operations? A need for further conceptualization. *Human Development, 26,* 91–105.

Luria, A.R., Pribram, K.H., & Homskaya, E.D. (1964). An experimental analysis of the behavioral disturbance produced by a left frontal arachnoid endothelioma (meningioma). *Neuropsychologia, 4,* 257–280.

Malmo, R.B. (1942). Interference factors in delayed response in monkeys after removal of frontal lobes. *Journal of Neurophysiology, 5,* 295–308.

McGuinness, D., Pribram, K.H., & Pirnazar, M. (1988). Upstaging the stage model. In C.N. Alexander & E. Langer (Eds.), *Beyond formal operations: Alternative endpoints to human development* (pp. 97–113). Oxford, England: Oxford University Press

Miller, G.A., Galanter, E.H., & Pribram, K.H. (1960). *Plans and the structure of behavior.* New York: Holt, Rinehart & Winston.

Milner, B. (1974). Hemispheric specialization: Scope and limits. *Neurosciences, 4,* 75–89.

Mishkin, M. (1966). Visual mechanisms beyond the striate cortex. In R.W. Russell (Ed.), *Frontiers in physiological psychology* (pp. 93–119). New York: Academic Press.

Morrell, F. (1961). Effect of anodal polarization on the firing pattern of single cortical cells. In F.N. Furness (Ed.), *Pavlovian inference on higher nervous activity* (pp. 813–1198). New York: New York Academy of Sciences.

Newell, A. (Ed.). (1961). *Information processing language V manual.* Englewood Cliffs, NJ: Prentice Hall.

Newell, A., Shaw, J.C., & Simon, H.A. (1958). Elements of a theory of human problem solving. *Psychological Review, 65,* 151–166.

Nissen, W.H. (1951). Phylogenetic comparison. In S.S. Stevens (Ed.), *Handbook of experimental psychology* (pp. 347–386). New York: John Wiley & Sons.

Petrides, M., & Milner, B. (1982). Deficits on subject-ordered tasks after frontal- and temporal-lobe lesions in man. *Neuropsychologia, 20,* 249–262.

Piaget, J., & Inhelder, B. (1966). *The psychology of the child.* New York: Basic Books.

Poppen, R., Pribram, K.H., & Robinson, R.S. (1965). The effects of frontal lobotomy in man on performance of a multiple choice task. *Experimental Neurology, 11,* 218–229.

Pribram, K.H. (1960). The intrinsic systems of the forebrain. In H.W. Magoun (Ed.), *Handbook of physiology: Sect. 1. Neurophysiology* (Vol. II, pp. 1323–1344). Washington, DC: American Physiological Society.

Pribram, K.H. (1961). A further experimental analysis of the behavioral deficit that follows injury to the primate frontal cortex. *Experimental Neurology 3,* 432–466.

Pribram, K.H. (1969). The neurobehavioral analysis of limbic forebrain mechanisms: Revision and progress report. In D.S. Lehrman, R.A. Hinde, & E. Shaw (Eds.), *Advances in the study of behavior* (pp. 297–332). New York: Academic Press.

Pribram, K.H. (1971). *Languages of the brain: Experimental paradoxes and principles in neuropsychology.* Englewood Cliffs, NJ: Prentice Hall.

Pribram, K.H. (1986). The hippocampal system and recombinant processing. In R. Isaacson & K.H. Pribram (Eds.), *The hippocampus* (Vol. 4, pp. 329–370). New York: Plenum.

Pribram, K.H. (1987). The subdivisions of the frontal cortex revisited. In E. Perecman (Ed.), *The frontal lobes revisited* (pp. 11–39). New York: IRBN Press.

Pribram, K.H. (1991). *Brain and perception: Holonomy and structure in figural processing.* Hillsdale, NJ: Lawrence Erlbaum Associates.

Pribram, K.H., Ahumada, A., Hartog, J., & Roos, L. (1964). A progress report on the neurological processes disturbed by frontal lesions in primates. In S.M. Warren & K. Aker (Eds.), *The frontal granular cortex and behavior* (pp. 28–55). New York: McGraw-Hill.

Pribram, K.H., Gardner, K.W., Pressman, G.L., & Bagshaw, M.H. (1962). An automated discrimination apparatus for discrete trial analysis (DADTA). *Psychological Reports, 11,* 247–250.

Pribram, K.H., Konrad, K., & Gainsburg, D. (1966). Frontal lesions and behavioral instability. *Journal of Comparative and Physiological Psychology, 62,* 123–214.

Pribram, K.H., Plotkin, H.C., Anderson, R.M., & Leong, D. (1977). Information sources in the delayed alternation task for normal and "frontal" monkeys. *Neuropsychologia, 15,* 329–340.

Riegel, K.F. (1973). Dialectic operations: The final stage of cognitive development. *Human Development, 16,* 346–370.

Riegel, K.F. (1975). Toward a dialectic theory of development. *Human Development, 18,* 50–64.

Rusinov, U.S. (1956). Electrophysiological research in the dominant area in the higher parts of the central nervous system. *Abstracts of the 20th International Physiology Conference,* 785–786.

Schneider, W., & Shiffrin, R.N. (1977). Controlled and automatic human information processing: I. Detection, search and attention. *Psychological Review, 34,* 1–66.

Stamm, J.S. (1963). Function of prefrontal cortex in timing behavior of monkeys. *Experimental Neurology 7,* 87–97.

Stamm, J.S. (1969). Electrical stimulation of monkeys' prefrontal cortex during delayed response performance. *Journal of Comparative and Physiological Psychology, 67,* 535–546.

Sullivan, H.S. (1953). *The interpersonal theory of psychiatry.* New York: Norton.

Thatcher, R.W. (1994a). Cyclic cortical reorganization during early childhood development. *Brain and Cognition, 20,* 24–50.

Thatcher, R.W. (1994b). Cyclic cortical reorganization: Origins of human cognitive development. In G. Dawson & K.W. Fischer (Eds.), *Human behavior and the developing brain* (pp. 232–266). New York: Guilford Press.

Treisman, A.M. (1969). Strategies and models of selective attention. *Psychological Review, 76,* 282–299.

Tucker, D.M., Liotti, M., Potts, G.F., Russell, G.S., & Posner, M.I. (1994). Spatiotemporal analysis of brain electrical fields. In *Human Brain Mapping 1* (pp. 134–152).

Ukhtomski, A.A. (1927). Concerning the condition of excitation in dominance. *Novoe y refteksologie I fiziologii nervnoisystemry, 2,* 3–15.

Wilson, W.A., Jr. (1962). Alternation in normal and frontal monkeys as a function of response and outcome of the previous trial. *Journal of Comparative Physiological Psychology, 55,* 701–704.

Development of the Prefrontal Cortex: Evolution, Neurobiology, and Behavior
edited by Norman A. Krasnegor, Ph.D., G. Reid Lyon, Ph.D.,
and Patricia S. Goldman-Rakic, Ph.D.
copyright © 1997   Paul H. Brookes Publishing Co., Inc.
Baltimore • London • Toronto • Sydney

Index

Page numbers followed by "t" or "f" indicate tables or figures, respectively.